Essential Quick Review
PERIODONTICS

Essential Quick Review

PERIODONTICS

Editor-in-Chief

Priya Verma Gupta MDS FPFA
Professor
Department of Pedodontics and Preventive Dentistry
Divya Jyoti College of Dental Sciences and Research
Ghaziabad, Uttar Pradesh, India

Co-Author

Vinita Ashutosh Boloor MDS
Associate Professor
Department of Periodontics
Yenepoya Dental College
Yenepoya University, Derelakatte
Karnataka, Mangalore, India

JAYPEE *The Health Sciences Publisher*
New Delhi | London | Philadelphia | Panama

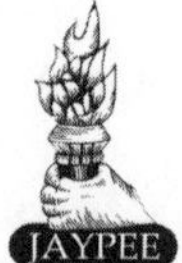

Jaypee Brothers Medical Publishers (P) Ltd

Headquarters

Jaypee Brothers Medical Publishers (P) Ltd
4838/24, Ansari Road, Daryaganj
New Delhi 110 002, India
Phone: +91-11-43574357
Fax: +91-11-43574314
Email: jaypee@jaypeebrothers.com

Overseas Offices

J.P. Medical Ltd
83 Victoria Street, London
SW1H 0HW (UK)
Phone: +44 20 3170 8910
Fax: +44 (0)20 3008 6180
Email: info@jpmedpub.com

Jaypee-Highlights Medical Publishers Inc.
City of Knowledge, Bld. 235, 2nd Floor, Clayton
Panama City, Panama
Phone: +1 507-301-0496
Fax: +1 507-301-0499
Email: cservice@jphmedical.com

Jaypee Medical Inc.
325 Chestnut Street
Suite 412, Philadelphia, PA 19106, USA
Phone: +1 267-519-9789
Email: support@jpmedus.com

Jaypee Brothers Medical Publishers (P) Ltd
17/1-B Babar Road, Block-B, Shaymali
Mohammadpur, Dhaka-1207
Bangladesh
Mobile: +08801912003485
Email: jaypeedhaka@gmail.com

Jaypee Brothers Medical Publishers (P) Ltd
Bhotahity, Kathmandu, Nepal
Phone: +977-9741283608
Email: kathmandu@jaypeebrothers.com

Website: www.jaypeebrothers.com
Website: www.jaypeedigital.com

Inquiries for bulk sales may be solicited at: jaypee@jaypeebrothers.com

Essential Quick Review: Periodontics

First Edition: **2016**

ISBN: 978-93-86056-18-4

Printed at Rajkamal Electric Press, Plot No. 2, Phase-IV, Kundli, Haryana.

<h1 align="right">Editorial Board</h1>

Preface

I am very pleased to introduce you to the first edition of Essential Quick Review; A series for final year undergraduate students.

The series will be available in eight subjects. I.e., Periodontics, Pedodontics, Prosthodontics, Endodontics and Conservative Dentistry, Oral Surgery, Oral Medicine Radiology and Public Health Dentistry covering essential parts of each subject. It will not only help the student to attain the knowledge, but will also give an idea how to attempt a question during the examination, covering entire syllabus in a limited period of time.

The book gives a complete outline for writing an essay type, a short answer type or a viva voce type of question. The language used is very simple enabling a better understanding with well-illustrated diagrams wherever possible. Each book also carries a section that contains recently asked questions covering majority of the universities in India.

What makes it different from other books is, that it is supported with a supplementary booklet for each subject that contains three sections, i.e., definitions, classifications and viva voce covering the entire syllabus enabling the student to undergo a quick revision.

The study material provided in this book is an attempt to provide an additional help to students for easy retention and reproduction of subject in the examination. This book is in no way a replacement to standard text books.

I thank all my subject matter experts for their valued suggestions and contributions. A very special word of thanks to my family for being the source of constant encouragement. I profusely thank Shri Jitender P Vij (CEO), Mr Ankit Vij (Group President), and production team of M/S Jaypee Brothers Medical Publishers (P) Ltd, New Delhi for their enthusiasm and constant efforts in bringing out this book.

Priya Verma Gupta

Contents

Section 2 Recently Asked Questions

SECTION 1

PERIODONTICS

CHAPTER 1

Gingiva

Question 1

Define gingiva. Enumerate the zones of oral mucosa. What are the different parts of gingiva? Explain in detail about the microscopic features of gingiva.

Answer

According to Glickman, gingiva is defined as "that part of oral mucosa that covers the alveolar processes of the jaws and surrounds the necks of the teeth in a collar-like fashion."

There are Three Zones of Oral Mucosa

1. Masticatory mucosa, e.g. Gingiva and covering of the hard palate.
2. Specialised mucosa, e.g. dorsum of the tongue.
3. Lining mucosa, e.g. oral mucous membrane lining the remainder of the oral cavity.

Gingiva is divided into three parts viz. marginal, attached and interdental (**Fig. 1.1**).

1. Marginal gingiva

a. It is also called as unattached gingiva, which is loosely bound and surrounds the teeth in a collar like manner.
b. It is differentiated from the attached gingiva by a mild/small (shallow) depression, which is called as free gingival groove.
c. Gingival sulcus: It is a V-shaped crevice around the tooth which is bounded by marginal gingiva on one side and tooth on the other side.
e. Normal depth of gingival sulcus is 1.3 mm. In pristine condition the depth of sulcus is 0 mm.
f. Gingival crevicular, fluid (GCF) is found in the gingival sulcus.

2. Attached gingiva

a. It begins after marginal gingiva and is tightly bound to the underlying periosteum of the alveolar bone (**Fig. 1.2**).
b. Attached gingiva is separated from the loosely bound alveolar mucosa by mucogingival junction.
c. It is maximum in the incisal region approx. 3.5–4.5 mm (maxilla) and 3.3–3.9 mm (mandible) and minimum is the posterior region i.e. 1.9 mm (maxilla) and 1.8 mm (mandible).

3. Interdental gingiva

a. It is found between the adjacent teeth, occupying the gingival embrasure.

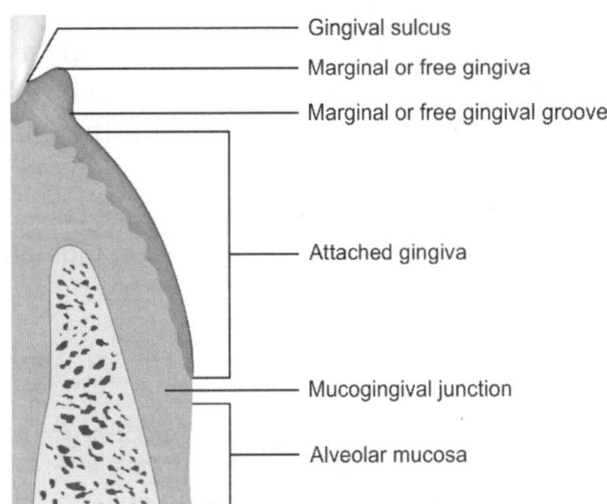

Fig. 1.1: Anatomic landmarks of gingiva.

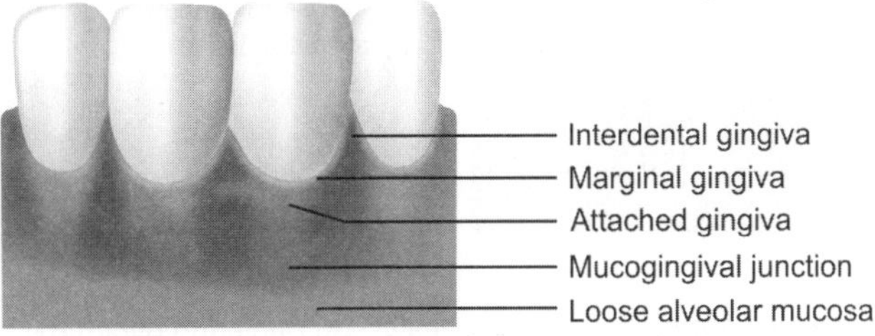

Fig. 1.2: Diagram depicting attached gingiva.

b. It forms a pyramidal shape when the teeth are in close contact (**Fig. 1.3A**), however in cases of diastema the pyramidal shape is lost (**Fig. 1.3B**).
c. Underneath the facial and the lingual papillae, there is a valley like depression known as Col.

Microscopic Features of Gingiva

Gingiva is microscopically divided into two parts, viz., gingival epithelium and gingival connective tissue.

Gingival Epithelium

- The epithelium not only provides a physical barrier to various infections but also plays an important role in host defence mechanisms
- Gingival epithelium protects the deep structures which are achieved by proliferation and differentiation of keratinocytes
- Proliferation occurs by mitosis in basal cell layer
- Few cells remain in the basal cell layer to act as proliferative compartment while majority of the cells move towards the surface
- Differentiation occurs during this movement of the cells to the surface, they undergo biochemical and morphologic changes, thus differentiating into keratinocytes. This process is called as keratinisation
- Keratinocytes form the bulk of the gingival epithelium.
- Other cells like Langerhans cells, Merkel cells and melanocytes are seen in small numbers. These cells are together called as non-keratinocytes
  - *Melanocytes:* These are specialised cells which synthesize melanin and cause melanin pigmentation which is occasionally seen on the gingiva
    - ➤ They are derived from neural crest cells and are located in stratum basale
    - ➤ Melanin is produced as melanosomes which is present in the cytoplasm of melanocytes and keratinocytes.
  - *Langerhans cells:* They are dendritic cells seen in suprabasal region. They play a role in immune reaction as they act as antigen presenting cells for lymphocytes. They also have G-specific granules known as Birbeck's granules
  - *Merkel cells:* These are present in deeper layers containing nerve endings and therefore have a sensory function.
- The epithelium is connected to the underlying connective tissue by a basal lamina which is approximately 300–400 Å thick
- It consists of lamina densa and lamina lucida. Hemidesmosomes are attached to the lamina lucida composed mainly of glycoprotein laminin. Type IV collagen forms the bulk of lamina densa.

Gingival epithelium is of three types:

1. Oral epithelium.
2. Sulcular epithelium.
3. Junctional epithelium.

Oral Epithelium

- It is also known as the outer epithelium that covers the outer surface of the keratinised gingiva, i.e. the marginal gingiva and attached gingiva
- It is composed of four layers viz., stratum basale, stratum spinosum, stratum granulosum and stratum corneum
- Keratinisation varies in different areas of the oral cavity, i.e. it is maximum in the palate, gingiva, ventral aspect of tongue, cheeks in the descending order
- The outer epithelium loses its keratinisation if it contacts a tooth.

Sulcular Epithelium

- It is a non-keratinised stratified squamous epithelium that lines the gingival sulcus
- It extends from the crest of the gingival margin till the coronal portion of the junctional epithelium. It lacks stratum granulosum and corneum
- It has the capacity to keratinise in certain conditions like:
  - Upon exposure to oral cavity
  - Upon complete elimination of inherent bacterial flora.

Junctional Epithelium

- It is also referred to as attachment epithelium which is stratified, squamous and non-keratinising in nature.

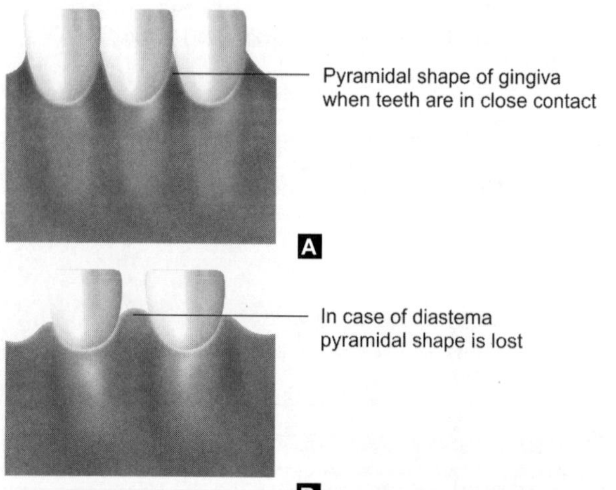

Fig. 1.3A & B: Interdental gingiva : (A) Depicting pyramidal shape. (B) Pyramidal shape lost in diastema.

It is found at cemento-enamel junction in healthy conditions. The width of JE is 10–29 cells coronally and 1–2 cells apically. The length of the junctional epithelium is approximately 0.25–1.35 mm

- It is formed by confluence of outer epithelium and reduced enamel epithelium during tooth eruption
- Junctional epithelium exhibits ribosomes, Golgi bodies and cytoplasmic vacuoles. The junctional epithelium is attached to the tooth by internal basal lamina and to the connective tissue by external basal lamina
- The epithelial attachment of junctional epithelium consists of internal basal lamina which consists of lamina densa that is adjacent to the enamel and lamina lucida to which hemidesmosomes are attached
- Hemidesmosomes help in cell-to-cell attachment and also take part in gene expression regulation, cell proliferation and cell differentiation
- The junctional epithelium and the gingival fibres together are referred as dentogingival unit because the attachment of the junctional epithelium to the tooth is reinforced by the gingival fibres.

Thus it could be concluded that junctional epithelium has various functions such as:

- JE forms an epithelial barrier against plaque bacteria as it is firmly attached to the tooth surface

- It also acts as a semipermeable membrane as it allows access of gingival fluid, inflammatory cells and immunologic components of host defence mechanism to the gingival sulcus
- It helps in rapid repair of the damaged tissue as cells of junctional epithelium exhibit rapid turnover.

Gingival Connective Tissue

It is also referred as lamina propria and it consist of two layers:

1. Papillary layer adjacent to epithelium.
2. Reticular layer adjacent to the periosteum of the alveolar bone.

- Connective tissue is mainly composed of collagen fibres which are about 60% by volume, fibroblasts (5%), and remaining 35% is formed by vessels, nerves and matrix
- It also consists of a ground substance which occupies the space between fibres and cells along with high water content. Ground substance is mainly composed of proteoglycans like hyaluronic acid, chondroitin sulphate and glycoproteins, mainly fibronectin
- Connective tissue consists of three types of fibres, i.e. collagen, reticular and elastic. Type I collagen is the main fibre seen in lamina propria and provides tensile strength. Elastic fibre is composed of elaunin, elastin and oxytalan fibres distributed among collagen fibres.

SHORT ESSAYS

Question 1

What is attachment epithelium? What is epithelial attachment?

Answer

Junctional epithelium is also referred to as attachement epithelium which is stratified, squamous and non keratinizing in nature. It is found at cemento–enamel junction in healthy conditions.

- Its width is 10- 29 cells coronally and 1- 2 cells apically.
- The length of the junctional epithelium is approxiametely 0.25 – 1.35 mm
- It is formed by confluence of outer epithelium and reduced enamel epithelium during tooth eruption
- It can be completely formed after surgery or instrumentation
- Junctional epithelium exhibits ribosomes, golgi bodies and cytoplasmic vacuoles. Lysosome- like bodies are seen

in this epithelium. There is absence of keratinosomes which is also referred as Odland bodies and also acid phosphatase is related to lower degree of differentiation , which reflects weak defence mechanism against bacteria in d dental plaque

- Poly morphonuclear leucocytes (PMN) are commonly found , but its number increases considerably at the time of bacterial attack to fight against infection **(Fig. 1.4)**.

Epithelial Attachment

- The junctional epithelium is attached to the tooth by internal basal lamina and to the connective tissue by external basal lamina
- The epithelial attachment of junctional epithelium consists of internal basal lamina which consists of lamina densa which is adjacent to the enamel and lamina lucida to which hemidesmosomes are attached

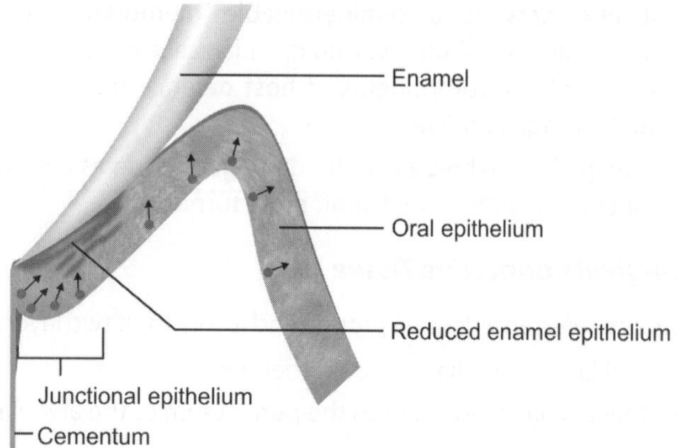

Fig. 1.4: Development of junctional epithelium and gingival sulcus.

- Hemidesmosomes help in cell-to-cell attachment and also take part in gene expression regulation, cell proliferation and cell differentiation
- The junctional epithelium and the gingival fibres together are referred as dentogingival unit because the attachment of the junctional epithelium to the tooth is reinforced by the gingival fibres
- Thus it could be concluded that junctional epithelium has various functions like:
  ○ It forms an epithelial barrier against plaque bacteria as junctional epithelium is firmly attached to the tooth surface
  ○ It acts as a semipermeable membrane as it allows access of gingival fluid, inflammatory cells and immunologic components of host defence mechanism to the gingival sulcus
  ○ It helps in rapid repair of the damaged tissue as cells of junctional epithelium exhibit rapid turnover.

Question 2

Describe in detail about gingival connective tissue.

Answer

Gingival Connective Tissue

It is also referred as lamina propria and it consists of two layers:

1. Papillary layer adjacent to epithelium.
2. Reticular layer adjacent to the periosteum of the alveolar bone.
- Connective tissue is mainly composed of collagen fibres which are about 60% by volume, fibroblasts (5%), and remaining 35% is formed by vessels, nerves and matrix
- It also consists of a ground substance which occupies the space between fibres and cells and has a high-water content

- Ground substance is mainly composed of proteoglycans like hyaluronic acid and chondroitin sulphate and glycoproteins, mainly fibronectin
- Connective tissue consists of three types of fibres, i.e. collagen, reticular and elastic
- Type I collagen is the main fibre seen in lamina propria and provides tensile strength
- Elastic fibre is composed of elaunin, elastin and oxytalan fibres distributed among collagen fibres
- Connective tissue is highly collagenous, containing bundles of fibres known as gingival fibres consisting of collagen type I. They serve the following functions:
  ○ It holds the marginal gingiva tightly against the tooth
  ○ Provides strength to withstand the masticatory forces
  ○ Unites the marginal gingiva with the cementum and attached gingiva of the adjacent tooth.
- Group of principal gingival fibres are:
  ○ Dentogingival group
  ○ Alveologingival group
  ○ Dentoperiosteal group
  ○ Circular group
  ○ Transseptal group.
- Group of secondary fibres are:
  ○ Periosteogingival group
  ○ Inter-papillary group
  ○ Trans-gingival group
  ○ Inter-circular group
  ○ Inter-gingival group
  ○ Semi-circular group.

Cellular Composition of Gingival Connective Tissue

- Fibroblast is the main cell type of gingival connective tissue. Fibroblasts are responsible for synthesising collagen, elastic fibres, glycoproteins and glycosaminoglycans. They also play an important role in development, maintenance and repair
- Mast cells, fixed macrophage and histiocytes are present in gingival connective tissue
- Also seen are adipose cells and eosinophils, which are less in number. Leucocytes and lymphocytes are also seen.

Question 3

Explain in detail about gingival sulcus.

Answer

Gingival sulcus is also referred to as gingival crevice.

- It is a V-shaped shallow crevice around the tooth which is surrounded by gingiva on one side and tooth on another side
- Normal depth of gingival sulcus is 1–3 mm. In pristine condition the depth of sulcus is 0 mm

- Depth of the gingival sulcus can be measured with the help of periodontal probe. Gingival crevicular fluid (GCF) is found in gingival sulcus.

Development of Gingival Sulcus

- When the tooth erupts into the oral mucosa, the reduced enamel epithelium combines with the oral epithelium forming, the junctional epithelium **(Fig. 1.4)**
- Further this united epithelium becomes condensed along the crown and ameloblasts gradually transform into squamous epithelial cells
- This transformation moves in an apical direction. This epithelium continuously renews itself by mitotic activity and moves in a coronal direction to the gingival sulcus, where they are shedded
- Gingival sulcus formation takes place when the tooth erupts into the oral cavity **(Fig. 1.5)**.

Gingival Crevicular Fluid

- Gingival crevicular fluid can be a transudate or an exudate which contains a wide range of biochemical factors which can be used as a potential diagnostic biomarker of the biologic state of the periodontium in health and disease
- Gingival crevicular fluid is mainly composed of epithelium, connective tissue, serum, inflammatory cells and microbial flora
- In the state of health GCF is present in small quantities whereas in inflammation, GCF increases and resembles an inflammatory exudate.
- Functions of GCF are as follows:
  - It has a cleansing action.
  - It provides adhesion of the gingival epithelium to the tooth as it contains plasma proteins.

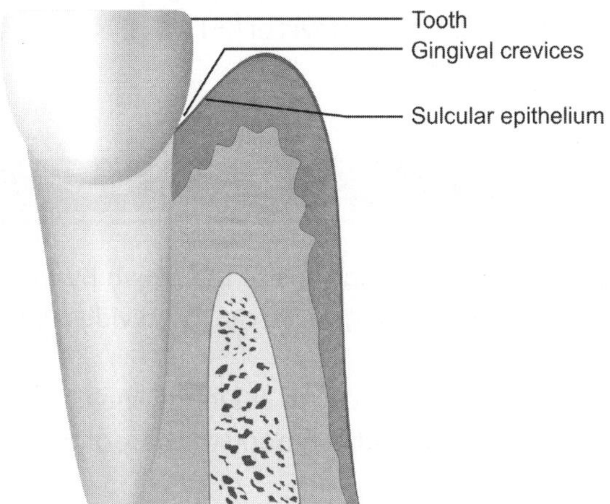

Fig. 1.5: Gingival crevice.

- It has anti-microbial action.
- It acts as gingival defence mechanism as it possesses antibody activity.
- Various methods of collecting GCF:
  - Filter paper strips.
  - Micro-capillary tubes.
  - Crevicular washing methods.
  - Twisted threads.
  - GCF samples can be measured on a blotter or a perio paper on an electronic transducer called as periotron.
  - Ninhydrin staining method.
  - Isotope dilution method.

Dento-gingival Junction

- Attachment of junctional epithelium to the tooth is reinforced by gingival fibre, therefore junctional epithelium and gingival fibres together is referred to as dento-gingival unit.
- The gingival fibres are highly collagenous consisting of collagen fibres mainly Type I collagen. Principal fibres of gingival connective tissue are:
  - Dento-gingival group
  - Alveolo-gingival group
  - Dento-periosteal group
  - Circular group
  - Transseptal group.
- Group of secondary fibres are:
  - Periosteoa-gingival group
  - Inter-papillary group
  - Trans-gingival group
  - Inter-circular group
  - Inter-gingival group
  - Semi-circular group.
- These fibres originate from cementum and are inserted into connective tissue of gingiva and periosteum of the alveolar bone.
- They provide stabilization and maintain the position of teeth in the arch by securing them.

Question 4

Correlate various clinical and microscopic features of gingiva.

Answer

Various clinical features of gingiva are:

- Colour
- Size
- Contour
- Shape
- Consistency
- Surface texture

❑ Position

❑ **Colour:** Normal colour of gingiva is pink. There are three factors on which the colour of gingiva is dependent, i.e. vascularity, degree of keratinisation, and pigment containing cells.

○ *Vascularity:* If the vascularity increases, the colour of gingiva becomes red. It is seen in cases of inflammation, but in absence of inflammation the vascularity is normal, and the colour of gingiva appears as coral pink.

○ *Degree of keratinisation:* More the keratinisation lesser would be the redness in gingiva. Therefore a highly keratinized gingiva would appear as pale pink, whereas if the keratinisation is low, gingiva would appear as reddish. Since the attached gingiva and marginal gingiva are keratinised, it appears as pink, whereas alveolar mucosa which is non-keratinised, appears red, smooth and shiny.

○ *Pigmentation containing cells:* Melanin is a brown coloured pigment which is responsible for normal pigmentation. But if these pigment containing cells increase in number, then the gingiva appears brownish-black in colour **(Fig. 1.6)**.

❑ **Size:** Size of gingiva depends upon the total amount of cellular and intercellular content of gingiva. In cases of gingival inflammation, size is enlarged, otherwise in normal conditions it is not enlarged.

❑ **Contour:** Contour of gingiva is dependent on various factors like alignment of teeth in the arch, shape of the teeth, location, size of the proximal contact and size of the gingival embrasure. In normal conditions the gingiva follows a scalloped contour, but in cases of inflammation, mostly it becomes a scalloped. In relatively flat teeth, the gingival contour is flat. If there is pronounced mesio-distal convexity or if there is gingival recession, the scalloping along the teeth becomes more accentuated.

❑ **Shape:** Shape of the gingiva depends upon the proximal

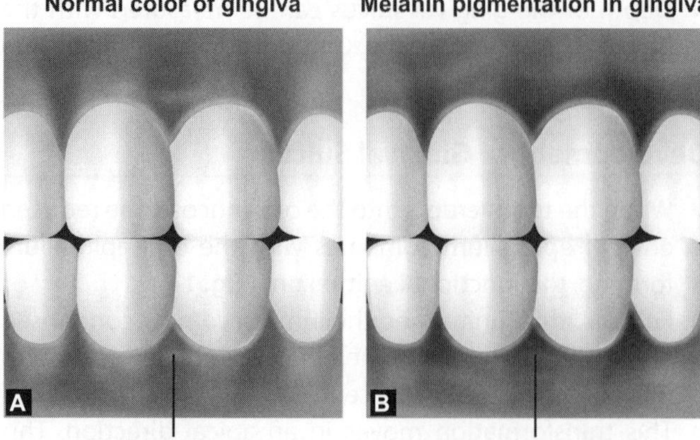

Fig. 1.6A & B: Gingiva : (A) Normal colour of gingiva and. (B) Melanin pigment in gingiva.

teeth contacts and shape of teeth. If the teeth are in tight contact and teeth are narrow mesio-distally, gingiva exhibits a pyramidal shape, e.g. in case of anterior teeth, but if the teeth are not in close contact the shape of the interdental gingiva becomes flattened. If the teeth are wide mesio-distally, that means if the teeth are broad, e.g. in posterior region, then the interdental gingiva exhibits a broader shape.

❑ **Consistency:** In normal conditions, gingiva is firm and resilient, but in cases of inflammation it becomes soft and oedematous.

❑ **Surface texture:** In health, gingiva exhibits an orange peel-like appearance referred to as stippling. Stippling is an adaptive specialisation or reinforcement of function produced by alternate rounded depressions and protuberances in gingiva. In this state of disease stippling becomes absent.

❑ **Position:** The normal position of gingiva is at cemento-enamel junction (CEJ). In disease, this position is either above CEJ or below the level of CEJ which is also referred to as gingival recession.

SHORT NOTES

Question 1

What is continuous tooth eruption?

Answer

There are two types of eruption viz., active and passive eruption.

1. Active eruption is referred as the eruption of the teeth in an occlusal direction.

2. Passive eruption is exposure of the crown by the apical migration of the gingiva. It can be divided into four stages:

a. **Stage 1:** In this the teeth are in the line of occlusion. The junctional epithelium and the base of the gingival sulcus are at the enamel.

b. **Stage 2:** In this stage there is an apical proliferation of the junctional epithelium such that one part is on

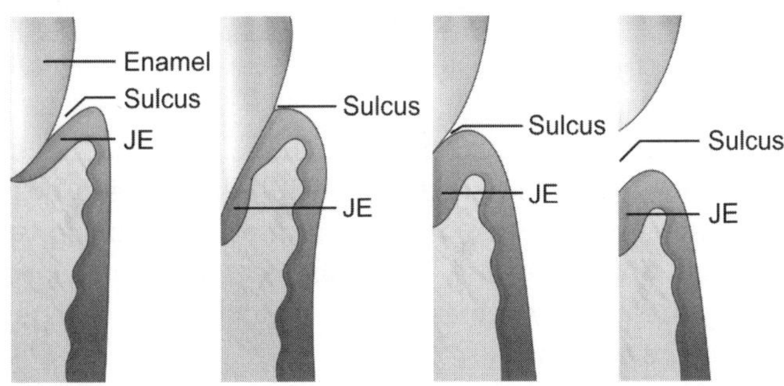

Fig. 1.7: Position of the gingiva in health and disease.

cementum while other part is on enamel. Whereas, the base of the gingival sulcus is still on the enamel.

c. **Stage 3:** In this the junctional epithelium completely rests on the cementum and the base of the sulcus is at cemento-enamel junction.

d. **Stage 4:** Both junctional epithelium and the base of the gingival sulcus are present on the cementum such that some part of the cementum is exposed (**Fig. 1.7**).

Question 2

Define is gingival col and what is its significance?

Answer

It is a valley like depression connecting the facial and lingual papillae and conforms to the shape of the interproximal contact. The interproximal space consists of interdental gingiva that occupies the gingival embrasure.

Significance of col: Since col is formed of non-keratinised epithelium, it is very prone to infections and inflammation and is the most prone site for disease initiation.

Question 3

What is attached gingiva? How is it measured? What is its significance?

Answer

It is that part of the gingiva that starts immediately after marginal gingiva and extends till mucogingival junction. It is separated from the marginal gingiva by a very shallow groove known as marginal groove and it is separated from adjacent loose alveolar mucosa by mucogingival junction.

It can be measured using a periodontal probe by subtracting the sulcular depth from the total distance between the marginal gingiva and the mucogingival junction.

It can also be measured using Schiller's potassium iodide solution which stains the keratinised gingiva.

Significance of attached gingiva are as follows:

- It helps in protection against microbes and other foreign bodies as it is tightly bound to the periosteum
- Since it is keratinised, it aids in bearing the masticatory forces
- It helps in proper placement of the toothbrush head
- It also enhances the aesthetics.

Question 4

Discuss the blood supply, lympatics and nerve supply of gingiva?

Answer

Blood Supply

- Supraperiosteal arterioles present along the surface of the alveolar bone that also pass through surrounding tissue.
- Periodontal ligament vessels, which extend into the gingiva and anastomose with the capillaries in the sulcular area.
- Arteries that emerge from the interdental septa and are extended parallel to the crest of the bone to anastomose with the vessels of the periodontal ligament.

Lymphatic Drainage

Gingiva brings in the lymphatic vessels of connective tissue papillae. It progresses to the periosteum of the alveolar process and then to the regional lymph nodes, mainly sub-maxillary group.

Nerve Supply

Neural system of gingiva is very extensive and is distributed throughout the gingiva. Neural innervation is derived from the nerves in the periodontal ligament and from the labial, buccal and palatal nerves. Nerve structures which are present in the connective tissue are:

- Meshwork of terminal argyrophilic fibres
- Meissner-type tactile corpuscles
- Temperature receptors, i.e. Krause type end bulbs
- Encapsulated spindles.

Question 5

What are clear cells?

Answer

Non-keratinocytes (melanocytes, Langerhans cells and Merkel cells) are referred to as clear cell because in the histologic section, the zone around their nuclei appears lighter than in the zone around the keratin producing cells.

Question 6

What is the difference between keratinised gingiva and attached gingiva?

Answer

Keratinised gingiva consists of both loose marginal gingiva and firmly adherent attached gingiva but, attached gingiva does not contain any movable mucosa.

Question 7

What are Stillman's cleft?

Answer

According to Carranza, they are defined as apostrophe-shape indentations extending from and into gingival margin of varying distances on facial surface. They are narrow V-shaped gingival recessions.

Quesiton 8

What are McCall's festoons?

Answer

These are rolled thickened margins of gingiva seen near the canines when recession reaches upto the mucogingival junction. These are also called as life preserver-shaped enlargement. They represent the inflammatory changes seen in the gingiva.

Question 9

What is mucogingival junction?

Answer

It is a junction which demarcates the firm attached gingiva from the loosely bound alveolar mucosa. Its position remains consistent throughout life.

CHAPTER 2

Periodontal Ligament

Question 1

Define periodontal ligament (PDL)? Discuss in detail about periodontal ligament and describe in detail about its functions.

Answer

According to Carranza, PDL is a complex vascular and highly cellular connective tissue that surrounds the tooth root and connects it to inner wall of the alveolar bone.

❑ Principal fibres are the most important component of periodontal ligament. They are collagenous in nature, arranged in the form of a bundle and follow a wavy course.

❑ Sharpey's fibres are the terminal portions of the principal fibres whose one end is embedded in to cementum and other end is embedded into the bone.

❑ There are six groups of principal fibres namely transseptal, alveolar crest, horizontal, oblique, apical and lastly the interradicular (**Fig. 2.1**).

1. **Transseptal group:** They are found in inter-proximal areas over the alveolar bone crest, embedded into the cementum of adjacent teeth. In cases of periodontal destruction, these fibres are reconstructed. Since these fibres do not have any osseous attachment, they can be considered as a part of gingival fibres.

2. **Alveolar crest group:** These fibres are extended in an oblique direction from the cementum just below the junctional epithelium into the alveolar bone crest. These fibres resist the lateral tooth movement and also prevent the tooth extrusion.

3. **Horizontal group fibres:** These fibres extend horizontally at right angles from cementum to the bone.

4. **Oblique group:** They are the largest group of periodontal fibres. They extend from the cementum in a coronal direction towards the bone. They have the capacity to tolerate the masticatory forces and transform them into tension on the alveolar bone.

5. **Apical group:** These are found at the apex of the tooth radiating in an irregular manner from the cementum into the bone. They are not present on incompletely formed roots.

6. **Inter-radicular group:** These are found in the furcation areas of the multi-rooted tooth from the cementum into the bone.

❑ In the PDL, 2 immature fibres are seen viz. oxytalan and eluanin fibres. The oxytalan fibres in a vertical direction running parallel to each other and bend to attach to the cementum in the cervical third of the root. They regulate the vascular flow.

❑ Along with these fibres small group of collagen fibres have been found which, run in all direction forming a plexus known as indifferent fibre plexus.

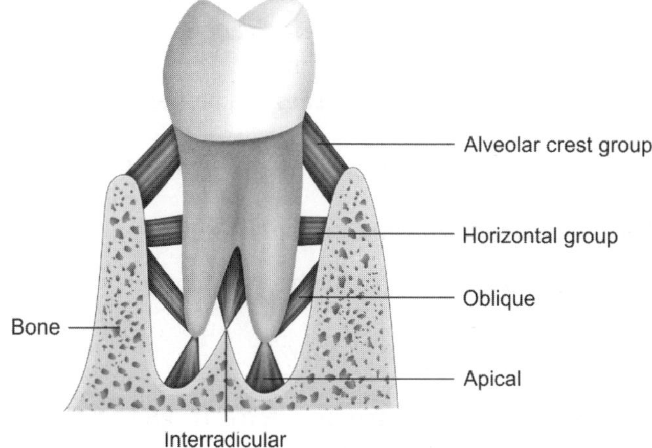

Fig. 2.1: Fibres of Periodontal Ligament.

Cellular Elements

There are four types of cells:

1. Connective tissue cells.
2. Epithelial rest cells.
3. Immune system cells
4. Cells associated with neurovascular elements.

- **Connective tissue cells:** e.g. fibroblasts, cementoblasts and osteoblasts.
- **Epithelial rest cells:** e.g. epithelial rests of Malassez which appear as isolated clusters of cells or interlacing strands.
- **Immune system cells:** e.g. neutrophils, lymphocytes, macrophages, mast cells and eosinophils.

Ground Substance

- It consists of glycosaminoglycans and glycoproteins.
- Hyaluronic acid and proteoglycans are the main glycosaminoglycans wheras, fibronectin and laminin are the main glycoproteins.
- Seventy percent of water content is found in the ground substance. It may also contain calcified mast cells known as cementicles.

Functions of Periodontal Ligament

- Physical.
- Formative and remodelling.
- Nutritional.
- Sensory.

Physical Functions

- It provides a soft tissue casing which protects the nerves and vessels from injury due to any mechanical force.
- It transmits the occlusal force to the bone.
- It attaches the teeth to the bone.
- It maintains the gingival tissues in a proper relationship with the teeth.
- It also acts as shock absorber for the occlusal forces.

Shock Absorber for the Occlusal Forces

There are two theories pertaining to this function:

1. Tension theory.
2. Viscoelastic theory.

- **Tension theory:** Whenever a force is applied to the tooth the principal fibres first unfold and then straighten that further transmit the forces to the bone **causeing**
the elastic deformation of the bony socket. Once the alveolar bone reaches its limit, the force is then transmitted to the basal bone.
- **Viscoelastic theory:** This theory is based on fluid movement, with fibres having just a secondary role. When the force is applied to the tooth, the extracelluar fluid is passed from the periodontal ligament into the marrow spaces of the bone through the cribriform plate. Thus the force is transferred to the cancellous portion of the alveolar bone. Once there is fluid depletion, the fibres bundles absorb the slack and tighten up which leads to the stenosis of the blood vessels. This further leads to ballooning of the vessels and passage of the blood is ultrafiltrated into the tissues causing the replenishment of the tissue fluids.

Transmission of Occlusal Forces to the Bone

- Whenever a horizontal or a tipping force is applied, two phases of tooth movement can be seen.
- First is within the confines of the PDL and second causes the displacement of the buccal and the lingual plates. The tooth would rotate about an axis that may change as the force is increased. In areas of tension, the periodontal fibres are taut whereas in areas of pressure, the fibres are in a compressed state causing the tooth to displace leading to distortion of bone.
- In single-rooted teeth, the axis of rotation is situated in between the apical-third and middle-third of the root whereas in a multi-rooted tooth, the axis of rotation is situated in the and furcation area.

Formative and Remodelling Functions

The periodontal ligament is always in a constant state of remodelling. Old cells and the fibres breakdown at a regular interval and are replaced by new cells and fibres. The mitotic activity can be seen in fibroblasts and endothelial cells.

Nutritional and Sensory Functions

Periodontal ligament provides the nutrition to gingiva, cementum and bone through the blood vessels. The periodontal ligament is also supplied with sensory nerve fibres which are capable of transmitting tactile, pain and pressure sensations. There are four types of nerve endings seen in periodontal ligament, viz. free endings carrying pain sensation, Ruffini-like mechanoreceptors, Meissner's corpuscles and spindle like pressure and vibration endings.

SHORT ESSAYS

Question 1

Discuss the composition and structure of collagen.

Answer

Collagen is a type of protein mainly responsible for maintaining the framework of the tissues. There are about 19 species of collagen. It is composed of various amino acids, most importantly are glycine, proline, hydroxylysine and hydroxyproline. Fibroblasts are the main cell type responsible for collagen synthesis. Tropocollagen molecule is formed within the fibroblast which combine together to form microfibril with a periodicity of 64 nm. These microfibrils are packed together to form fibrils and they again aggregate to form fibre and these fibres associate to form a bundle. The principal fibres are composed mainly of type I collagen. Type III collagen forms reticular fibres and type IV collagen forms basal lamina **(Fig. 2.2)**.

Diagram showing collagen microfibrils, fibrils, fibers and bundle

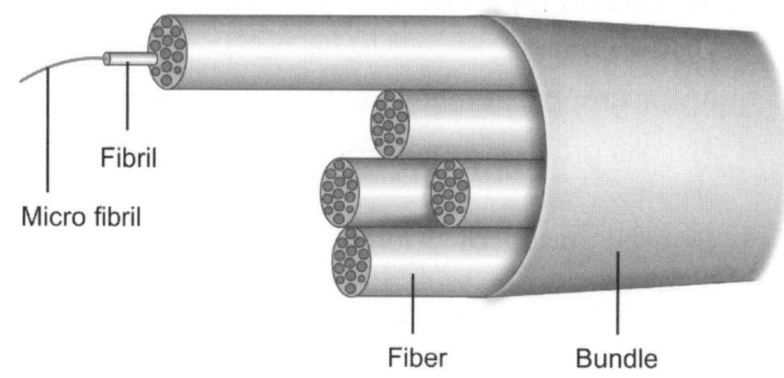

Fig. 2.2: Structure of collagen.

Functions of Collagen

- Provides flexibility and strength to the tissue because of its high tensile strength.
- Responsible for maintaining the framework of tissues.

SHORT NOTES

Question 1

Write short note on oxytalan fibres.

Answer

- Oxytalan fibres are one of the immature fibres found in PDL, other one being the elaunin.
- They run in a vertical direction parallel to the root surface and bend to attach to the cementum in the cervical third of the root.
- These fibres regulate the vascular flow since they are associated with the blood vessels and nerves of the periodontal ligament.
- There is an elastic meshwork of oxytalan and elaunin fibres in the periodontal ligament.
- Oxytalan fibres develop from the beginning in the regenerated PDL.

Question 2

Write short note on Sharpey's fibres.

Answer

- Sharpey's fibres are the terminal portions of the principal fibres which are embedded in to cementum in one end and the other end is embedded into the bone.
- They constitute the bulk of cementum and are mainly composed of type I collagen.
- Once they are embedded into the wall of the alveolus, they get calcified.
- They are also associated with some non-collagenous proteins found in bone and cementum, i.e. bone sialoprotein and osteopontin.

Question 3

Write short note on indifferent fibre plexus.

Answer

- Along with the mature and immature fibres of PDL, small group of collagen fibres have been found which run in all direction forming a plexus known as indifferent fibre plexus.

Question 4

What is the blood supply of periodontal ligament?

Answer

- Main blood supply to PDL is through superior and inferior alveolar arteries.
  - Apical group of arteries—vessels of the pulp.
  - Alveolar group of arteries—also known as perforating arteries.
  - Gingival group of arteries—vessels supplying the gingiva.

Question 5

Enumerate principal fibres of periodontal ligament?

Answer

There are six groups of principal fibres of PDL:

1. Transseptal group.
2. Alveolar crest group.
3. Horizontal group.
4. Oblique group.
5. Apical group.
6. Interradicular group.

CHAPTER 3

Alveolar Process

Questiuon 1

Define alveolar bone. What are the parts and composition of alveolar bone? Discuss in detail about remodelling.

Answer

According to Carranza, it is defined as "the portion of the maxilla and mandible that forms and supports the tooth socket". When the tooth erupts to provide the osseous attachment to the forming periodontal ligament (PDL) that is the time when alveolar process is formed. When the tooth is lost, the alveolar process also disappears gradually. Alveolar processes are the tooth-dependent bony structures, because the alveolar process develops and remodels with the tooth formation and eruption. Therefore, the morphology of alveolar process is dependent upon size, shape, location, and function of the teeth. Parts of alveolar process are as follows:

- **External cortical bone:** It is formed by compact bone lamellae and haversian bone.

- **Alveolar bone proper:** It is the inner socket wall which is made up of thin compact bone. It is also known as lamina dura in the radiographs. It contains a number of openings because of the cribriform plate, through which the neurovascular bundles passes and connects the PDL with the alveolar bone.

- **The cancellous bone:** Cancellous trabeculae act as supporting alveolar bone present between two compact bones. The interdental bone consists of cancellous bone present between compact bones.

Besides the above mentioned bones, the jaws also contain basal bone which is situated apically and is also not related to teeth **(Fig. 3.1)**.

Most facial and lingual portions of the socket are formed by compact bone.

Cells and Inter-cellular Matrix

Osteoblasts produce the organic matrix of the bone. It is formed during foetal growth through intra-membranous ossification and consists of calcified matrix. Osteocytes are enclosed in spaces called lacunae. Osteocytes extend their processes into canaliculi which radiates from the lacuna. The canaliculi forms an anastomosing system through an inter-cellular matrix of bone, which brings oxygen and nutrients to the osteocytes through the blood and also removes metabolic waste products. Blood vessels branch extensively and traverse through periosteum. The endosteum lies close to the marrow vasculature. The haversian system, also known as osteons are the internal mechanisms that bring a vascular supply to the bones. They are many found in the outer cortical plate and alveolar bone proper.

Composition of Bone

Two-third inorganic matter and one-third of organic matter.

Inorganic matter

It consists of minerals like calcium, phosphate, along with hydroxyl, carbonate, citrate, and trace amounts of other ions, e.g sodium, magnesium, and fluorine. These salts are

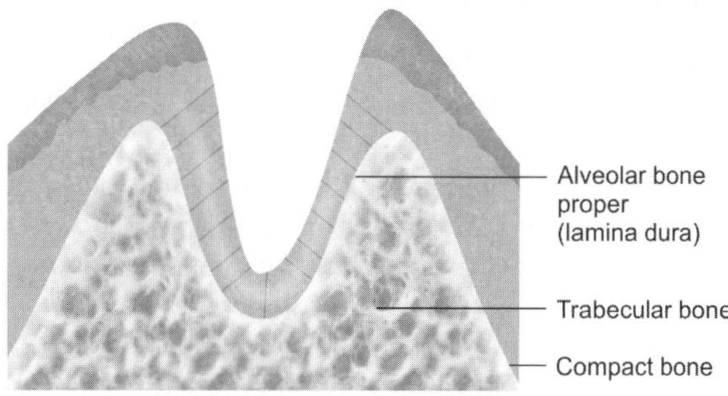

Fig. 3.1: Alveolar bone.

in the form of hydroxyapatite crystals which are of ultra-microscopic size and bone constitute two-thirds of these crystals.

Organic matter

Main component of organic matter is type I collagen which is around 90%. Along with it, small amounts of non-collagenous proteins are present such as osteocalcin, osteonectin, bone morphogenic protein, phosphoproteins and proteoglycans. Some paracrine factors are also present such as cytokines, chemokines and growth factors.

Remodelling

- Bone remodelling is a process that involves change in shape, resistance to forces, repair of wounds and calcium and phosphate homeostasis in the body. It also includes bone formation and bone resorption. Coupling of bone deposition and bone resorption constitutes one of the fundamental principles by which bone is remodelled throughout life.
- Bone remodelling includes cells of distinct lineages, i.e. osteoblasts and osteoclasts. Osteoblasts and osteoclasts form and resorb the mineralised connective tissues bone respectively. Number of osteoblasts decreases with age, whereas no change is seen in the number of osteoclasts.
- Bone remodelling is a complex process which involves hormones and local factors which act in an autocrine and paracrine manner on the production and function of differentiated bone cells.

- The bone consists of 99% of body's calcium. Therefore, whenever there is a decrease in the levels of blood calcium levels, the bone calcium is released. This process is monitored by parathyroid gland.
- There are receptors present on the chief cells parathyroid gland, which get activated in case of decrease in blood calcium levels. These receptors start producing parathyroid hormone (PTH).
- This PTH stimulates the osteoblasts to produce Interleukin-1 (IL-1), and IL-6, which further stimulates monocytes to migrate into the area of bone.
- Osteoblasts also secrete leukaemia inhibitory factor (LIF), which coalesces monocytes into multi-nucleated osteoclasts, which causes bone resorption, and helps in release of calcium ions from hydroxyapatite into the blood.
- When the blood levels of calcium becomes normal, through a feedback mechanism, the secretion of PTH stops.
- On the other hand osteoclasts have resorbed the organic as well as inorganic content of bone which causes breakdown of collagen. Due to this breakdown, certain osteogenic substrates are released, which bind to collagen, and this results in stimulation of osteoblasts, which ultimately deposit the bone.
- Therefore resorption and deposition of bone goes side by side. And this interdependency of osteoblasts and osteoclasts in bone remodelling is referred to as "coupling".

SHORT ESSAYS

Question 1

Discuss alveolar bone in healthy and diseased.

Answer

In Health Condition

Parts of alveolar process are as follows:

- **External cortical bone:** It is formed by compacted bone lamellae and haversian bone.
- **Alveolar bone proper:** It is the inner socket wall which is made up of thin compact bone. It is also known as lamina dura in the radiographs. It contains a number of openings because of the cribriform plate, through which the neurovascular bundles pass and connect the periodontal ligament with the alveolar bone.

- **The cancellous bone:** Cancellous trabeculae act as supporting alveolar bone present between two compact bones. The interdental bone consists of cancellous bone present between compact bone.

Besides the above mentioned bones, the jaws also contains basal bone which is situated apically and is also not related to teeth.

Most facial and lingual portions of the socket are formed by compact bone.

Composition of Bone

Two-third of inorganic matter and one-third f organic matter:

Inorganic Matter

It consists of minerals like calcium, phosphate, along with hydroxyl, carbonate, citrate, and trace amounts of other ions, e.g. sodium, magnesium, and fluorine. These salts are in the form of hydroxyapatite crystals which are of ultramicroscopic size and bone constitutes two-thirds of these crystals.

Organic Matter

Main component of organic matter is type I collagen which is around 90%. Along with it, small amounts of non-collagenous proteins are present such as osteocalcin, osteonectin, bone morphogenic protein, phosphoproteins and proteoglycans. Some paracrine factors are also present such as cytokines, chemokines and growth factors.

Remodelling

- Bone remodelling is a process that involve changes in shape, resistance to forces, repair of wounds and calcium and phosphate homeostasis in the body. It also includes bone formation and bone resorption. Coupling of bone deposition and bone resorption constitutes one of the fundamental principles by which bone is remodelled throughout life.
- Bone remodelling includes cells of distinct lineages, i.e. osteoblasts and osteoclasts. Osteoblasts and osteoclasts form and resorb the mineralised connective tissues bone respectively. Number of osteoblasts decreases with age, whereas no change is seen in the number of osteoclasts.
- Bone remodelling is a complex process which involves hormones and local factors which act in an autocrine and paracrine manner on the production and function of differentiated bone cells.
- The bone consists of 99% of body's calcium. Therefore, whenever there is a decrease in the levels of blood calcium levels, the bone calcium is released. This process is monitored by parathyroid gland.
- There are receptors present on the chief cells of parathyroid gland, which get activated in case of decrease in blood calcium levels. These receptors start producing PTH.
- This PTH stimulates the osteoblasts to produce IL-1, and IL-6, which further stimulates monocytes to migrate into the area of bone.
- Osteoblasts also secrete LIF, which coalesces monocytes into multinucleated osteoclasts, which causes bone resorption, and helps in release of calcium ions from hydroxyapatite into the blood.
- When the blood levels of calcium becomes normal, through a feedback mechanism, the secretion of PTH stops.
- On the other hand osteoclasts have resorbed the organic as well as inorganic content of bone which causes breakdown of collagen. Due to this breakdown, certain osteogenic substrates are released, which bind to collagen, and this results in stimulation of osteoblasts, which ultimately deposit the bone.
- Therefore resorption and deposition of bone goes side by side. And this interdependency of osteoblasts and osteoclasts in bone remodelling is referred to as "coupling".

In Disease Condition

- **Fenestrations:** They are the isolated areas in which the root is denuded of the bone and the root surface is covered only by the periosteum and the overlying gingiva. In these areas the marginal bone is intact.
- **Dehiscence:** When the denuded areas extend through the marginal bone, such defects are termed as dehiscence.

Such kind of defects are seen in approximately in 20% of teeth. These are more commonly seen on facial bone as compared to the lingual bone. They are most often found on anterior teeth than of posterior teeth and they are bilateral frequently. The possible causes for these kinds of defects can be prominent root contours, malposition, and labial protrusion of the tooth combines with the thin bony plate.

These defects are important because they might complicate the outcome of periodontal surgery.

There are other bony defects also, like one wall defect, two wall defect, three wall defect, reverse architecture, lipping, ledges, craters, horizontal bone defect, and vertical bone defects.

SHORT NOTES

Question 1

What are paracrine factors and what are their functions?

Answer

Cytokines, chemokines and various growth factors are referred to as paracrine factors. They are responsible for the local control of mesenchymal condensations that occur at the start of organogenesis. These factors also play an important role in the development of the alveolar processes.

Question 2

What is the function of bone sialoprotein and osteopontin?

Answer

These are non-collagenous proteins referred to as cell-adhesion proteins which are responsible for cell to cell adhesion of both osteoclasts and osteoblasts.

Question 3

What is osteoid?

Answer

Osteoid is a non-mineralised bone matrix which is laid down by osteoblasts. As the new osteoid deposits, the older osteoid located below the surface becomes mineralised as the mineralisation front advances.

Question 4

What is the origin of osteoclast and how are they formed?

Answer

Osteoclast originates from hematopoietic tissue and are formed by the fusion of mononuclear cells of asynchronous populations.

Question 5

Explain bone resorption.

Answer

Bone resorption is a complex process. It appears as eroded rough surface referred to as Howship's lacunae and also there is involvement of large multi-nucleated cells known as osteoclasts. Osteoclasts originate from hematopoietic tissue and are formed by the fusion of mononuclear cells of asynchronous populations. When these osteoclasts are active, they develop a ruffled border from which hydrolytic enzymes are secreted, which digest the organic matter of the bone. The activity of osteoclasts can be modified by hormones, e.g. PTH and calcitonin which have the receptors on the osteoclasts membrane.

There is another mechanism of bone resorption in which an acidic environment is created on the bone surface which leads to dissolution of the minerals of the bone. This can be produced by different conditions including a proton pump through the cell membrane of the osteoclasts, bone tumours, and local pressure which are translated through the secretary activity of the osteoclasts.

Ten Cate has also described sequence of events in the process of bone resorption, which are as follows:

- Attachment of osteoclast to the mineralised bone surface.
- Creation of a sealed acidic environment through action of the proton pump, which demineralises bone and exposes the organic matrix.
- Degradation of the exposed organic matrix to its constituent amino acids by the action of released enzymes such as acid phosphatase and cathepsins.
- Sequestering of mineral ions and amino acids within the osteoclasts.

Question 6

What is scalable processor architecture (SPARC)?

Answer

It is a secreted protein, acidic and rich in cysteine. This protein plays an important role in bone remodelling.

Question 7

What is bundle bone?

Answer

It is the bone adjacent to the periodontal ligaments which contain a large number of Sharpey's fibres. It is characterised by a thin lamella which is arranged in layers parallel to the root along with intervening appositional lines. Bundle bone is located within the alveolar bone proper or lamina dura. Some of the Sharpey's fibres are completely calcified, but most contain an uncalcified central core within a calcified outer layer.

Bundle bone is also found throughout the skeletal system wherever muscles and ligaments are attached.

Question 8

What is periosteum and endosteum?

Answer

Tissue covering the outer surface of the bone is referred to as periosteum whereas the tissue lining the internal bone cavities in called as endosteum

- The periosteum consists of an inner layer and an outer layer:
    - The inner layer is composed of osteoblasts which are surrounded by osteoprogenitor cells. These cells have the potential to differentiate into osteoblasts.
    - The outer layer is rich in blood vessels and nerves and is composed of collagen fibres and fibroblasts.
- The endosteum is composed of a single layer of osteoblasts and sometimes a small amount of connective tissue may also be found. The outer layer is the fibrous layer whereas the inner layer is the osteogenic layer.

Question 9

What is fenestration and dehiscence?

Answer

- **Fenestrations:** They are the isolated areas in which the root is denuded of the bone and the root surface is covered only by the periosteum and the overlying gingiva. In these areas the marginal bone is intact.
- **Dehiscence:** When the denuded areas extend through the marginal bone, such defects are termed as dehiscence.

    Such kinds of defects are seen in approximately in 20% of teeth. These are more commonly seen on facial bone as compared to the lingual bone. They are most often found on anterior teeth than of posterior teeth and they are bilateral frequently. The possible causes for these kinds of defects can be prominent root contours, malposition, and labial protrusion of the tooth combines with the thin bony plate.

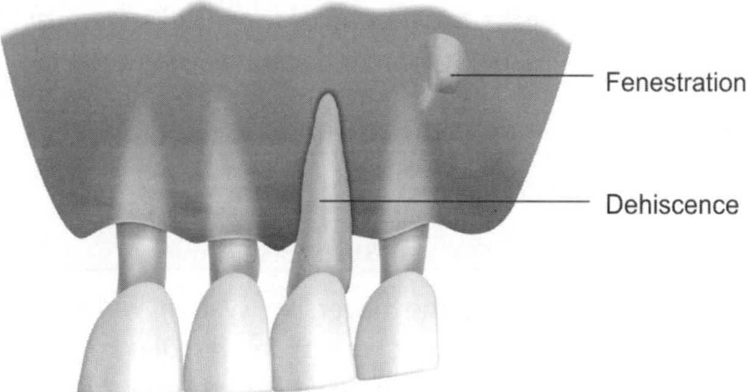

Fig. 3.2: Fenestrations and Dehiscence.

These defects are important because they might complicate the outcome of periodontal surgery (**Fig. 3.2**).

Question 10

What is the attachment apparatus?

Answer

Cementum, periodontal ligament and alveolar bone all together form the attachment apparatus.

Question 11

What is physiological migration of the teeth.

Answer

Tooth movement continues even after active eruption phase. With time because of the wear and tear, the proximal contacts of the teeth are flattened and therefore, the teeth tend to migrate mesially. This is referred to physiological migration. Alveolar bone remodels in compliance with the physiological migration of the teeth. Bone resorption increases in the areas of pressure along the mesial surface of the tooth and new layers are deposited in the areas of tension along the distal surface of the tooth.

Question 12

What is bone remodelling?

Answer

- Bone remodelling is a process that involve change in shape, resistance to forces, repair of wounds and calcium and phosphate homeostasis in the body. It also includes bone formation and bone resorption. Coupling of bone deposition and bone resorption constitutes one of the fundamental principles by which bone is remodelled throughout life.
- Bone remodelling includes cells of distinct lineages, i.e. osteoblast and osteoclasts. Osteoblasts and osteoclasts form and resorb the mineralised connective tissues bone respectively. Number of osteoblasts decreases with age, whereas no change is seen in the number of osteoclasts.
- Bone remodelling is a complex process which involves hormones and local factors which act in an autocrine and paracrine manner on the production and function of differentiated bone cells.
- The bone consists of 99% of body's calcium. Therefore, whenever there is a decrease in the levels of blood calcium levels, the bone calcium is released. This process is monitored by parathyroid gland.

- There are receptors present on the chief cells of parathyroid gland, which get activated in case of decrease in blood calcium levels. These receptors start producing PTH.
- This PTH stimulates the osteoblasts to produce IL-1, and IL-6, which further stimulates monocytes to migrate into the area of bone.
- Osteoblasts also secrete LIF, which coalesces monocytes into multinucleated osteoclasts, which causes bone resorption, and helps in release of calcium ions from hydroxyapatite into the blood.
- When the blood levels of calcium becomes normal, through a feedback mechanism, the secretion of PTH stops.
- On the other hand osteoclasts have resorbed the organic as well as inorganic content of bone, which causes breakdown of collagen. Due to this breakdown, certain osteogenic substrates are released, which bind to collagen, and this results in stimulation of osteoblasts, which ultimately deposit the bone.
- Therefore resorption and deposition of bone goes side by side. And this interdependency of osteoblasts and osteoclasts in bone remodelling is referred to as "coupling".

Question 13

What is coupling?

Answer

- The bone consists of 99% of body's calcium.Therefore, whenever there is a decrease in the levels of blood calcium levels, the bone calcium is released. This process is monitored by parathyroid gland.
- There are receptors present on the chief cells parathyroid gland , which get activated in case of decrease in blood calcium levels. These receptors start producing PTH.
- This PTH stimulates the osteoblasts to produce IL-1, and IL-6, which further stimulates monocytes to migrate into the area of bone.
- Osteoblasts also secrete LIF, which coalesces monocytes into multinucleated osteoclasts, which causes bone resorption, and helps in release of calcium ions from hydroxyapatite into the blood.
- When the blood levels of calcium becomes normal, through a feedback mechanism, the secretion of PTH stops.
- On the other hand osteoclasts have resorbed the organic as well as inorganic content of bone which causes breakdown of collagen. Due to this breakdown, certain osteogenic substrates are released, which bind to collagen, and this results in stimulation of osteoblasts, which ultimately deposit the bone.
- Therefore resorption and deposition of bone goes side by side. And this interdependency of osteoblasts and osteoclasts in bone remodelling is referred to as "coupling".

Question 14

Discuss the development of alveolar bone.

Answer

Just prior to mineralisation, matrix vesicles are produced by the osteoblasts. These vesicles are rich in enzymes like alkaline phosphatase that help in jump starting the seeding of hydroxyapatite crystals. These hydroxyapatite crystals grow into coalescing bone nodules. These nodules along with rapidly-developing non-oriented collagen fibres from the basic structure of the woven bone and thus first bone is formed in the alveolus. This woven bone transforms itself into mature lamellar bone by the process of bone deposition, remodelling and orientation of collagen fibres into layers.

In the mature lamellar bone, the hydroxyapatite crystals align themselves parallel to the collagen fibres along the long axis and are deposited on and within the fibres. This kind of layout helps the bone matrix to bear the heavy mechanical stresses and strains during various functions. It is seen that the alveolar bone develops around the dental follicle during the development of a tooth. When a deciduous tooth is shed, the alveolar bone accompanying it also gets resorbed and is succeeded by new alveolar bone formation along with the permanent tooth follicle. As the root formation of the permanent tooth occurs and the surrounding tissue develops, the alveolar bone merges with the basal bone. Thus forming a continuous entity (alveolar bone and the basal bone). Both basal bone and the alveolar bone are derived from neural crest ectomesenchyme.

Mineralisation of the mandibular basal bone begins from the mental foramen at the exit of the mental nerve whereas mineralisation of the basal bone of the maxilla starts at the exit of infraorbital nerve from infraorbital foramen.

Question 15

What is an osteon?

Answer

Osteon is referred as the haversian system which is the internal mechanisms that brings a vascular supply to the bones, specially the bones which are took hick to be supplied by only surface vessels. They are many found in the outer cortical plate and alveolar bone proper.

CHAPTER 4

Cementum

Questiuon 1

Define cementum? Discuss in details the types, classification, composition and functions of cementum.

Answer

According to Carranza, cementum is defined as the calcified, avascular mesenchymal tissue that forms the outer covering of the anatomic root.

There are basically two types of cementum:

1. Acellular cementum.
2. Cellular cementum.

Acellular Cementum

It is also known as primary cementum since it is the first-formed cementum. It covers cervical third or half of the root and as the name suggests, it does not contain cells. It is formed before the teeth reaches occlusal plane. Its thickness is between 30–230 µm. The main component of the acellular cementum is Sharpey's fibres which plays an important role in supporting the tooth.

Cellular Cementum

It is formed after the tooth reaches the occlusal plane and as name suggests it contains cells, i.e. cementocytes, that are present in individual spaces known as lacunae which communicates with each other through a system of anastomosing canaliculi. This cementum is less calcified as compared to acellular cementum. Sharpey's fibres are found less in number in cellular cementum.

Classification of Cementum

According to Schroeder, cementum has been classified as follows:

- **Acellular afibrillar cementum (AAC):** This type of cementum neither contains cells nor collagen fibres. It consists of mineralised ground substance. It is produced by cementoblasts with a thickness of 1–15 µm.
- **Acellular extrinsic fibre cementum (AEFC):** It consists of mainly Sharpey's fibres and does not contain any cells. It is produced by fibroblasts and cementoblasts, commonly found in the apical third of the roots. Its thickness is around 30–230 µm.
- **Cellular mixed stratified cementum (CMSC):** It consists of both extrinsic and intrinsic fibres and also consists of cells. It is produced by fibroblasts and cementoblasts. It is found in the apical third of the roots, apex and in furcation areas.
- **Cellular intrinsic fibre cementum (CIFC):** It consists of cells and intrinsic fibres, but does not contain extrinsic fibres. It is formed by cementoblasts.
- **Intermediate cementum:** It consists of cellular remnants of Hertwig's epithelial sheath which is embedded in a calcified ground substance. It is seen near the cemento-dentinal junction.

Composition of Cementum

It consists of an organic portion and an inorganic portion:

- **Organic portion:** The organic matrix of cementum is basically of collagen. Out of which 90% is Type I and 5% Type III collagen. There are two main sources of collagen in cementum:
  1. **Sharpey's fibres** are also known as extrinsic fibres. They are the embedded portions of the principal fibres of the periodontal ligament (PDL). They are produced by fibroblasts.
  2. **Intrinsic fibres:** They belong to the cemental matrix and are produced by cementoblasts.

Sharpey's fibres form the major bulk of cementum and is composed of Type I collagen. Type III collagen coats the Type I collagen of Sharpey's fibres. Ground substance consists of proteoglycan, glycoproteins and phosphoproteins.

- **Inorganic portion:** It is around 45–50% and is mainly composed of hydroxyapatite. Inorganic component of cementum is less than bone, enamel and dentine.

Functions of Cementum

- Cementum provides anchorage to the tooth in its socket.

The ends of PDL fibres are embedded into the cementum, which helps in achieving this.

- Cementum helps in maintain the occlusal relationships. Whenever there is attrition, the incisal or the occlusal surface gets abraded, because of which the tooth is supra-erupted, to compensate for this occlusal discrepancy. Cementum gets deposited at the apex of the tooth, in such situations.

- It also maintains the integrity of root surface, by acting as a reparative tissue for the root.

SHORT ESSAYS

Question 1

What is cemento-enamel junction (CEJ)?

Answer

It is that junction where the cementum and enamel meet. There are three types of CEJ:

1. Cementum overlapping the enamel: It is seen in 60–65% cases.

2. Edge to edge contact: It is also referred as butt joint. It is seen in 30% of cases.

3. Gap between cementum and enamel: In this case the cementum and enamel do not meet. It is seen in 5–10% cases (**Fig. 4.1**).

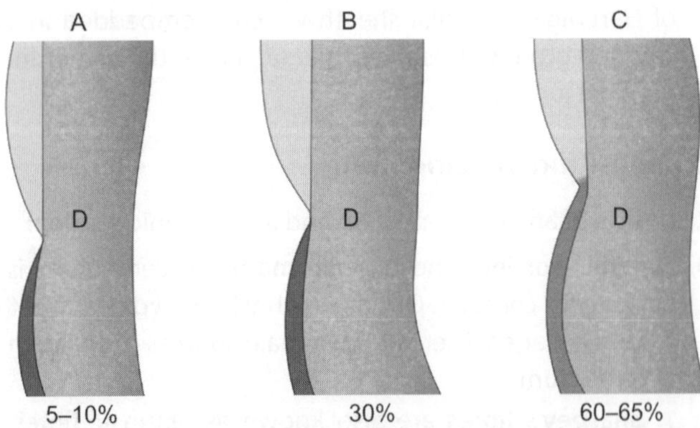

Fig. 4.1: Normal variations in tooth morphology at cemento-enamel junction. (A) Space between enamel and cementum with dentin (D); (B) End-to end relationship of enamel and cementum and (C) cementum overlapping the enamel.

Question 2

What is cemento-dentinal junction (CDJ) ?

Answer

- The part of cementum, which joins to the internal root canal dentine is referred to as CDJ.

- The width of CDJ remains almost constant throughout life.

- It is around 2–3 µm wide.

- It consists significant amount of proteoglycans, and the fibrils inter-mingle between the cementum and the dentine (**Fig. 4.1**).

Question 3

What is cementum attachment protein (CAP)?

Answer

- It is a cementum-derived collagenous protein.

- It promotes spreading and adhesion of mesenchymal cell types.

- Osteoblasts and fibroblasts shows better adhesion than keratinocytes and gingival fibroblasts.

Question 4

What is cementum derived growth factor (CGF)?

Answer

- It is an insulin like growth factor like molecule.

- It helps in proliferation of PDL cells and gingival fibroblasts.

Question 5

What are the functions of cementum?

Answer

- Cementum provides anchorage to the tooth in its socket. The ends of PDL fibres are embedded into the cementum, which helps in achieving this.

- Cementum helps in maintain the occlusal relationships. Whenever there is attrition, the incisal or the occlusal surface gets abraded, because of which the tooth is supra-erupted, to compensate for this occlusal discrepancy. Cementum gets deposited at the apex of the tooth, in such situations.

- It also maintains the integrity of root surface, by acting as a reparative tissue for the root.

Question 6

What is cementum resorption and repair?

Answer

- Cementum of erupted as well as unerupted teeth undergoes some amount of cemental resorption that may be of microscopic proportion.

- There are various local and systemic factors that are responsible for cemental resorption.

- Various local factors responsible for cemental resorption are as follows:
  - Trauma from occlusion
  - Orthodontic tooth movement
  - Pressure from mal-aligned erupting teeth
  - Cysts and tumours
  - Teeth without functional antagonists
  - Embedded teeth
  - Re-planted and transplanted teeth
  - Periapical disease
  - Periodontal disease.

- Various systemic factors responsible for cemental resorption are as follows:
  - Calcium deficiency
  - Hypothyroidism
  - Hereditary fibrous osteodystrophy
  - Paget's disease.

- Microscopically cementum resorption appears as bay like concavities in the root surface.

- Multi-nucleated giant cells and large mononuclear macrophages are seen adjacent to cementum undergoing resorption.

- Several resorption sites coalesce to form large areas of destruction.

- Resorption may extend into dentine and pulp, but is generally painless.

- Resorption may not always be continuous, but it may alternate with periods of repair, with deposition of cementum.

- The newly formed cementum may be demarcated by a deeply staining irregular line, referred to as reversal line.

- Embedded fibres of PDL forms a functional relationship with new cementum.

- Viable connective tissue is required for cementum repair.

- Cementum repair can take place in vital as well as non vital teeth.

Question 7

What are reversal lines?

Answer

- In periods of repair of cementum, the newly formed cementum is differentiated from the root by a deeply staining irregular line, which is known as reversal line. Reversal line consists of few collagen fibrils and a high content of proteoglycans with glycosaminoglycans.

- Fibril intermingling takes place in between reparative cementum and resorbed cementum or dentin. This takes place only at few places.

- Embedded fibres of the PDL re-establishes a functional relationship with the newly formed cementum.

Question 8

What is hypercementosis?

Answer

- Hypercementosis is also referred to as cemental hyperplasia.

- It is thickening of the cementum.

- It is mainly an age related process, and it may effect a single tooth or the entire dentition.

❑ It appears as a nodular enlargement at the apical one-third or appear as spike like excrescences because of fusion of cementicles to the root or because of calcification of periodontal fibres which are embedded into cementum.

Causes of Hypercementosis

There can be two types of hypercementosis:

1. **Localised:** It is seen in teeth without antagonist to keep pace with active eruption. It is believed to be a compensatory mechanism to counteract the destruction of fibrous attachment of the tooth.
2. **Generalised:** It can be due to hereditary reasons or patients having Paget's disease. Acromegaly, arthritis, calcinosis, rheumatic fever and thyroid goitre are some of the systemic conditions associated with generalized hypercementosis.

Radiographic Features

❑ Lamina dura appears radiopaque and periodontal appears radiolucent, as it is seen in normal situation.

❑ Periapical cemental dysplasia, condensing osteitis, and focal periapical osteoporosis can be differentiated from hypercementosis that the above mentioned conditions fall outside the shadow of periodontal and lamina dura.

Clinical Significance

❑ Treatment is not required in cases of hypercementosis

❑ Extraction in such conditions can create a problem. In cases of multirooted teeth, sectioning of the tooth should be done before extraction procedure.

Question 9

Define ankylosis?

Answer

❑ Fusion of cementum with bone with obliteration of PDL is referred as ankylosis.

❑ Ankylosis may be seen in following situations.

○ It is a feature of abnormal repair as it occurs in teeth with cemental resorption.
○ After chronic periapical inflammation.
○ Tooth replantation.
○ Occlusal trauma
○ Around embedded teeth.

❑ Diagnostic sign for ankylotic resorption are:
○ Lack of physiologic mobility.
○ Upon percussion, there is usual a metallic sound.
○ Teeth would be in infra-occlusion, if the ankylotic process continues.

❑ Proprioception is lost in ankylosed teeth, since PDL is replaced by bone. The pressure receptor in the PDL is deleted or does not function.

❑ Also due to absence of periodontium, the physiologic drifting and movement of teeth does not take place.

❑ Resorption lacunae are filled with bone, and the periodontal space is absent.

❑ Treatment options for ankylosed teeth are as follows:
○ Restorative intervention.
○ Surgical extraction of the affected tooth.

Question 10

Enumerate the various differences between cellular and acellular cementum.

Answer

Acellular cementum	Cellular cementum
• It is also known as primary cementum.	• It is also known as secondary cementum.
• It is formed before the teeth reaches the occlusion.	• It is formed after the teeth has reached occlusion.
• It is devoid of cells.	• It contains cementocytes.
• Sharpey's fibre make up the bulk.	• Sharpey's fibre are found in smaller proportions.
• Seen at the coronal portion	• Seen at apical portion.
• Slow formation.	• Rapid formation.
• Collagen fibres are more organised.	• Collagen fibres are irregularly arranged.

CHAPTER 5

Age-related Changes in Periodontium

Question 1

What are the effects of ageing on periodontium?

Answer

Cellular ageing is the cause for periodontal tissues ageing. Basis for the intrinsic changes are the cellular ageing. Every tissue is not affected in the same way in the process of ageing, e.g. epithelial tissue renews very fast which is the primary component of the periodontium, on the other hand, nerve tissue and muscle tissue undergo very minimal renewal.

Intrinsic Changes

- In the process of ageing, the regenerative capacity of tissues is slowed down because the cell renewal takes place at a very slow pace.
- There are very few cells left to renew, the dead cells as the progenitor cells wear out and die gradually. This effect is characteristic of the age related changes and biological changes that occur with ageing.
- The protein synthesis is also slowed down, because of all these effects, the epithelium becomes thin because of reduced keratinisation process.

Stochastic Changes

- Stochastic changes occurring within the cells affect the tissues. Morphological and physiological changes occur in the process of glycosylation and cross linking.
- Structures become stiffer due to reduced elasticity and increase in mineralisation.
- Structures become more thermally stable and become less soluble as there is a loss of regenerative power.
- There are structurally-altered protein and decrease in protein synthesis because of somatic mutations.

- There is presence of free radicals because of which there is an accumulation of waste in the cell.
- There is a decline in the physiologic processes of tissues because of all these factors.
- Maximum changes are because of ageing, but few are secondary to the physiologic deterioration, for example loss of elasticity and increase in tissue resistance may cause decrease in permeability, decrease in nutrient and also the accumulation of waste in cells.
- Therefore, vascular peripheral resistance, i.e. decrease in blood supply may decrease in cellular function.

Physiologic Changes

- There is a reduction in tissue elasticity because of decrease in number of collagen fibres.
- There is a decrease in production of mucopolysaccharides, due to decreased vascularity.
- With ageing, alveolar bone shows a decrease in the bone density, an increase in resorption of bone, and also a decrease in vascularity. However, in contrast cementum shows cemental thickness.

Functional Changes

- There is decrease in mitotic activity of the oral epithelium and the periodontal ligament. Also, there is a decrease in the metabolic rate of the tissues.
- Immune system is also found to be affected. As the healing capacity of the tissues also declines.
- Inflammation, develops very rapidly and more severely.
- There is a high susceptibility to fungal and viral infections because of abnormality in function of T cells.
- Functional changes are associated with reduced efficiency of mastication. This efficacy is lost due to missing teeth, poorly fitting prosthesis, or non-compliance of the patient, who may refuse to wear prosthetic appliances.

Compensatory Changes

- Compensatory changes occur, due to ageing or disease.
- These changes affect the periodontium in the following ways:
  - Bone height is reduced and there is presence of gingival recessions.
  - Attrition is also seen as a compensatory change which acts as a stabilizer between loss of bony support and excessive leveraging from occlusal forces imposed on teeth.
  - There is a reduction in overjet of the teeth, manifesting as an increase in the edge-to-edge contact to the approximal wear of the posterior teeth.
  - There is an increase in food table area, with loss of sluiceways and in the mesial migration.

Effect of Ageing on Periodontal Tissues

Gingiva

Gingival Epithelium

- There is thinning and decrease in keratinization of gingival epithelium because of which there is epithelial permeability to bacterial antigens and a decreased resistance to functional trauma.
- Rete pegs gets flattened and cellular density is also altered.
- Stippling is reduced or is unchanged.
- Width of attached gingiva is increased.
- Inter-cellular substances are increased.

Gingival Connective Tissue

- Connective tissue becomes coarser and denser due to increase in rate of conversion of insoluble collagen into soluble collagen, increase in mechanical strength, and increased denaturing temperature.

Periodontal Ligament

- Fibroblasts are reduced and their structure becomes irregular.
- Organic matrix production and epithelial cells are reduced but elastic fibres are increased.
- Width of periodontal ligament may increase or decrease.
- The periodontal ligament width is increased because of less number of teeth supporting the entire functional load.
- The periodontal ligament width is decreased because of reduced strength of the masticatory musculature and continues deposition of cementum and bone.

Cementum

- There is an increase in width of cementum, which is a common finding, since deposition continues after tooth eruption.
- Because of accumulation of resorption bays, there is an increase in surface irregularity.

Alveolar Bone

- There is decrease in vascularity.
- Osteoporosis is seen.
- There is a decrease in healing capacity and reduction in metabolic rate.
- Rate of bone deposition is decreased, whereas rate of bone resorption is increased.
- Alveolar bone facing periodontal ligament shows irregularities. Because of irregular periodontal surface of bone, there is an irregular insertion of collagen fibres.

SHORT ESSAYS

Question 1

What is the nature of periodontal diseases in older age group?

Answer

Chronic periodontitis is the disease of periodontal tissues seen mainly in older adults.

- Chronic periodontitis seen in older adults is due to accumulation of disease over time. Therefore, it is chronic.
- One of the theory states that many sites of advanced periodontitis, resulted in tooth loss, early in life, which suggests that old age is not a risk factor for periodontal disease.
- Factors which can modify the relationship between periodontal disease and age are general health status, immune status, diabetes, nutrition, smoking, genetics, medications, mental-healthstatus, salivary flow, functional deficits, and finances.
- Gingival tissues can also be altered by medications prescribed for older adults, e.g. in post-menopausal women who are receiving steroids, steroid-induced gingivitis can be seen. Drugs like cyclosporins, calcium channel blockers, and anticonvulsants can induce gingival overgrowth. This gingival enlargement can further decrease an individual ability to maintain proper oral hygiene.

Question 2

What is bruxism and what are its effects on the periodontium?

Answer

Bruxism can be defined as diurnal or nocturnal parafunctional activity that includes clenching, bracing, gnashing and grinding of teeth.

Effects of Bruxism on Periodontium

- They are tooth mobility, tooth fracture, tooth wear, periodontal and muscular pain. Bruxism can be managed by a stabilization appliance like a night guard.

Question 3

What are the age changes seen in gingiva?

Answer

Gingival Epithelium

- There is thinning and decrease in keratinization of gingival epithelium because of which there is epithelial permeability to bacterial antigens and a decreased resistance to functional trauma.
- Rete pegs gets flattened and cellular density is also altered.
- Stippling is reduced or is unchanged.
- Width of attached gingiva is increased.
- Intercellular substances are increased.

Gingival Connective Tissue

- Connective tissue becomes coarser and denser due to increase in rate of conversion of insoluble collagen into soluble collagen, increase in mechanical strength, and increased denaturing temperature.

Question 4

What are the age changes in periodontal ligament?

Answer

Age changes in periodontal ligament are as follows:

- Fibroblasts are reduced and their structure becomes irregular.
- Organic matrix production and epithelial cells are reduced and elastic fibres are increased.
- Width of periodontal ligament may increase or decrease.
- The periodontal ligament width is increased because of less number of teeth supporting the entire functional load.
- The periodontal ligament width is decreased because of reduced strength of the masticatory musculature and continues deposition of cementum and bone.

Question 5

What are the age changes in cementum?

Answer

Age changes in cementum are as follows:

- There is an increase in width of cementum, which is a common finding, since deposition continues after tooth eruption.
- Because of accumulation of resorption bays, there is an increase in surface irregularity.

Question 6

What are the age changes seen in alveolar bone?

Answer

Age changes seen in alveolar bone are as follows:

- There is decrease in vascularity.
- Osteoporosis is seen.
- There is a decrease in healing capacity and reduction in metabolic rate.
- Rate of bone deposition is decreased, whereas rate of bone resorption is increased.
- Alveolar bone facing periodontal ligament shows irregularities. Because of irregular periodontal surface of bone, there is an irregular insertion of collagen fibres.

CHAPTER 6

Classification of Periodontal Diseases

Question 1

What is the 1999 International workshop for classification of periodontal diseases and conditions?

Answer

Gingival Diseases

Dental Plaque Induced

- Associated with dental plaque only with or without other local contributing factors.
- Gingival diseases modified by systemic factors:
  - Associated with endocrine system: Puberty - associated gingivitis, menstrual-cycle associated gingivitis, pregnancy associated gingivitis, pyogenic granuloma and diabetes mellitus associated gingivitis.
  - Associated with blood dyscrasias: Leukaemia associated gingivitis and others.
- Gingival diseases modified by medications:
  - Drug- induced gingival enlargements
  - Drug- influenced gingivitis, e.g. oral contraceptives, etc.
- Gingival diseases modified by malnutrition, e.g. vitamin C and others.

Non-plaque-induced Gingival Lesions

- **Specific bacterial origin:** Neisseria gonorrhoeae, Treponema pallidum, streptococcal species and others.
- **Viral origin:** Herpes virus infections and others.
- **Fungal origin:** Candida species infections, linear gingival erythema, histoplasmosis and others.
- **Genetic origin:** Hereditary gingival fibromatosis and others.
- Manifestations of systemic conditions:
  - Mucocutaneous disorders: Lichen planus, pemphigus, pemphigoid, etc.
  - Allergic reactions:
    - Dental restorative materials—mercury, acrylic, etc.
    - Reactions attributed to toothpastes/dentifrices, mouth rinses/washes, chewing gum additives, food and additives.
    - Others.
- **Traumatic lesions:** Chemical, physical, thermal, factitious, iatrogenic, accidental.
- Foreign body reactions.
- Not otherwise specified (NOS).

Chronic Periodontitis

It is based on clinical radiographic, historic and laboratory characteristics:

- Localized (< 30% of sites involved)
- Generalized (> 30% of sites involved).

Aggressive Periodontitis

Otherwise clinically healthy individuals, rapid attachment and bone loss, not consistent with local deposits, familial aggregation.

- Localized (circumpubertal onset, first molar or incisor has proximal attachment loss, robust serum antibody response to infective agents).
- Generalized (affects below 30 years of age, generalized proximal attachment loss, poor serum antibody response to infective agents, episodic nature of periodontal disease).

Periodontitis as a Manifestation of Systemic Disease

- Associated with haematological disorders: Acquired neutropenia, leukaemia, and others.

❑ Associated with genetic disorders: Leukocyte adhesion deficiency (LAD) syndromes and others.

Necrotizing Periodontal Diseases

NUG, NUP.

Abscesses of the Periodontium

Gingival, periodontal, pericoronal abscesses.

Periodontitis Associated with Endodontic Lesions

Combined periodontal-endodontic lesion.

Developmental or Acquired Deformities and Conditions

❑ Localized tooth related factors that modify or predispose to plaque induced gingival diseases/periodontitis.
  ○ Tooth anatomic factors.
  ○ Dental restorations/appliances.
  ○ Root fractures.
  ○ Cervical root resorption and cemental tears.
❑ Mucogingival deformities and conditions around teeth
  ○ Gingival/soft tissue recession on facial/lingual/interproximal/papillary.
  ○ Lack of keratinized gingiva.
  ○ Decreased vestibular depth.
  ○ Aberrant frenum/muscle position.
❑ Gingival excess.
❑ Pseudo pockets, inconsistent gingival margin, excessive gingival display, gingival enlargement, abnormal colour, mucogingival deformities and conditions on edentulous ridges.
  ○ Vertical and/or horizontal ridges deficiency.
  ○ Lack of gingival/keratinized tissue.
  ○ Gingival/soft tissue enlargement.
  ○ Aberrant frenum/muscle position.
  ○ Decreased vestibular depth.
  ○ Abnormal colour.
❑ Occlusal trauma
  ○ Primary occlusal trauma.
  ○ Secondary occlusal trauma.

What is the American Academy of Periodontology (AAP) 1999 classification of periodontal diseases? Describe in detail.

It is based upon clinical, radiographic, historical and laboratory characteristics, periodontitis can be classified as:

❑ Chronic periodontitis.
❑ Aggressive periodontitis.
❑ Periodontitis as a manifestation of systemic disease.

Chronic Periodontitis

Following characteristics can be seen in a patient of chronic periodontitis:

❑ Prevalent in adults, but can occur in children.
❑ Amount of destruction consistent with local factors.
❑ Associated with a variable microbial pattern.
❑ Subgingival calculus frequently found.
❑ Slow to moderate rate of progression with possible periods of rapid progression.
❑ **Possible modified by or associated with the following:**
  ○ Systemic diseases such as diabetes mellitus and human immunodeficiency virus (HIV) infection.
  ○ Local factors predisposing to periodontitis.
  ○ Environmental factors such as cigarette smoking and emotional stress.

Chronic periodontitis may be further subclassified into localized and generalized forms and characterized as slight, moderate, or severe based on the common features:

❑ Localized form: Less than 30 % of sites involved.
❑ Generalized form: More than 30 % of sites involved.
❑ Slight: 1–2 mm of clinical attachment loss.
❑ Moderate: 3–4 mm of clinical attachment loss.
❑ Severe: > = mm of clinical attachment loss.

Aggressive Periodontitis

Following characteristics can be seen in the patient suffering from aggressive periodontitis:

❑ Otherwise clinically healthy patient.
❑ Rapid attachment loss and bone destruction.
❑ Amount of microbial deposits inconsistent with disease severity.
❑ Familial aggregation of diseased individuals.

The following characteristics are common but not universal:

❑ Diseased sites infected with Actinobacillus actinomycetemcomitans.

- Abnormalities in phagocyte function.
- Hyper-responsive macrophages, producing increased prostaglandin E2 (PGE2) and interleukin-1 beta.
- In some cases, self-arresting disease progression.

Aggressive periodontitis may be further classified into localized and generalized forms based upon the common features described here and the following specific features.

Localized Form

- Circumpubertal onset of disease.
- Localized first molar or incisor disease with proximal attachment loss on at least two permanent teeth, one of which is a first molar.
- Robust serum antibody response to infecting agents.

Generalized Form

- Usually affecting persons under 30 years of age (however, may be older).
- Generalized proximal attachment loss affecting at least three teeth other than first molars and incisors.
- Pronounced episodic nature of periodontal destruction.
- Poor serum antibody response to infecting agents.

Periodontitis as a Manifestation of Systemic Disease

Periodontitis may be observed as a manifestation of the following systemic disease:

- Haematologic disorders:
  - Acquired neutropenia.
  - Leukaemias.
  - Others.
- Genetic disorders:
  - Familial and cyclic neutropenia.
  - Down syndrome.
  - Leucocyte adhesion deficiency syndromes.
  - Papillon-Lefevre syndrome.
  - Histiocytosis syndromes.
  - Glycogen storage disease.
  - Infantile genetic agranulocytosis.
  - Chediak-Higashi syndrome.
  - Cohen syndrome.
  - Ehlers-Danlos syndrome (types IV and VII AD).
  - Hypophosphatasia.
  - Others.
- Not otherwise specified.

SHORT ESSAYS

Question 1

What are the various developmental or acquired deformities and conditions?

Answer

Various developmental or acquired deformities and conditions are as follows:

- Localized tooth-related factors that modify or predispose to plaque-induced gingival diseases or periodontitis.
  - Tooth anatomic factors
  - Dental restorations or appliances
  - Root fractures
  - Cervical-root resorption and cemental tears.
- Mucogingival deformities and conditions around teeth.
  - Gingival or soft tissue recession
    - Facial or lingual surfaces
    - Interproximal (papillary)
  - Lack of keratinized gingiva
  - Decreased vestibular depth
  - Aberrant frenum or muscle position
  - Gingival excess?
    - Pseudopocket
    - Inconsistent gingival margin
    - Excessive gingival display
    - Gingival enlargement
    - Abnormal colour
- Mucogingival deformities and conditions on edentulous edges.
  - Vertical and/or horizontal ridge deficiency
  - Lack of gingiva or keratinized tissue
  - Gingival or soft tissue enlargements
  - Aberrant frenum or muscle position
  - Decreased vestibular depth
  - Abnormal colour
- Occlusal trauma.
  - Primary occlusal trauma
  - Secondary occlusal trauma.

Question 2

What are the various classifications of various forms of Periodontitis?

Answer

Various classifications of various forms of periodontitis are as follows:

- According to American Academy of Periodontology (AAP) world workshop in clinical periodontics (year 1989).
- European Workshop in Periodontology (year 1993).
- According to American Academy of Periodontology International Workshop for Classification of Periodontal Diseases (year 1999).
  - Chronic periodontitis.
  - Aggressive periodontitis.
  - Periodontitis as a manifestation of systemic disease.

Forms of periodontitis	Disease characteristics
1. Adult periodontitis	Age of onset more than 35 years, slow rate of disease progression, no defect in host defences
2. Early-onset periodontitis (may be prepubertal, juvenile, or rapidly progressive)	Age of onset less than 35 years, rapid rate of disease progression, defect in host defences, associated with specific microflora
3. Periodontitis associated with systemic disease	Systemic disease that predispose to rapid rates of periodontitis. Diseases are: diabetes, Down's syndrome, human immunodeficiency virus (HIV) infection, Papillon-Lefevre syndrome
4. Necrotizing ulcerative periodontitis	Similar to acute necrotizing ulcerative gingivitis but with associated clinical attachment loss
5. Refractory periodontitis	Recurrent periodontitis that does not respond to treatment

Forms of periodontitis	Disease characteristics
1. Adult periodontitis	**Age of onset:** 4th decade of life, slow rate of disease progression, no defects in host response
2. Early-onset periodontitis	**Age of onset:** Before 4th decade of life, rapid rate of disease progression, defect in host defence
3. Necrotizing periodontitis	Tissue necrosis with bone and attachment loss

CHAPTER 7

Epidemiology of Gingival and Periodontal Diseases

SHORT ESSAYS

Question 1

Discuss about the community periodontal index of treatments needs (CPITN) PROBE.

Answer

It is also termed as WHO probe.

- It serves three goals:
  1. Measures pocket depth.
  2. Detects subgingival calculus.
  3. Manipulate the sensitive soft tissues around the tooth.
- The probe has a ball and tip of 0.5 mm diameter that allows detection of subgingival calculus and gingival bleeding without causing trauma to the tissues.
- Probe has a black band beginning at 3.5 mm from the tip and ending at 5.5 mm [CPITN-E (epidemiological)].
- Probe has two additional markings of 8.5 mm and 11.5 mm [CPITN-C (clinica)].

Question 2

What is Russell's periodontal index?

Answer

- This index was proposed by Russell in 1950s.
- This index requires a light source, mouth mirror and explore.
- Supporting tissues of each tooth has scored according to progressive scale that gives little importance to gingival inflammation and higher weightage to advanced periodontal disease.
- An individual score is the sum of the tooth scores divided by the number of teeth examined.

Scoring Criteria

- **0 = negative:** There is neither overt inflammation in the investing tissues nor loos of function due to destruction of supporting tissues
- **1 = mild gingivitis:** There is an overt area of inflammation in the free gingiva but this area does not circumscribe the tooth.
- **2 = gingivitis:** Inflammation completely circumscribes the tooth, but there is no apparent break in the epithelial attachment.
- **6 = gingivitis with pocket formation:** The epithelial attachment has been broken and there is a pocket (not merely a deepened gingival crevice caused by swelling in the free gingiva). There is no interference with normal masticatory function; the tooth is firm in its socket and has not drifted.
- **8 = advanced destruction with loss of masticatory function:** The tooth may be loose, may be drifted, may sound dull on percussion with metallic instrument and may be depressible in its socket.
- **Russell's rule:** When in doubt assign a lower score.
- The value obtained by calculating individual score is interpreted as follows:
  - 0– 0.2—clinically normal supportive tissue.
  - 0.3–0.9—simple gingivitis.
  - 1–1.9—beginning of destructive periodontal disease.
  - 2–4.9—established destructive periodontal disease.
  - 5–8—terminal disease.

Question 3

What is periodontal disease index (given by SP Ramfjord, 1959)?

Answer

- In this index six pre-selected teeth in the mouth are examined, viz.:
    1. Maxillary right first molar.
    2. Maxillary left central incisor
    3. Maxillary left first premolar
    4. Mandibular left first molar
    5. Mandibular right central incisor
    6. Mandibular right first premolar
- In this index cemento-enamel junction (CEJ) is used as a fixed landmark for measuring periodontal attachment loss.
- To begin the assessment, the examiner dries the area around the six teeth.
- Then the examiner assesses the severity of gingival inflammation and gives the following scores:
    - G0 = Absence of inflammation
    - G1 = Mild to moderate inflammatory gingival changes, not extending all around the tooth
    - G2 = Mild to moderate severe gingivitis extending around the tooth
    - G3 = Severe gingivitis characterized by marked redness, tendency to bleed and ulceration.

Recording of Pocket

- The distance from the CEJ to the bottom of the gingival sulcus is the measurement of periodontal attachment loss.
- If the gingival sulcus does not extend apically to the CEJ, in any of the measured areas the periodontal disease index (PDI) score for the tooth is the gingival score.
- If the gingival sulcus extends below the CEJ in any of the measured areas by 3 mm or less the PDI score is 4.
- If the sulcus measurement is between 3 mm and 6 mm the PDI score is 5. If it is more than 6 mm, the PDI score is 6.
- If the free gingival margin is on the cementum, it distance from CEJ is recorded as a negative number.

What is Silness-löe Index?

This is also known as plaque index.
- The purpose of this index is to assess the thickness of plaque only at gingival surface.
- Instruments used are mouth mirror, dental explorer and light source.
- The teeth selected are: 16, 12, 24, 36, 32, 44.
- Only plaque at the cervical third of the tooth is evaluated and no attention is given to the plaque that has extended above that.
- Scoring criteria:
    - 0 = No plaque in the gingival area
    - 1 = A film of plaque adhering to free gingival margin at the adjacent area of tooth. The plaque may be recognized only after the application of disclosing agent.
    - 2 = Moderate accumulation of soft deposits within the gingival pocket on the gingival margin which can be seen by the naked eye.
    - 3 = Abundance of soft matter within the gingival pocket and/or on the gingival margin and on the adjacent tooth surface.
- Plaque index score of each tooth equals to total score of each tooth divided by four.
- Plaque index for individual = total of plaque index of each tooth divided by number of teeth examined.
- Interpretation:
    - 0—excellent
    - 0.1–0.9—good
    - 1.0–1.9—fair
    - 2.0–3.0—poor.

What is oral hygiene index-simplified (OHI-S) ?

- It was given by Greene and Vermillion in the year 1964.
- This index measures the surface area of the tooth that is covered by debris and calculus.
- It consist of two components: (1) debris index-simplified (DI-S) and (2) calculus index-simplified (CI-S).
- Scoring criteria for DI-S:
    - 0 = No debris or stain present.
    - 1 = Soft debris covering not more than one-third of the tooth surface or the presence of extrinsic stains without other debris regardless of surface area covered.
    - 2 = Soft debris covering more than one-third but not more than two-third of the exposed tooth surface
    - 3 = Soft debris covering more than two-thirds of the exposed tooth surface.
- Scoring criteria for CI-S:
    - 0 = No calculus present.

- ○ 1 = Supragingival calculus not covering more than one-third of the exposed tooth surface.
- ○ 2 = Supragingival calculus covering more than one-third but not more than two-third of the exposed tooth surface or the presence of individual flex of subgingival calculus around the cervical portion of the tooth or both.
- ○ 3 = Supragingival calculus covering more than two-third of the exposed tooth surface or a continuous heavy band of subgingival calculus around the cervical portion of the tooth or both.
- ❑ Debris index simplified score per person is obtained by totalling debris scores per tooth surface and dividing it by the number of surfaces examined.

- ❑ Calculus index simplified scores per person is obtained by totalling the calculus scores per tooth surface and dividing it by the number of surfaces examined.
- ❑ The OHI-S scores per person is the sum total of DI-S and CI-S scores per person.
- ❑ Interpretation of DI-S/CI-S scores:
  - ○ 0.0–0.6—good
  - ○ 0.7–1.8—fair
  - ○ 1.9–3—poor.
- ❑ The Interpretation of OHI-S scores:
  - ○ 0.0–1.2—good
  - ○ 1.3–3.0—fair
  - ○ 3.1–6.0—poor.

CHAPTER 8

Periodontal Microbiology

LONG ESSAYS

Question 1

Define dental plaque. Explain in detail about plaque as a biofilm.

Answer

Dental plaque is a specific but highly variable structural entity, resulting from sequential colonisation of microorganisms on tooth surfaces, restorations and other parts of oral cavity, composed of salivary components like mucin, desquamated epithelial cells, debris and microorganisms, all embedded in extracellular gelatinous matrix (WHO, 1961).

Plaque as a Biofilm

- Bacteria in a biofilm are not distributed evenly. They are grouped in microcolonies surrounded by an enveloping intermicrobial matrix.
- Dental plaque biofilm is heterogeneous in structure, with open fluid-filled channels running through the plaque mass (act as circulatory system). The matrix is penetrated by fluid channels that conduct the flow of nutrients, waste products, enzymes, metabolites, and oxygen. These microcolonies have micro-environments with differing pH, nutrient availability, and oxygen concentrations.
- The bacteria in a biofilm communicate with each other by sending out chemical signals. These chemical signals trigger the bacteria to produce potentially harmful proteins and enzymes.

Plaque Formation at an Ultrastructural Level

Process of plaque formation divided into three major phases (**Fig. 8.1**):

1. The formation of pellicle on tooth surface.
2. Initial adhesion and attachment of bacteria.
3. Colonisation and plaque maturation.

Formation of the Pellicle

All surfaces of the oral cavity are coated with a pellicle.

Acquired Pellicle

Within nanoseconds after vigorous polishing of the teeth, a thin saliva derived layer, called the acquired pellicle, covers the tooth surface.

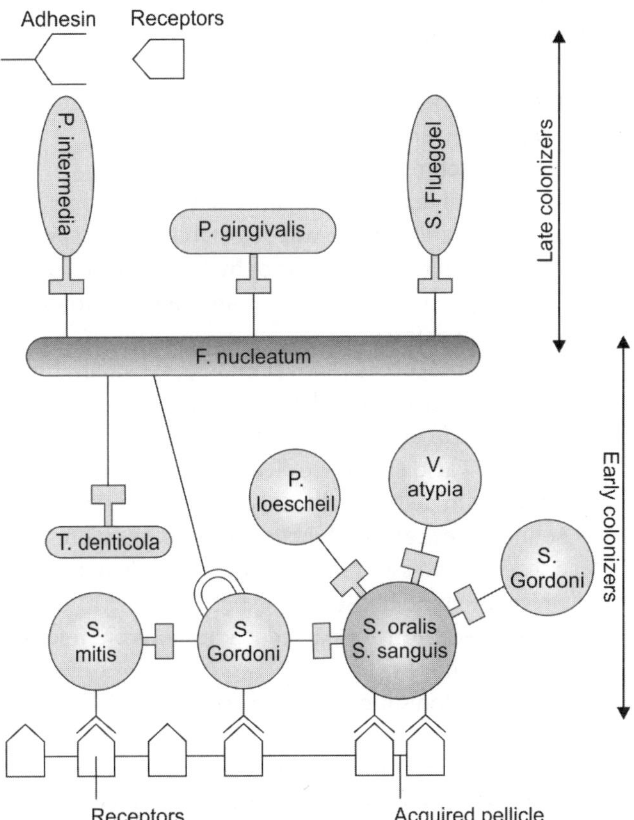

Fig. 8.1: Diagram showing plaque formation

Composition of the Pellicle

- Glycoproteins (mucin).
- Proline-rich proteins.
- Phosphoproteins (e.g. statherin).
- Histidine-rich proteins.
- Enzymes (α-amylase) and other molecules that can function as adhesion sites for bacteria.
- Bacteria can colonise tooth surface only when this pellicle is in place for some hours.

Study of early (2 hourly) enamel pellicle reveal that its amino acid composition differs from that of saliva.

Mechanism involved

- Electrostatic.
- Van der waals.
- Hydrophobic forces.

Initial Adhesion and Attachment of Bacteria

This situation is very complex. The microbial adhesion to surfaces in an aquatic environment as a four stage sequence.

- **Phase 1:** Transport to the surface:
  - Random contact may occur through Brownian motion (40 μm/hr) causing sedimentation of microorganisms, via liquid flow or chemotactic activity.
- **Phase 2:** Initial Adhesion:
  - Reversible adhesion of the bacterium, initiated by the interaction between the bacteria and the surface from a certain distance.
- **Phase 3:** Attachment:
  - After initial adhesion, a firm anchorage between bacterium and surface will be established by specific interactions (covalent, ionic or hydrogen bonding).
  - On rough surface, bacteria are better protected against shear forces.
  - Each streptococcus and actinomyces strain binds specific salivary molecules.
  - *Streptococcus sanguinis*, the principle early coloniser bind to acidic proline-rich proteins and other receptors in pellicle such as α-amylase and sialic acid.
  - Actinomyces can also function as primary colonisers.
  - Viscosus possesses fimbriae which contain adhesions which also bind to the proline rich-layer.
  - Hidden receptors for bacterial adhesions are referred to as cryptitopes.
- **Phase 4:** Colonisation of the surface and biofilm formation:
  - Firmly attached microorganisms start growing and bacterial clusters are formed, then microcolonies or a biofilm can develop.
  - Therefore intrabacterial connections occur.

- Eighteen genera from the oral cavity show some form of co-aggregation.
- Co-aggregation is the cell-to-cell recognition of genetically distinct partner cell type.
- All oral bacteria possess surface molecules (protein or carbohydrate molecules) that foster some type of cell interaction.
- Fusobacteria co-aggregate with all other human oral bacteria; whereas veillonellae, capnocytophage and prevotella bind to streptococci and actinomyces.
- Most co-aggregations among strains of different genera are mediated by lectin like adhesins and inhibited by lactose and other galactosides.

Early Coloniser

Each strain of early coloniser is coated with distinct molecules. Identical cells coated with a specific salivary molecule may agglutinate, leading to microconcentration and juxta-positioning of a particular strain.

- *Secondary colonisers* interact with early colonisers, co-aggregation of fusobacterium nucleatum with S. sanguinis.
- *Prevotella loescheii* with *Actinomyces viscosus*.
- *Capnocytophaga ochracea* with *Actinomyces viscosus*.
- Co-aggregation has focussed on interactions among different Gram positive species and between Gram positive and Gram negative species.
- Both Actinomycetes and Streptococci are facultative anaerobes, doubling times for microbial populations during first 4 hours of development is less than 1 hour.

Secondary Coloniser

- *Prevotella intermedia*.
- *P. loescheii*.
- *Capnocytophaga*.
- *F. nucleatum*.
- *Porphyromonas gingivalis*.

In the later stages of plaque formation, co-aggregation between different Gram negative species is likely to predominate, e.g. "Corncob" formation. Streptococci adhere to filaments of *Bacterionema matruchotii* or *Actinomyces specis* and the "test tube brush" composed of filamentous bacteria to which Gram negative rods adhere.

Secondary Colonisers fall Into **(Fig. 8.2)**

- **Green complex:** *Eikenella corrodens, Actinobacillus actinomycetemcomitans* serotype A and Capnocytophaga species.
- **Orange complex:** Fusobacterium, Prevotella, and Campylobacter.

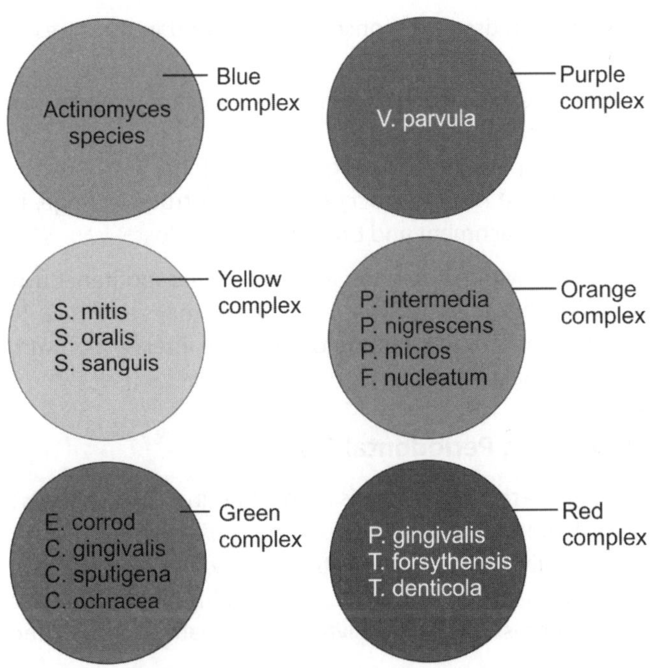

Fig. 8.2: Various bacterial complexes.

- **Red complex:** *P. gingivalis, Tannerella forsythia* and *Treponema denticola.*
- **Yellow complex:** *Streptococcus specis.*
- **Purple complex:** *Actinomyces odontolyticus.*

Question 2

Describe various microorganisms associated with specific periodontal diseases.

Answer

The total number of bacteria, determined by microscopic counts per gram of plaque was twice as high in periodontally diseased sites than in healthy sites.

More motile rods and spirochetes are found. Fewer coccal cells are present.

Periodontal Health

Bacteria associated with periodontal health are Gram positive facultative species and members of the genera Streptococcus and Actinomyces (e.g. *S. sanguinis, S. mitis, A. viscosus, A. naeslundii*). Small proportions of Gram negative species *P. intermedia, F. nucleatum,* Capnocytophaga, Neisseria and Veillonella species. Few spirochetes and motile rods are also present.

Species beneficial to host are:

- *S. sanguinis, Veillonella parvula* and *Capnocytophaga ochraceus.*

- *S. sanguinis*–hydrogen peroxide lethal to cells of Actinomycetemcomitans.
- *C. ochraceus* and *S. sanguinis* are associated with greater gain in attachment after therapy.

Gingivitis

After 8 hours without oral hygiene, bacteria may be found at concentrations of 10^3 to $10^4/mm^2$ of tooth surface and will increase in number by a factor of 100–1,000 in the next 24-hours period. After 36 hours, the plaque becomes clinically visible.

The transition to gingivitis is evident by inflammatory changes and is accompanied first by the appearance of Gram-negative rods and filaments, spirochetal and motile microorganisms.

Microbiota of Dental-plaque-induced Gingivitis (Chronic Gingivitis)

It consist of the following:

- Gram positive (*S. sanguis, S. mitis, S. intermedius, S. oralis, A. viscosus, A. naeslundii,* and *P. micros*).
- Gram negative (*F. nucleatum, P. intermedia,* and *V. parvula,* Haemophilus, Capnocytophaga, and Campylobacter species), facultative and anaerobic microorganisms.

Pregnancy-associated Gingivitis

It is an acute inflammation of the gingival tissues associated with pregnancy. *P. intermedia* is associated with this gingivitis. It is accompanied by increase in steroid hormones in crevicular fluid and increases in the levels of growth factors.

Chronic Periodontitis

Bacteria seen are:

- *P. gingivalis, T. forsythia, P. intermedia, C. rectus, E. corrodens, F. nucleatum, A. actinomycetemcomitans, P. micros, Treponema* and *Eubacterium* species.
- Recent studies shown that presence of subgingival Epstein-Barr virus type 1 (EBV-1) and human Cytomegalovirus (HCMV) are associated with high levels of putative bacterial pathogens, i.e. *P. gingivalis, T. forsythia, P. intermedia,* and *T. denticola.*

Microbial Shift during Disease

Comparing the microbiota in health, gingivitis, and periodontitis, the following microbial shifts can be identified:

- From gram positive to gram negative

- From cocci to rods (and at a later stage to spirochetes)
- From non-motile to motile organisms
- From facultative anaerobes to obligate anaerobes
- From fermenting to proteolytic species.

Localised Aggressive Periodontitis

- Localised aggressive periodontitis (previously referred to as localised juvenile periodontitis) develops around the time of puberty, is observed in females more often than in males and affects.
- The first symptom of localised aggressive periodontitis (detectable in deciduous) dentition is periodontal destruction around canines and second molars.
- Microbiota: Gram negative, capnophilic and anaerobic rods.
- *A. actinomycetemcomitans* compose 90% of the microbiota. *A. actinomycetemcomitans* can be classified into six distinct serotypes (A to F) based on the surface polysaccharides located on the O side chains of lipopolysaccharides.
- *P. gingievalis, E. corrodens, C. rectus, F. nucleatum, B. capillus, Eubacterium brachy*, Capnocytophaga species and spirochetes.
- Herpes virus, including EBV-1 and HCMV play important roles in the aetiopathogenesis of severe types of periodontitis.
- HCMV associated periodontal sites also tend to harbour elevated levels of bacteria including *P. gingivalis, T. forsythia, T. denticola*, Campylobacter rectus and *A. actinomycetemcomitans*.
- A high prevalence of HCMV and EBV type-1 DNA revealed in aggressive periodontitis sites compared to healthy sites.
- Mechanical debridement with antibiotics are necessary to control the levels of *A. actinomycetemcomitans*.

Generalised Aggressive Periodontitis

- Generalised aggressive periodontitis (GAP) affects individuals under the age of 30, but older patients may be affected.
- Characterised by generalised interproximal attachment loss affecting at least three permanent other than first molars and incisors.
- The destruction occurs episodically, with periods of advanced destruction followed by weeks to months or years.
- Small amount of plaque associated with the affected teeth.
- *P. gingivalis, A. acintomycetemcomitans*, and *T. forsythia* are detected in the plaque that is present.

Two gingival tissue responses can be found in the cases of GAP:

- One is severe, acutely inflamed tissue, often proliferating, ulcerated and fiery red.
- Bleeding may occur by slight stimulation
- This tissue response occurs in the destructive stage, in which attachment and bone are actively lost.

Patients with the diagnosis of GAP arrested spontaneously or after the therapy, whereas others may continue to progress inexorably to tooth loss, despite intervention with conventional treatment.

Necrotising Periodontal Disease

- Characterised by necrosis of the marginal gingival tissue and interdental papillae
- Clinically associated with stress or HIV infection
- Accompanied by mal-odour, pain, and systemic symptoms including lymphadenopathy, fever and malaise
- High levels of *P. intermedia*, and spirochetes are found in ulcerative gingivitis lesions
- Spirochetes are found to penetrate necrotic tissue and unaffected connective tissue.

Abscesses of the Periodontium

- Acute lesions that result in very rapid destruction of the periodontal tissues.
- Occur in patient with untreated periodontitis or during maintenance phase.
- May occur in the absence of periodontitis, associated with impaction of foreign material.
- **Clinical symptoms:** Pain, swelling, suppuration, bleeding on probing, and mobility of the involved teeth. Systemic involvement including cervical lymphadenopathy and WBC count.
- **Pathogens include:** *F. nucleatum, P. intermedia, P. micros*, and *T. forsythia* are present.

Periodontitis as Manifestation of Systemic Disease

- Demonstrates varied immune deficiency, neutrophil defects and leucocyte adhesion defects.
- **Recent studies:** Some cases of severe periodontal destruction are associated with a mutation in the cathepsin C gene in affected children.
- Increased host susceptibility resulting from systemic disease.

Peri-implantitis

- It is an inflammatory process that affects the tissues around an already osseo-integrated implant and resulting in loss of supporting bone.
- Healthy peri-implant is pocket characterized high proportions of coccoid cells, a low-ratio anaerobic or aerobic species, a low number of Gram-anaerobic species and low detection frequencies for periodontal pathogens.
- Peri-implantitis reveal a complex microbiota. A. *actinomycetemcomitans, P. gingivalis, T. forsythia, P. micros, Campylobacter rectus,* Fusobacterium and Capnocytophaga are isolated from failing sites.
- *Pseudomonas aeruginosa,* enterobacteriaceae, *Candida albicans,* and staphylococci are frequently detected around implants.
- High proportions of *Staphylococcus aureus* and S. *epidermidis* on oral implants have also been reported.

Question 3

What are the various key characteristics of specific pathogens?

Answer

Actinobacillus Actinomycetemcomitans

- Size varies from 0.4–1 μm.
- Straight or curved rods with rounded ends.
- It is non-motile and Gram negative.
- **Forms:** Five serotypes (a-e).

Culture Condition and Identification

- Grows as a white, translucent, smooth, non-haemolytic colony on blood agar, because of its low density.
- A. actinomycetemcomitans is preferably identified on a specific growth medium (with vancomycin and bacitracin as antibiotic to suppress other species) under 5–10% carbon dioxide where it appears white, translucent colony with a star-shaped internal structure.
- It possesses a number of virulence factors including lipopolysaccharide (endotoxin), a leucotoxin collagenase and a protease.

Tannerella Forsythia

It is a non-motile, spindle shaped, highly polymorphic rod and a Gram negative obligate anaerobe.

Culture Conditions and Identification

It grows slowly only under anaerobic conditions and need several growth factors from other species.

Pathogenicity

This species produces several proteolytic enzymes that are able to destroy immunoglobulin and factors of complement system. It also induces apoptotic cell death.

Porphyromonas Gingivalis

P. gingivalis is a non-motile, pleomorphic rod and Gram –ve obligate anaerobe. *Its form based on the capsule type.*

Culture Conditions and Identification

It grows anaerobically with dark pigmentations on blood agar. *L. Porphyromonas gingivalis* has a strong proteolytic activity.

Specific Pathogenic Characteristics

- Aggressive periodontal pathogen. Its fimbriae mediate adhesion, and its capsule defends against phagocytosis.
- Produces series of virulence factors, including proteases, haemolysin and a collagenase.
- Also inhibit migration of PMNs across an epithelial barrier and affects the production or degradation of cytokines by mammalian cells.
- *P. gingivalis* also has the capacity to invade soft tissues.

Prevotella Intermedia and Prevotella Nigrescens

Prevotella group are short, round-ended, non-motile, Gram negative rods. Its forms *P. intermedia* and *P. nigrescens* are the most pathogenic.

Culture Condition and Identification

Grow anaerobically, with dark pigmentation on blood agar.

Special Pathogenic Characteristics

Prevotella species are less virulent and less proteolytic than *P. gingivalis.*

Campylobacter Rectus

- It is one of the rare motile organisms involved.
- It is Gram negative, short rod, curved or helical.
- The motility results from the polar flagellum.

Culture Conditions and Identification

Grows anaerobically with dark pigmentation. Sulphide is added → FeS, giving a grey stain.

Special Pathogenic Characteristics

Produces a leucotoxin.

C. rectus is less virulent and less proteolytic than *P. gingivalis.*

Fusobacterium Nucleatum

It is a Gram negative, cigar shaped bacillus with pointed ends.

Its forms are *F. nucleatum ss nucleatum, F. nucleatum ss polymorphum, F. nucleatum ss vincentii,* and *F. periodonticum.*

Culture Conditions and Identification

Grows anaerobically on blood agar and can easily be identified on a specific medium.

Special Pathogenic Characteristics

- Induc apoptotic cell death in mononuclear and polymorphonuclear cells and can trigger the release of cytokines, elastase, and oxygen radicals from leucocytes.
- Believed to be important bridging organisms.

Peptostreptococcus Micros

This is one of the rare cocci in periodontitis. This species is Gram +ve and grows obligate anaerobically.

Eubacterium Species

- Gm positive, obligate anaerobic, small pleomorphic rod.
- **Forms:** E. nodatum, E. brachy, and E. timidum.

Culture Conditions and Identification

Grow anaerobically, but with difficulty on standard blood agar.

Spirochaetes

- Represent a diverse group of spiral, motile organisms.
- They are helical rods 5–15 μm long with a diameter of 0.5 μm.
- **Forms:** Treponema denticola, Treponema vincentii, Treponema socranskii (often associated with periodontitis), and Treponema pallidum (associated with secondary syphilis).

Culture Conditions and Identification

Extremely difficult to grow and need strict anaerobic conditions and a specific medium.

Special Pathogenic Characteristics

- Ability to travel through viscous environments enables them to migrate within the gingival crevicular fluid and to penetrate both the epithelium and the connective tissue.
- Degrade collagen and dentin.
- *T. denticola* produces proteolytic enzymes and can destroy (IgA, IgM, IgG) or complement factors.

What is the composition of plaque? What is the classification of plaque?

Plaque is mainly composed of microorganisms:

- One gram of plaque approximately contains 10^{11} bacteria.
- Non-bacterial microorganisms like yeast, mycoplasma, protozoa, and viruses are also present in small amounts.
- Cells like host cells, e.g. epithelial cells, macrophages and leucocytes are also present.
- Organic matter of plaque consists of mainly polysaccharide protein produced by plaque microorganisms. Proteins such as albumin are present. Levans, glucans, galactose, and methyl pentose are some carbohydrates produced by bacteria. Small amounts of lipids found in plaque are derived from the disrupted cell walls of gram negative bacteria.
- The main inorganic matter of dental plaque consists of calcium, and phosphorous along with small amounts of magnesium, sodium and potassium.

Classification of Dental Plaque

It is majorly classified as:

- Supragingival **(Fig. 8.3)**.
- Subgingival.
- Supragingival plaque is further classified as :
  - Coronal plaque: It is in contact with only the tooth surface.
  - Marginal plaque: It is in contact with tooth surface at the margin of gingiva.
- Subgingival plaque is further classified as:
  - Attached plaque.
  - Unattached plaque.

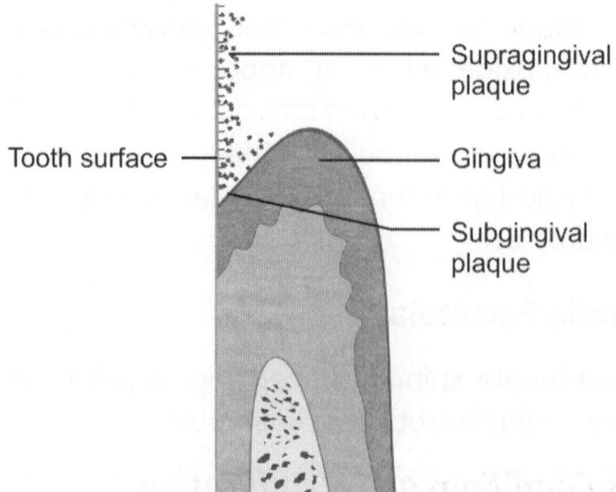

Fig. 8.3: Diagram showing supragingival and subgingival plaque.

Attached plaque is further classified as tooth associated, epithelium associated or connective tissue associated.

Supragingival Plaque

- ❑ It basically consists of Gram positive cocci and Gram negative rods and filaments.
- ❑ It is adherent to the tooth surface.
- ❑ It is found at or above the gingival margin.
- ❑ When it is in contact with gingival margin, it is referred as marginal plaque.
- ❑ It has stratified organisation of a multi-layered accumulation of bacterial morpho-types.
- ❑ The morphological arrangements of the flora in supragingival plaque are referred to as "corn cob" formations.
- ❑ Corn cob consists of rod-shaped bacterial cells e.g., Fusobacterium nucleatum and coccal cells mainly streptococci.

Subgingival Plaque

- ❑ This plaque is found below the gingival margin, between tooth and gingival pocket epithelium.

- ❑ This plaque mainly consists of filaments with flagella and also spirochetes.
- ❑ This is because of the local availability of blood products and a low oxidation reduction (redox) potential.

There are three kinds of subgingival plaque (**Fig. 8.4**):

1. Tooth associated which is similar to supragingival plaque.
2. Tissue associated which is associated with flagellated bacteria without a well-defined extracellular matrix and numerous bristle brush formations. This arrangement is also known as test tube brush formation.
3. Unattached plaque is seen in between the tooth and tissue associated plaque (**Fig. 8.5**).

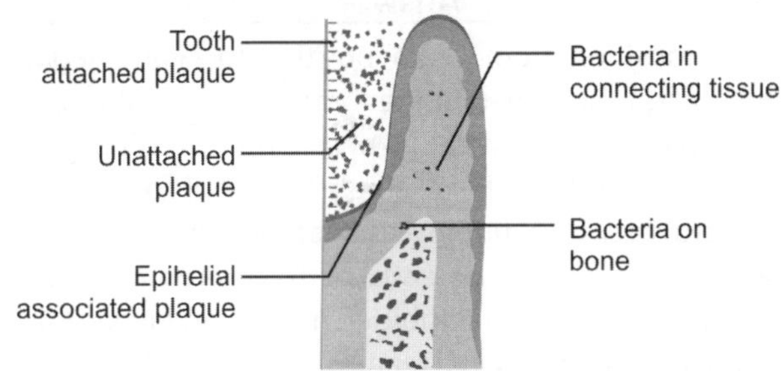

Fig. 8.4: Diagram showing.

SHORT ESSAYS

Question 1

What is meant by commensal relationship?

Answer

Bacteria and host cells are the two parties which form a commensal relationship. Generally in this kind of relationship, both the sides get benefit from each other, e.g. the host's oral epithelial cells produce glucose, which is utilised by lactobacilli bacteria colonised in the oral cavity, which in turn produces acid. Lowering of pH would prevent the colonisation of many other deleterious effects of other bacterias. Therefore in this manner both the parties get the benefit from each other.

Question 2

Define biofilm. What is the significance of biofilm?

Answer

Biofilm: A collection of microorganisms, extracellular polymeric products, and organic matter located at the interface in solid-liquid, gas-liquid, or liquid-liquid biphasic systems.

Significance of Biofilms

- ❑ Contributing to host-tissue damage:
  - ○ Sessile bacterial cells release antigens, which results in antibodies stimulation which further results in immune-complex activation.
  - ○ Extracellular polymeric substances mainly polysaccharides are released which cause constant irritation to macrophages (frustrated macrophages).
- ❑ Resistance to antimicrobial agents:
  - ○ 1,000-fold greater than planktonic cells.
  - ○ Failure of an agent to penetrate the full depth of the biofilm
  - ○ Cells in a biofilm experience nutrient limitation and therefore exist in a slow-growing or starved state
  - ○ Oral biofilms are more resistant to chlorhexidine, amine fluoride, amoxycillin, doxycycline, and metronidazole than planktonic cells.
- ❑ Potential to spread:
  - ○ Seeding dispersal: Programmed detachment of planktonic bacterial cells caused by local hydrolysis of the extracellular polysaccharide matrix, and conversion of a subpopulation of cells into motile planktonic cells

○ Clumping dispersal: A physical detachment pathway in which a fragment of a microcolony, simply detaches from the biofilm and is carried by the bulk until it lodges in a new location and initiates a new sessile population.

Question 3

What are the physiologic properties of dental plaque?

Or

Describe the metabolic interactions among different species of bacteria in plaque and between host and plaque bacteria.

Answer

❑ The transition from Gram positive to Gram negative microorganisms seen in the formation of dental plaque goes hand in hand with the physiologic transition in the developing plaque. For example the initial colonisers, i.e. streptococci or Actinomyces species utilise the oxygen and lower the redox potential of the environment, which in turn makes the anaerobic environment, favouring the growth of anaerobic bacteria.

❑ The metabolic by-products of actinomycetes and streptococci are lactate and formate, which can be further utilised by other plaque microorganisms for their metabolism.

❑ *C. ochraceus* produces succinate and *Campylobacter rectus* produces protoheme, and both succinate and protoheme are utilised by *P. gingivalis* for its growth.

❑ The host can also function as an important source of nutrients to the bacterial plaque. For example, the bacterial enzymes which are responsible for the degradation of host proteins, causes the release of

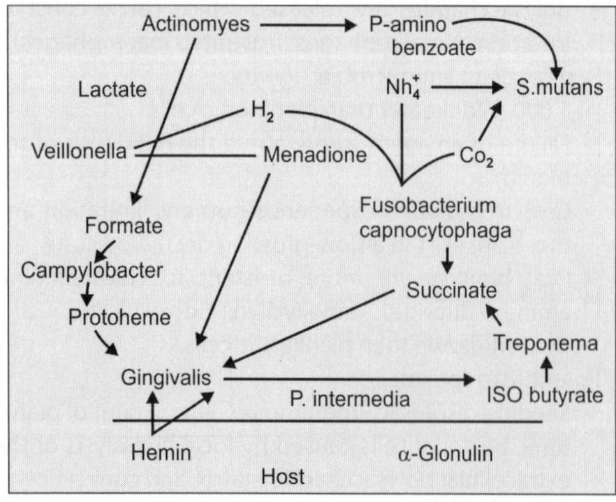

Fig. 8.5: Physiologic properties of dental plaque.

ammonia, which can be further utilised by the bacteria as the nitrogen source.

❑ Breakdown of host haemoglobin results in production of haemin, which can be used by *P. gingivalis* for its metabolism (**Fig. 8.5**).

❑ Increase in steroid hormone is associated with increase in proportions of *P. intermedia* present in sub-gingival plaque.

Question 4

What are nutritional interdependencies? What is its significance?

Answer

There are physiologic interactions which occur in between various species of plaque bacteria and between host and plaque bacteria. Both release certain by-products which can be utilised by each other for their growth and metabolism. This is referred to as nutritional interdependencies. For example, initial colonisers, i.e. streptococci or actinomyces species utilise the oxygen and lower the redox potential of the environment, which in turn makes the anaerobic environment, favouring the growth of anaerobic bacteria.

The metabolic by-products of actinomycetes and streptococci are lactate and formate, which can be further utilised by other plaque microorganisms for their metabolism.

Capnocytophaga ochraceus produces succinate and *C. rectus* produces protoheme, and both succinate and protoheme are utilized by *P. gingivalis* for its growth.

The host can also function as an important source of nutrients to the bacterial plaque. For example, the bacterial enzymes which are responsible for the degradation of host proteins, causes the release of ammonia, which can be further utilised by the bacteria as the nitrogen source.

Breakdown of host haemoglobin result in production of haemin, which can be used by *P. gingivalis* for its metabolism.

Increase in steroid hormone is associated with increase in proportions of *P. intermedia* present in subgingival plaque.

Significance

❑ These nutritional interdependencies are very important in the growth and survival of microorganisms present in dental plaque.

❑ It is responsible for evolution of highly specific structural interactions among various bacterias (**Fig. 8.6**).

Question 5

What are the various tests done for the microbial analysis?

Answer

Various microbial tests are:

- **Culture methods:** Qualitative measurement of all viable microorganisms. Antibiotic sensitivity is determined. But costly, time-consuming and difficult.
- **Immunodiagnostic methods:** Methods like enzyme-linked immunosorbent assay (ELISA), immunofluorescence etc., less time consuming and less expensive. Disadvantage is that cross reaction is more.
- **DNA probes:** It entails segments of single-stranded DNA, labelled with an enzyme or radioisotope that can locate and bind to their complementary nucleic acid sequence. No cross reaction seen.
- **Polymerase chain reaction (PCR):** Amplification of a region of DNA flanked by a selected primer pair specific for the target species. More specific real time PCR is an advanced version where quantitative measurement is also possible.

Question 6

What are the special bacterial behaviour in biofilms?

Answer

The bacteria present in a liquid environment, i.e. planktonic state behaves differently as compared to bacteria present in a biofilm.

- Organisms in a biofilm are 1,000–1,500 times more resistant to antibiotics than in their planktonic state.
- The mechanism of increased resistance depends upon species to species, antibiotic to antibiotic, and for biofilms growing in different environment.
- Another reason for increased resistance of bacteria to antibiotics is slow growth rate of bacteria in a biofilm, which makes them less susceptible to many antibiotics.
- Extracellular enzymes such as beta lactamase, formaldehyde-lyase and formaldehyde dehydrogenase may become trapped and concentrated in extracellular matrix, thus inactivating some antibiotics.
- Recently super-resistant bacteria have been identified in a biofilm. These cells have multi-drug-resistant pumps that can extrude antimicrobial agents from the cell.
- In a biofilm, bacteria have the capacity to communicate with each other through quorum sensing. This involves the regulation of expression of specific genes through the accumulation of signalling compounds that mediate intercellular communication. When these signalling compounds reach a threshold level (quorum cell density), gene expression can be activated.
- The high density of bacterial cells in a biofilm also facilitates the exchange of genetic information among cells of the same species and across species and also genera.

Question 7

What are the reasons for drug resistance in a biofilm?

Answer

- Organisms in a biofilm are 1,000–1,500 times more resistant to antibiotics than in their planktonic state.
- The mechanism of increased resistance depends upon species to species, antibiotic to antibiotic, and for biofilms growing in different environment.
- Another reason for increased resistance of bacteria to antibiotics is slow growth rate of bacteria in a biofilm, which makes them less susceptible to many antibiotics.
- Extracellular enzymes such as beta lactamase, formaldehyde-lyase and formaldehyde dehydrogenase may become trapped and concentrated in extracellular matrix, thus inactivating some antibiotics.
- Recently super resistant bacteria have been identified in a biofilm. These cells have multi-drug-resistant pumps that can extrude antimicrobial agents from the cell.
- Conjugation (exchange of genes through a direct inter-bacterial connection formed by a sex pilus), transformation (movement of small pieces of DNA from the environment into the bacterial chromosome), plasmid transfer, and transposon transfer have all been seen in a biofilm.

Question 8

What is corn cob structure and test tube formation?

Answer

Marginal plaque has stratified organisation of a multi-layered accumulation of bacterial morpho-types **(Fig. 8.6)**.

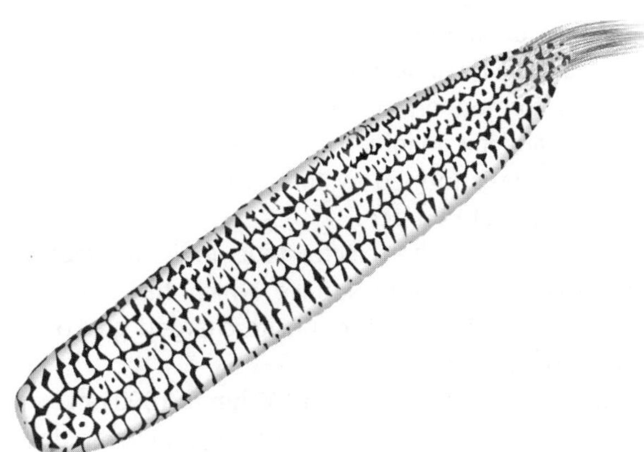

Fig. 8.6: Corn-cob structure.

The morphological arrangements of the flora in supragingival plaque are referred to as corn cob formations.

Corn cob consists of rod shaped bacterial cells for example Fusobacterium nucleatum and coccal cells mainly streptococci which attach along the surface of the rod shaped cells.

Tissue associated plaque is associated with flagellated bacteria without a well-defined extracellular matrix and numerous bristle brush formations. This arrangement is also known as test tube brush formation. Large filaments are seen in the test tube brush formation that form the long axis, and short filaments or Gram negative rods embedded in an amorphous matrix **(Fig. 8.7)**.

Question 9

What are the Socransky's modification of Koch's postulates?

Answer

Sigmund Socransky gave the criteria by which the pathogenicity of microorganisms can be detected.

Socransky's criteria based on Koch's postulates are as follows:

- A potential pathogen associated with disease should be increased in number at diseased sites.
- After treatment it should be decreased in number at sites that show clinical improvement.
- It should produce some form of cellular or humoral immune response in the host.
- When experimentally inoculated into animal models, it should be capable of causing the same disease.

Question 10

What is dental pellicle?

Answer

Within nanoseconds of brushing and polishing of teeth, all the oral surfaces, both hard and soft tissues of the oral-cavity are coated with a pellicle.

- Pellicle is formed on surfaces of teeth and artificial prosthesis and it is an initial organic structure.
- Dental pellicle is formed by the adsorption of salivary proteins to apatite surfaces.
- This results from the electrostatic ionic interaction between hydroxyapatite surface which has negative charge that interacts with opposite charged groups in the salivary macromolecules.
- Thickness of pellicle varies from 100 nm to 1000 nm.
- Pellicle gets converted into dental plaque quite rapidly.

Question 11

What is acquired pellicle?

Answer

Acquired pellicle is a thin saliva derived layer which covers the tooth surface and consists of glycoproteins, proline-rich proteins, phosphoproteins, histidine-rich proteins, enzymes and other molecules which function as adhesion sites for bacteria

This process involves adsorption of positively-charged salivary, crevicular fluid and other environmental macromolecules to negatively charged hydroxyapatite surfaces of teeth.

Various kinds of energies are involved in this process like electrostatic force, van der Waals forces and hydrophobic forces.

Pellicle is protective in nature. Along with this it provides lubrication and prevents tissue desiccation. It provides a base for colonisation and proliferation of microorganisms.

Question 12

What are the differences between dental plaque and materia alba?

Answer

Characteristic	Materia alba	Dental plaque
Colour	White	Greyish yellow
Removal	Easy	Difficult
Organisation	Poorly organised	Well organised
Bacterial count	Less	More
Presence of living organisms	Less	More
Distribution of micro organisms	Similar	Similar
Pathogenicity	Less	More

Question 13

What are the methods of detection of plaque?

Answer

There are various methods of plaque detection:

- Direct vision:
  - If the plaque is very thin, it will not be visible with naked eye.
  - Plaque may acquire extrinsic stain, because of which it becomes visible.
  - Thick layer of plaque is visible and appears as dull and dizzy in colour.

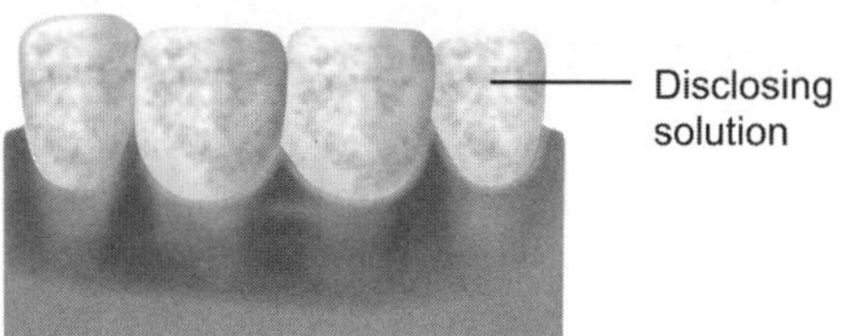

Fig. 8.7: Color of plaque changes upon application of disclosing soluion.

- ❑ Use of explorer:
  - ❍ By tactile sensation.
  - ❍ By removal of plaque with explorer.
- ❑ By use of a curette.
- ❑ Using a disclosing solution: It stains the plaque, because of which it is easily visualised **(Fig. 8.7)**
- ❑ By recording indices and comparing it.

Question 14

What are the differences between supragingival and sub-gingival plaque?

Answer

		Supragingival plaque	*Subgingival plaque*
1.	Location	Located above the margin of gingiva	Located below the margin of the gingiva
2.	Origin	Salivary glycoproteins for acquired pellicle. Microorganisms attach to this pellicle	Down growth of bacteria from supragingival plaque and gingival crevicular fluid (GCF)
3.	Distribution	Proximal surfaces, cracks, pits, fissures, over-hanged margin restoration, artificial crowns, orthodontic bands etc.	Sulcus and periodontal Pockets
4.	Adhesion	Acquired pellicle, other bacteria, tooth surface	Tooth surface, sub-gingival pellicle, calculus
5.	Shape and size	Friction of tongue, cheeks and lips, limits the size and shape	Moulded by pocket wall
6.	structure	Adherent, densely packed microbial layer over pellicle on tooth surface with intermicrobial matrix	Tooth-attached, tissue attached, connective tissue-associated, un-attached plaque
7.	Microorganisms	Gram positive cocci, filamentous	Gram negative, spirochetes
8.	Source of nutrients	Saliva and ingested food	GCF, exudate and leucocytes
9.	Significance	Gingivitis and formation of supragingival calculus	Periodontitis and formation of subgingival calculus

Question 15

What are the various plaque hypothesis?

Answere

Non-specific Plaque Hypothesis

In mid-1900s, periodontal diseases were believed to result from an accumulation of plaque, along with a lower host response and increased host susceptibility with age. This is referred to as non-specific plaque hypothesis, where the quantity plaque is considered rather than quality of plaque.

Specific Plaque Hypothesis

According to this theory only specific bacteria in plaque are responsible for the disease. That means quality of plaque is more important than quantity of plaque. An increase in the number of specific bacteria would produce the disease because of release of certain virulent factors. This theory was given in 1976, by Loesche.

SHORT NOTES

Question 1

What is ecological plaque hypothesis?

Answer

Environmental perturbations lead to growth and development of pathologic flora, which is referred to as ecological plaque hypothesis.

This means that any change in the nutrients of pocket or chemical or physical change in the environment can lead to the overgrowth of pathogens. For example increase in levels of gingival crevicular fluid would lead to enrichment of proteolytic species, by providing nutrients to the pathogens.

Question 2

What is quorum sensing?

Answer

In a biofilm, bacteria have the capacity to communicate with each other through quorum sensing. This involves the regulation of expression of specific genes through the accumulation of signalling compounds that mediate intercellular communication. When these signalling compounds reach a threshold level (quorum cell density), gene expression can be activated.

Question 3

What is conjugation and transformation in a plaque biofilm?

Answer

Conjugation means exchange of genes through a direct inter-bacterial connection formed by a sex pilus.

Transformation means movement of small pieces of DNA from the environment into the bacterial chromosome.

Question 4

What is materia alba?

Answer

Material alba is a soft deposition of tissue and bacteria, lacking the organised structure of dental plaque. It can be easily displaced with a water spray.

Question 5

What is the difference between attached, unattached and tissue-associated plaque?

Answer

Attached plaque	Unattached plaque	Tissue associated plaque
It is attached to the tooth surface	It is present between attached plaque and tissue-associated plaque	It is attached to the epithelia of the pocket lining
Gram positive bacteria pre-dominate	Variable	Variable
Does not extend to junctional epithelium	Extend to junctional epithelium	Extend to junctional epithelium
Responsible for calculus formation and root caries	gingivitis	Gingivitis and periodontitis

Question 6

What is environmental plaque hypothesis?

Answer

In 1991, Haffajee and colleagues suggested that the entire subgingival microbial environment is the key to development of disease.

CHAPTER 9

Dental Calculus and Iatrogenic Factors

LONG ESSAYS

Question 1

Describe the structure and composition of calculus. What are the various theories of calculus formation?

Answer

Calculus is defined as an adherent calcified or calcifying amorphous mass that forms on the surface of natural teeth, restorations and dental prosthesis.

Structure of Calculus

- ❑ The most important feature of calculus is that its surface is covered with a layer of unmineralised plaque.
- ❑ Calculus is a very porous structure which contains several spaces within its calcified mass. These spaces can be uncalcified bacteria, or they may be seen around individual calcified organisms themselves.
- ❑ Supragingival calculus, microscopically, is heterogeneous in nature since it is a layered structure in which the degree of calcification varies from layer-to-layer.
- ❑ On contrary, subgingival calculus is homogeneous as it is built in layers with almost equal quality of minerals.

Composition

Calculus consists of an inorganic matter which accounts for 70–90% and an organic matter that accounts for 10–30%.

Inorganic Component

- ❑ Calcium phosphate: 75.9%
- ❑ Calcium carbonate: 3.1%
- ❑ Magnesium phosphate and other metals: Trace amounts
- ❑ Calcium: 39%
- ❑ Phosphorous: 19%
- ❑ Magnesium: 0.8%
- ❑ Sodium, zinc, bromine, copper, silicon, iron and fluorine: Trace amounts.

About two-third of the inorganic component is crystalline in structure and the four main crystal forms in which they exist are:

1. Hydroxyapatite: 58%, it appears as sand grain or rod like crystals.
2. Magnesium whitlokite: 21%, hexagonal (cuboidal, rhomboidal) crystals.
3. Octacalcium phosphate: 21%, they are platelet-like crystals.
4. Brushite: 9%.

Incidence of these crystals varies with age, and location of the calculus, therefore all these crystals do not appear at same frequency.

Hydroxyapatite and octacalcium phosphate are the most common crystals seen in supragingival calculus, while brushite is seen commonly in mandibular anterior region, magnesium whitlokite is seen more often in the posterior areas.

Organic Components

- ❑ Mixture of protein polysaccharide complexes, very little fractions of lipids, desquamated epithelial cells, leucocytes and various types of microorganisms.
- ❑ **Salivary proteins:** 5.9–8.2%, includes most of the amino acids.
- ❑ **Polysaccharides:** 1.9–9.1%. These are mainly derived from proteoglycans of bacteria, and salivary glycoproteins, e.g. galactose, glucose, rhamnose, mannose and galactosamine.
- ❑ **Lipids:** 0.2% of neutral fats, free fatty acids, cholesterol, cholesterol esters and phospholipids. These are mainly derived from the cell walls of bacteria that present within the calculus during the process of mineralisation.

Various Theories of Calculus Formation

Various theories of calculus formation are as follows:
- Precipitation theory: Booster mechanism.
- Epitactic concept/heterogeneous nucleation concept.
- Inhibition theory.

Precipitation Theory

Due to local rise in degree of saturation of calcium and phosphate ions, minerals gets precipitated.

Booster Mechanism

This the most important mechanism of precipitation, in which local rise in the degree of saturation of calcium and phosphate ions results in precipitation of calcium phosphate salts in the following ways:

- Increase in pH of saliva because of:
  - Loss of carbon dioxide.
  - Production of ammonia from dental plaque.
  - Precipitation of calcium and phosphate would result from protein degradation during stagnation by lowering the precipitation constant.
- Colloidal proteins in saliva bind calcium and phosphate ions and maintain a super-saturated solution. When saliva stagnates in the oral cavity, colloids settle down and super-saturated stage is no longer maintained. It results in the precipitation of calcium and phosphorus salts.
- Phosphate and esterases are two enzymes that play a very important role in precipitation of calcium and phosphate salts.
  - **Phosphates:** Dental plaque, desquamated epithelial cells and bacteria liberate phosphates that hydrolyse organic phosphates in saliva. Because of this there is increase in concentration of free phosphate ions that initiate the mineralisation of plaque.
  - **Esterases:** Dental plaque, bacteria, leucocytes, macrophages, desquamated epithelial cells hydrolyse fatty esters into free fatty acids. These fatty acids form soap with calcium and magnesium, which gets converted into less soluble calcium phosphate salts.

Epitactic Concept

- This is also known as heterogeneous nucleation concept.
- Epitactic means formation of crystals of a compound through a seeding mechanism. Formation of the initial crystal or nucleus is referred to as nucleation.
- According to this concept, calculus formation can be initiated through epitaxiy by organic complexes in the matrix.
- An intercellular matrix provides the architectural template for the initial hydroxyapatite crystal. This focus of calcification gets enlarged and coalesces to form a calcified mass.
- Intercellular matrix of plaque, plaque bacteria and lipid component of the organic matrix is believed to be the seeding or nucleating agent in calculus.
- These seeding agents form small foci of calcification. These foci get enlarged and coalesce to form calculus, therefore known as heterogeneous nucleation.

Inhibition Theory

- According to this theory, there is existence of an inhibiting mechanism present in calculus at non-calcifying site, therefore calcified mass occurs only at specific sites.
- The inhibitors are removed or altered when the calcification occurs.
- The most common inhibiting substance is pyrophosphate which inhibits calcification by preventing the initial nucleus from growing by poisoning the growth center of the crystal.

SHORT ESSAYS

Question 1

What is Epitactic concept in calculus formation?

Answer

Epitactic means formation of crystals of a compound through a seeding mechanism. Formation of the initial crystal or nucleus is referred to as nucleation.

According to this concept, calculus formation can be initiated through epitaxiy by organic complexes in the matrix.

An intercellular matrix provides the architectural template for the initial hydroxyapatite crystal. This focus of calcification gets enlarged and coalesces to form a calcified mass.

Intercellular matrix of plaque, plaque bacteria and lipid component of the organic matrix is believed to be the seeding or nucleating agents in calculus.

These seeding agents form small foci of calcification. These foci get enlarged and coalesce to form calculus, therefore known as heterogeneous nucleation.

Question 2

What is the classification of dental calculus? Explain in detail.

Answer

Calculus can be classified as according to its relation to the gingival margin as:

- Supragingival calculus.
- Subgingival calculus.

Supragingival Calculus

- As the name suggests, supragingival calculus is present above the level of gingival margin.
- It is also referred as salivary calculus as it is derived from the components of salivary secretions.
- It is visible in the oral cavity, clinically.
- It is can be white or yellowish-white in colour, and can be stained because of tobacco and food pigments.
- It hard and clay-like consistency.
- It is more on facial surfaces of maxillary molars and on the lingual surfaces of mandibular anterior teeth.
- It can be easily detached from the tooth.

Subgingival Calculus

- As the name suggests, subgingival calculus is present below the level of gingival margin.
- It is also referred to as serumal calculus or submarginal calculus as it is derived from gingival exudates.
- It is dark brown or green in colour, present as calcified deposit on the root surface of the tooth.
- It is present below the gingival sulcus or within the periodontal pocket.
- It is firmly attached to the tooth surface and is difficult to remove.
- It is initially seen on the inter-proximal areas where the supragingival calculus already exists.
- It can also be seen on the dentures, within the narrow grooves.

It can be diagnosed as by the following methods:

1. **Direct vision:**
   - By the help of an air spray, when the gingival margin is deflected, it can be visualised.
   - In cases of any gingival surgeries like gingivectomy or periodontal surgeries like flap surgeries.

2. **Indirect vision:**
   - When the gingival margin is dried either with the help of a cotton or an air spray, the dark-coloured subgingival calculus may be seen through the marginal tissue.
   - With the help of probing or exploring. A fine calculus probe (WHO 621) can be used to detect calculus subgingivally, also an explorer can be used to explore the calculus subgingivally.
   - Radiographs can also be an important tool for diagnosing subgingival calculus.
   - Transillumination.
   - Fiber optic transillumination probes to detect subgingival calculus are also available.

Question 3

Briefly explain inhibition theory of calculus formation.

Answer

According to this theory, there is existence of an inhibiting mechanism present in calculus at non-calcifying site, therefore calcified mass occurs only at specific sites.

The inhibitors are removed or altered when the calcification occurs.

The most common inhibiting substance is pyrophosphate which inhibits calcification by preventing the initial nucleus from growing by poisoning the growth center of the crystal.

Question 4

Describe briefly the formation of calculus.

Answer

Mineralised plaque is referred to as calculus.

- It is formed by the precipitation of mineral salts present in saliva or gingival crevicular fluid (GCF), which approximately starts between 1st and 14th day of plaque formation. Within first 2 days plaque can be 50% mineralised and within 12 days 60–90% mineralization can occur.
- Within the inner surface of plaque, the process of calcification starts in form of separate foci, which gradually increases in size and coalesce to form a solid mass of calculus.
- Early plaque of heavy calculus formers contains more calcium, thrice more phosphorus and less potassium. Phosphorous may be more critical than calcium in plaque mineralisation.
- Calculus formation continues until it reaches maximum levels in about 10 weeks and 6 months, after which there is a decline in its formation, due to mechanical wear from food and from the lips, cheeks and tongue. This process is referred to as reversal phenomenon.

Question 5

What are the differences between supragingival and sub-gingival calculus?

Answer

These are the following differences between supragingival and subgingival calculus:

S. No.	Features	Supragingival calculus	Subgingival calculus
1.	Location	It is seen above the level of gingival margin	It seen below the level of gingival margin
2.	Source	It is derived from the components of salivary secretions, therefore it is referred to as salivary calculus.	It is derived from the gingival-fluid exudates, therefore referred to as serumal calculus
3.	Distribution	It is arranged symmetrically on teeth, present more on facial surfaces of maxillary molars and lingual surfaces of mandibular anterior teeth	It is distributed within the pocket and more on proximal surfaces
4.	Visibility	It is visible with naked eye in the oral cavity	Not visible with naked eye or on routine oral examination. Can be detected by tactile exploration
5.	Colour	It is white, yellow in colour, can be stained by tobacco and food pigments	It can be dark brown or greenish-black in colour
6.	Consistency	Clay to hard consistency	Firm in consistency
7.	Composition	Calcium phosphate ratio is less than subgingival calculus. Sodium content is less	Calcium phosphate ratio is more than supragingival calculus. Sodium increases with increase in depth of pocket, more magnesium whitlokite and less of brushite
8.	Ease of removal	Can be easily removed	Difficult to remove

Question 6

What are the iatrogenic factors other than plaque and calculus responsible for periodontal inflammation?

Answer

The word iatrogenic is derived from the Greek word, iatro which means physician and genic means induced by or produced by. The factors induced in a patient by a physician's manner, activity or therapy, are known as iatrogenic factors.

Deficiencies in the quality of dental restorations or prostheses are contributing factors to gingival inflammation and periodontal destruction. Inadequate dental procedures that contribute to the destruction of the periodontal tissues are referred to as iatrogenic factors. Various iatrogenic factors which lead to poor periodontal health are as follows:

- **Locations of margins of restorations:** Subgingival margins of restorations generally lead to irritation to the periodontal structures and also favour plaque accumulation. Equigingival or supragingival margins should be preferred.
- **Contours/open contacts:** It can lead to food impaction.

Food impaction is the forceful wedging of food into the periodontium by occlusal forces.

This can lead to plaque accumulation and inflammation subsequently.

- **Materials used in the restorations:** Plaque can be formed over the materials used for restoration. And its composition is similar to that formed over natural tooth.
- **Design of removable partial dentures:** Complex designing of removable partial dentures can favour plaque accumulation and further lead to periodontal destruction.
- **Restorative dentistry procedures:** Restorative procedures can themselves lead to impingement into the periodontal structures.
- **Potential complications caused due to endodontic therapy:** Endodontic therapy can also lead to periodontal destruction. For example at the time of biomechanical preparation in Randomized controlled trial, over instrumentation by an endodontic file can lead to extension of inflammation into the periodontal space through the apical foramen.

Other factors could be:

- Periodontal complications associated with orthodontic therapy.
- Extraction of impacted third molars.
- Chemical irritation.
- Radiation therapy.

CHAPTER 10

Inflammation and Immunity

LONG ESSAYS

Question 1

Define inflammation. What are the signs of inflammation? Describe the forms of inflammation in detail.

Answer

Inflammation can be defined as the local response of living tissues to injury due to any agent. It is the body's defence mechanism in order to eliminate or reduce the spread of injurious agent as well as to remove the consequent necrosed cells and tissues.

Agents Causing Inflammation

- Physical agents like heat, cold, radiation and mechanical trauma
- Chemical agents like organic and inorganic substances
- Infective agents and their toxins like from bacteria and viruses
- Immunological agents like cell-mediated and antigen-antibody reactions.

Various Signs of Inflammation

There are five cardinal signs of inflammation:

1. *Rubor* (redness).
2. *Calor* (heat).
3. *Dolor* (pain).
4. Tumour (swelling).
5. *Functio laesa* (loss of function).

Classification of Inflammation

Inflammation can be classified as acute and chronic.

Acute is of relatively short duration, lasting from a few minutes to a few days, and is characterized by fluid and plasma-protein exudation, and by mainly neutrophilic leukocyte accumulation.

On the other hand chronic inflammation is of longer duration (days to years) and is manifested by infiltration of lymphocytes and macrophages (**Fig. 10.1**).

Acute Inflammation

It is the immediate and early response to injury. The function is to deliver leukocytes to the site of injury, where they can help eradicate the causative agents (or other infectious agents) as well as degrade necrotic tissues resulting from the destruction. But, leukocytes themselves may also prolong inflammation and induce tissue damage by releasing enzymes, chemical mediators and toxic oxygen radicals.

Major Compounds

Acute inflammation has three major components:

1. Changes in vascular supply that lead to a local increase in blood flow (vasodilation).
2. Structural changes in the microvasculature that allows the plasma proteins to leave the circulation.

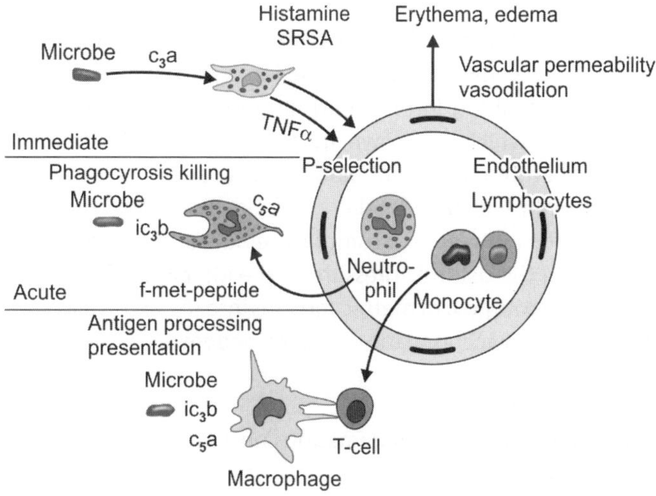

Fig. 10.1: Stages of Inflammation

3. Emigration of the leukocytes from the microcirculation and accumulation at the site of injury.

The changes in acute inflammation can be conveniently described in two steps:

1. Vascular events.
2. Cellular events.

Vascular Events

Alteration in the microvasculature (arterioles, capillaries and venules) is the earliest response to tissue injury. These alterations include—haemodynamic changes and changes in vascular permeability.

Haemodynamic Changes

The initial features of inflammatory response result from changes in the vascular flow of small blood vessels in the injured tissue. The sequence of these changes is as follows:

- In case of mild injury, the blood flow may be re-established in 3–5 seconds. While with more severe injury, the vasoconstriction may last for about 5 minutes.
- It is the persistent progressive vasodilation, which involves mainly the arterioles.
- Progressive vasodilation will elevate the local hydrostatic pressure resulting in transudation of fluid into the extra-swelling space.
- Next is the slowing or stasis of microvasculature.
- Stasis is followed by leukocytic margination or peripheral orientation of leukocytes (mainly neutrophils) along the vascular endothelium. The leukocytes stick to the vascular endothelium briefly, and then move and migrate through the gaps between spaces. This process is known as emigration.

Increased Vascular Permeability (Vascular Leakage)

In the earliest phase of acute inflammation, the vasodilation and increased blood flow increase intravascular hydrostatic pressure, resulting in increased filtration of fluid from the capillaries, which is known as transudate. Transudate is basically an ultrafiltrate of blood plasma and little protein. The movement of protein-rich fluid from the plasma reduces the intravascular osmotic pressure at the same time increasing the osmotic pressure of the interstitial fluid. The net result is outflow of matter and ions into the extravascular tissues, which accumulation is called oedema.

Cellular Events

The cellular events of inflammation consist of two processes:

1. Exudation of leukocytes.
2. Phagocytosis.

Exudation of Leukocytes

The escape of leukocytes from the lumen of microvasculature to the interstitial tissue is most important aspect of inflammatory response. In acute inflammation, polymorphonuclear neutrophils (PMNs) act as the first line of defence, later followed by monocytes and macrophages.

The sequence of events in the extravasation of leukocytes from the vascular lumen to extravascular space is divided into:

- Margination and rolling.
- Adhesion and transmigration.
- Migration in interstitial tissues toward a chemotactic stimulus.

- **Margination and rolling:** In normal blood flow, red blood cell and white blood cell (WBC) generally travel along the central axis, leaving a cell-poor layer of plasma in I contact with endothelium. As vascular permeability increases fluid exits the vascular lumen and blood flow slows. As a result, the leukocytes settle out of central column, marginating to the vessel periphery. Subsequently, the leukocytes stick to the endothelial surface, along the way and this process is called rolling.

- **Adhesion and trans endothelial migration:** Eventually the leukocytes firmly adhere to the endothelial surface (adhesion) before crawling between the cells and through the basement membrane into the extravascular space (diapedesis).

  The adhesion is largely mediated by endothelial adhesion molecules of immunoglobulin superfamily, binding to various integrins found on leukocyte cell surfaces. The endothelial adhesion molecules include intercellular adhesion molecule 1 (ICAM-1) and vascular cell adhesion molecule 1 (VCAM-1) both of which have increased surface expression after stimulation of endothelium by various cytokines **(Fig. 10.2)**.

- **Chemotaxis and activation:** After extravasation, leukocytes emigrate toward the site of injury along a chemical gradient, in a process called chemotaxis.

  Both exogenous and endogenous substance can act as chemotactic agents for leukocytes.

Chemotactic Agents Include

- Soluble bacterial products, particularly peptides with N-formylmethionine terminus.
- Components of complement system, particularly C5a.
- Products of the lipoxygenase pathway of arachidonic acid (AA) metabolism, particularly leukotriene B4 (LTB4).
- Cytokines especially those of the chemokine family [e.g. interleukin 8 (IL-8)].

Chemotactic agents bind to specific receptors on the leukocyte cell surface and induce an intracellular cascade of phospholipid metabolites, eventually culminating in increased intracellular calcium (Ca^{++}). The increased cytosolic Ca^{++} triggers the assembly of cytoskeletal contractile elements necessary for movements. The leukocytes move by extending pseudopods that anchor themselves to extracellular matrix and then pull the remainder of the cell after **(Fig. 10.3)**.

Besides stimulating locomotion, chemotactic factors also induce other leukocyte responses, generally referred as to leukocyte activation.

Phagocytosis

Phagocytosis is defined as the processes of engulfment of solid particulate material by the cells (cell-eating). The cells performing this function are called phagocytes. There are two main types of phagocytic cells.

1. Polymorphonuclear neutrophils, which are also called microphages.
2. Circulating monocytes and fixed tissue mononuclear phagocytes called as macrophages.

Phagocytosis Consists of three Distinct but Interrelated Steps

1. Recognition and attachment of the particle to the ingesting leukocyte.

2. Engulfment with subsequent formation of a phagocytic vacuole.
3. Killing or degradation of the ingested material.

Attachment stage (opsonisation):-

The phagocytic cells as well as microorganisms to be ingested have usually negative charged surface and thus they repel each other. In order to establish a bond between bacteria and the cell membrane of phagocytic cell the microorganism gets coated with opsonins, which are naturally occurring factors in the serum.

The two main opsonins present in serum and their corresponding receptors on the surface of phagocytic cells are as under:

1. Immunoglobulin G opsonins and its corresponding receptor on the surface of polymorphs and monocytes is Fc fragment of immunoglobulin.
2. C3b opsonin fragment of complement and its corresponding receptor for C3b on the surface of phagocytic cells.

Engulfment stage:-

The opsonised particles binding triggers engulfment. Pseudopods are extended around the object to be engulfed eventually forming a phagocytic vacuole. The lysosome of the cell fused with phagocytic vacuole and form phagolysosome or phagosome.

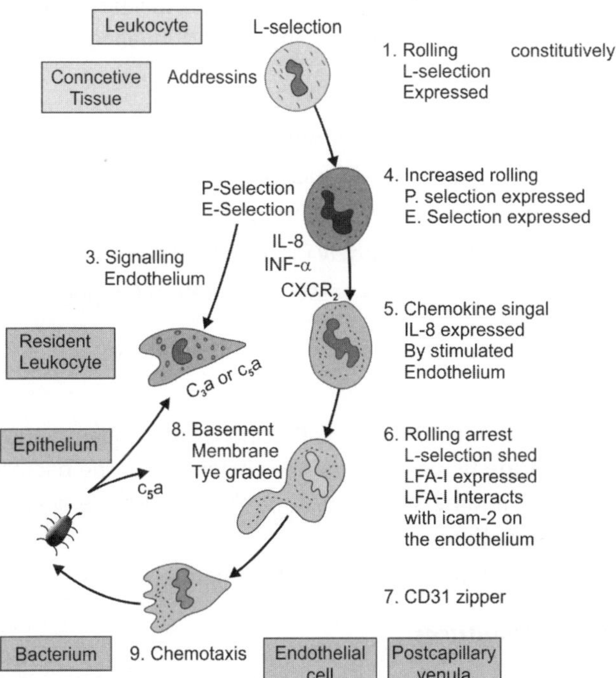

Fig. 10.2: Trans-endothelial migration.

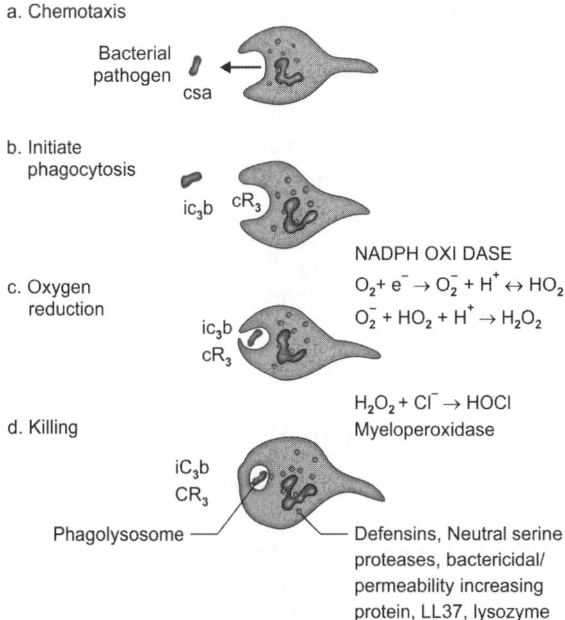

Fig. 10.3: Chemotaxis.

Secretion (Degranulation) Stage

- The preformed granules stored products of PMNs are discharged or secreted into the phagosome and extracellular environment.
- The ultimate step in phagocytosis of microbes is killing and degradation.
- The microorganisms after being killed by antibacterial substances are degraded by hydrolytic enzymes. However, the mechanism fails to kill and degrade same bacteria like tubercle bacilli.

The antimicrobial agents act by either of following mechanism:

- Oxygen-dependent bactericidal mechanism.
- Oxygen-independent bactericidal mechanism.
- Nitric oxide (NO) mechanism.

- **Oxygen-dependent mechanism:** Phagocytosis stimulates an oxidative burst characterised by a sudden increase in oxygen consumption, glycogen catabolism (glycogenolysis), increased glucose oxidation and production of reactive oxygen metabolites. The generation of the oxygen metabolites is due to rapid activation of leukocyte Nicotinamide adenine dinucleotide (NADH) oxidase, which oxidizes reduced nicotinamide adenine dinucleotide phosphate (NADPH) and in the process reduces oxygen to superoxide ion (O_2^-).

$$2O_2 + NADPH \longrightarrow 2O_2^- + NADP^+ + H^+$$

Superoxide is then converted mostly by spontaneous dismutation into hydrogen peroxide.

$$O^{2-} + 2H^+ \longrightarrow H_2O_2$$

This type of bacterial activity is carried out either via enzymes myeloperoxidase (MPO) present in granules of neutrophils or independent of enzyme MPO.

a. **MPO-dependent killing:** (H_2O_2-MPO-halide system): In this mechanism the enzyme MPO acts on H_2O_2 in the presence of halides (Cl^-, Br^-, I^-) to form hypohalous acid ($HOCl$, HOI, $HOBr$), which is more potent antibacterial agent than H_2O_2.

$$H_2O_2 \xrightarrow[\substack{Cl^-,\ Br^-,\ I^-}]{MPO} HOCl + H_2O$$
$$\text{(Hypochlorous acid)}$$

b. **MPO-dependent killing:** Mature macrophages lack the enzyme MPO and they carry OH^- ions and superoxide singlet oxygen (O') from H_2O_2 in presence of O_2' (Haber-Weiss reaction) or in Fe^{++} (Fenton reaction).

Tenton's Reaction

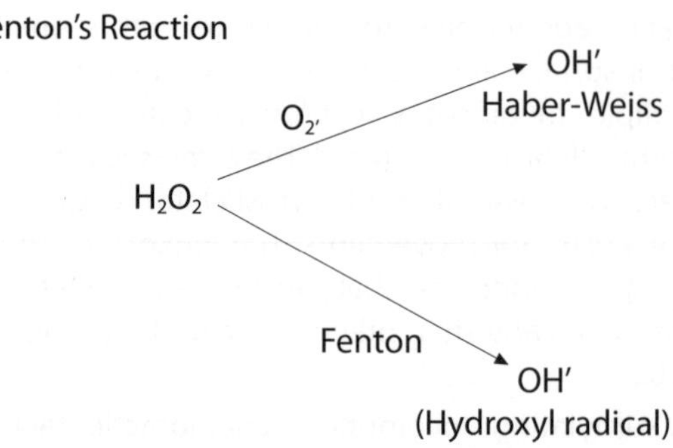

Reactive oxygen metabolites are particularly useful in eliminating microbial organism that grows within phagocytosis, e.g. *Mycobacterium tuberculosis, Histoplasma capsulatum.*

2. **Oxygen-independent bacterial mechanism:** Some agents released from granules of phagocytic cell do not need oxygen for bactericidal activity. These include lysosomal hydrolases, permeability increasing factors defensins and cationic.

3. **Nitric oxide mechanism:** In addition to others, the nitric oxide is produced by endothelial cells as well as by activated macrophages. In experimental animals, nitric oxide has been shown to have fungicidal and anti-parasitic action.

Chronic Inflammation

Chronic inflammation can be considered to be inflammation of prolonged duration (weeks to months to years) in which active inflammation, tissue injury and healing proceed simultaneously.

Chronic inflammation is characterized by

- Infiltration with mononuclear (chronic inflammatory) cells, including macrophages, lymphocytes and plasma cells.
- Tissue destruction largely induced by inflammatory cells.
- Repair involving new vessel proliferation (angiogenesis) and fibrosis.

Causes

- Chronic inflammation following acute inflammation: When the tissue destruction is extensive or the bacteria survive and persist in small numbers at the site of acute inflammation.
- Recurrent attacks of acute inflammation.

General Features

- **Mononuclear cell infiltration:** Chronic inflammation lesions are infiltrated by mononuclear inflammation cells like phagocytes and lymphoid cells. Macrophages compromise the most important cells in chronic inflammation.

- **Tissue destruction or necrosis:** These are common and are brought about by activated macrophages by release of variety of biologically-active substance.
- **Proliferative changes:** As a result of necrosis, proliferation of small blood vessels and fibroblasts is stimulated resulting in formation of inflammation granulation tissue.

Question 2

What are the various chemical mediators of inflammation?

Answer

The substances acting as chemical mediators of inflammation can be released from the cells, the plasma or damaged tissue itself. They are broadly classified into two groups:

1. Mediators released by cells.
2. Mediators originally from plasma.

Cell-Derived Mediators

Vasoactive Amines

Histamine is widely distributed in tissues, particularly in mast cells adjacent to vessels, as well as in circulating basophils and platelets. Performed histamine is present in mast cell granules that are released in response to a variety of stimuli.

- Physical injury such as trauma or heat.
- Immune reaction involving binding of Ig E antibodies to Fc receptors on mast cells.
- C3a and C5a fragments of complement so called anaphylatoxins.
- Leukocyte-derived histamine releasing proteins.
- Neuropeptides. (e.g. substance P).
- Certain cytokines. (e.g. IL-1 and IL-8).

In humans, histamine causes arteriolar dilation and is the principle mediator of the immediate phase of increased vascular permeability, causing endothelial contraction and widening of the inter-endothelial cell junctions. Soon after its release, histamine is inactivated by histaminase.

Serotonin (5-hydroxytryptamine) is also a vasoactive mediator with effects similar to histamine. It is found primarily within platelet-dense body granules (along with histamine, adenosine diphosphate and calcium) and release is stimulated by platelet aggregation.

Arachidonic Acid Metabolism

Product derived from the metabolism of AA affect a variety of biologic processes including inflammation and haemostasis.

Arachidonic acid is a 20-carbon polyunsaturated fatty acid (four double bonds) derived primarily from dietary linoleic acid and present in the body only in esterified form as a component of cell membrane phospholipids. arachidonic acid metabolism proceeds along one of the two major pathways, named for the enzymes that initiate the reactions.

1. Cyclooxygenase pathway.
2. Lipoxygenase pathway.

1. Cyclooxygenase Pathway

These include prostaglandin E_2 (PGE$_2$), PGD$_2$, PGF$_{2\alpha}$, PGI$_2$ (prostacyclin), and thromboxane (YTXA$_2$), each of which is derived by these enzymes has a restricted tissue distribution. For example, platelets contain the enzyme thromboxane synthesis, and hence TXA$_2$, a potent platelet-aggregating product in these cells. Endothelium, on the other hand, lacks thromboxane synthetase but possess prostacyclin synthetase, which leads to the formation of PGI2, a vasodilator and a potent inhibitor of platelet aggregation. Both TXA$_2$ and PGI$_2$ have an opposing action.

Prostaglandin D$_2$ is the major metabolic product of the cyclooxygenase (COX) pathway in most cells, along with PGE$_2$ and PGI$_{2\alpha}$ (which are more widely distributed), it causes vasodilation and potentiates oedema formation.

Aspirin and non-steroidal anti-inflammatory drugs (NSAIDS) such as ibuprofen inhibit all PG synthesis. Lipoxygenase however is not affected by these (NSAIDS).

Recent studies have revealed that there are two forms of COXs called COX-1 and COX-2 that are of interest, COX-1 but not COX-2 are expressed in the gastric mucosa. At this site the mucosal PG generated by action of COX-1 are protective because they prevent acid-induced damage.

2. Lipoxygenase Pathway

5-lioxygenase is the predominant AA-metabolising enzyme in neutrophils. 5-hydroperoxy derivative of AA, 5-hydroperoxyeicosatetraenoic acid (5-HPETE) is quite unstable and is either reduced to 5-HETE (chemotactic for neutrophils) or converted into a family of compounds collectively called leukotrienes. The first leukotriene generated from 5-HPETE is called leukotriene A4 (LTA4), which in turn gives rise to LTB4 by enzymatic hydrolysis or LTC4 and its subsequent metabolites LTD4 and LTE4, cause vasoconstriction, bronchospasm and increased vascular permeability.

Lysosomal Components

The inflammatory cells—neutrophils and monocytes contain lysosomal granules, which on release elaborate a variety of mediators of inflammation. These are as under:

- **Granules of neutrophils:**
  - Specific or secondary.
  - Azurophil or primary.

  The specific (secondary) granules—contain lactoferrin, lysozyme, alkaline phosphatase and collagenase while the large azurophil granules have myeloperoxidase, acid hydrolases and neutral proteases such as elastase, collagenase and proteinase.

  Acid proteases act within the cell to cause destruction of bacteria in the phagolysosome while neutral proteases attack on the extracellular constituents such as basement membrane, collagen, elastin, cartilage, etc.

- **Granules of monocytes and tissue macrophages:** These cells on degranulation also release mediators of inflammation like acid proteases, collagenases and plasminogen activator. However, they are more active in chronic inflammation than acting as mediators of acute inflammation.

Platelet Activating Factor

It is released from immunoglobulin E (IgE)-sensitized basophils or mast cells, other leukocytes endothelium and platelets. Apart from its action on platelet aggregation and release, the actions of platelet activating factor (PAF) as mediator of inflammation are:

- Increased vascular permeability.
- Vasodilatation in low concentration and vasoconstriction otherwise.
- Bronchoconstriction.
- Adhesion of leukocytes to endothelium.
- Chemotaxis.

Cytokines

- Cytokines are polypeptide substances produced by activated lymphocytes (lymphokines) and activated monocytes (monokines).
- Cytokines can act on the same cell that produces them (autocrine effect) on other cells in the immediate vicinity (paracrine) or systemically (endocrine effect).
- Currently main cytokines acting as mediators of inflammation are:
- Interleukin-1 (IL-1), tumour necrosis factor a (TNF-a) and b, interferon-a (IF-a) and chemokines [IL-8, platelet factor 4 (PF4)]. The actions of various cytokines as mediator of inflammation are as under:
  - Interleukin-1 and TNF a and b induce endothelial effects in the form of increased leukocytes adherence, thrombogenicity, elaboration of other cytokines, fibroblastic proliferation and acute phase reactions.
  - IF-a causes activation of macrophages and neutrophils and is associated with synthesis of nitric acid synthase.

Nitric Oxide and Oxygen Metabolites

Nitric oxide plays the following role in inflammation:

- Vasodilation.
- Anti-platelet activating agent.
- Possibly microbicidal action.
- Oxygen-derived metabolites are released from activated neutrophils and macrophages, their action in inflammation is:
  - Endothelial cell damage and thereby increased vascular permeability.
  - Activation of protease and inactivation of antiprotease causing tissue matrix damage.
  - Damage to other cells.

Plasma-derived Mediators (Plasma Proteases)

These include the various products derived from activation and interaction of four interlinked systems:
1. Kinin
2. Clotting
3. Fibrinolytic
4. Complement.

Hageman factor (factor XII) of clotting system plays a key role in interactions of four systems.

Kinin System

This system on activation is factor XIIa generates bradykinin, so named because of the slow contraction of smooth muscle it induces. First, kallikrein by the action of pre-kallikrein activator, which is a fragment of factor XIIa. Kallikrein then acts on high molecular weight kininogen to form bradykinin.

Bradykinin effects include:

- Smooth muscle contraction.
- Vasodilatation.
- Increased vascular permeability.
- Pain.

Clotting System

Factor XIIa initiates the cascade of the clotting system resulting in formation of fibrinogen to form fibrin and fibrinopeptides or fibrin split products.

Actions of fibroblast-specific protein (FSP) in inflammation are:

- Increased vascular permeability
- Chemotaxis for leukocyte
- Anticoagulant activity.

Fibrinolytic System

This system is activated by plasminogen activator. It acts on plasminogen present as component of plasma protein to form plasmin. Further breakdown of fibrin by plasmin forms fibrinopeptides or FSP.

Actions of plasmin are:

- Activation of factor XII to form prekallikrein activator that stimulates the kinin system to bradykinin.
- Splits off complement C3 to form C3a, which is a permeability factor.
- Degrades fibrin to form fibrin split product which to form fibrin split product which increase vascular permeability and are chemotactic to leukocytes.

Complement System

Complement system consists of cascade of plasma protein that plays an important role in both immunity and inflammation. They function in immunity primarily by generating a pore like membrane attack complex (MAC) that effectively punches holes in the membranes of invading microbes. In the process of generating the MAC, a number of complement fragments are produced, including C3a opsonins, as well as fragments that contribute to the inflammatory response by increasing vascular permeability and leukocyte chemotaxis.

Complement components (numbered C1–C9) are present in plasma in inactive forms. Briefly the most inactive step in the elaboration of the biological functions of complement is the activation of third complement C3. C3 cleavage can occur:

- Via classic pathway, triggered by fixation of C1 to antigen-antibody complexes or
- Through the alternative pathway, triggered by bacterial polysaccharides or aggregated IgA. Alternative pathway involves distinct set to serum components, including properdin and factors B and D.

Whichever pathway is involved, C3 convertase cleaves C3 to C3a and C3b.C3b then binds to C3b to C3 convertase complex to form C5 convertase, this complex cleaves C5 to generate C5a and initiate the final stages of assembly of the C5 to Ca MAC.

Phenomenon in acute inflammation

- Vascular effect: C3a and C5a (called anaphylaxins) increase vascular permeability and cause vasodilation by inducing mast cells to release their histamine. C5a also activates the lipoxygenase pathway of AA metabolism in neutrophils and monocytes causing further release of inflammatory mediators
- Leukocyte activation, adhesion and chemotaxis
- **Phagocytosis:** With fixed to a microbial surface C3b and C3bi act as opsonins, augmenting phagocytosis by cells bearing C3b receptors (neutrophils and macrophages).

SHORT ESSAYS

Question 1

What are the systemic effects of inflammation?

Answer

Various systemic effects of inflammation are defined below:

Pyrexia

Fever is only one of the more common obvious of the systemic effects of inflammation called as acute phase reaction.

These include slow-wave sleep, anorexia, and accelerated degradation of skeletal muscle hypotension, hepatic synthesis of acute-phase proteins (e.g. complement or coagulation protein) and alterations in the circulating WBC pool.

Cytokines

Interleukin-1, IL-6, and TNF are most important in acute-phase reaction. These are produced by leukocytes in response to infection, or to immune and toxic injury and are released systemically frequently in a short of cytokine cascade.

Tumour necrosis factor can induce production of IL-1 in turn induces production of IL-6 that stimulates the hepatic synthesis of several plasma proteins, most notably fibrinogen.

Elevated fibrinogen levels cause erythrocytes to agglutinate more readily. So higher erythrocyte sedimentation rate is associated with inflammation.

Leukocytosis

Especially in bacterial infection, it results from the release of cells from the bone marrow (caused by IL-1 and TNF) and is associated with an increase number of relatively immature neutrophils in the blood.

- ❑ *Neutrophilia*—increase in polymorphonuclear cells.
- ❑ *Eosinophilia*—in parasitic infection and allergic reactions.
- ❑ Lymphocytosis—in viral infection, such as mumps, and rubella.

Question 2

What is phagocytosis? Explain in detail with diagrams?

Answer

Phagocytosis is defined as the processes of engulfment of solid particulate material by the cells (cell-eating). The cells performing this function are called phagocytes. There are two main types of phagocytic cells:

1. Polymorphonuclear neutrophils, which are also called microphages.
2. Circulating monocytes and fixed tissue mononuclear phagocytes called as macrophages.

Phagocytosis consists of three distinct but interrelated steps:

1. Recognition and attachment of the particle to the ingesting leukocyte.
2. Engulfment with subsequent formation of a phagocytic vacuole.
3. Killing or degradation of the ingested material.

Attachment Stage (Opsonisation)

The phagocytic cells as well as microorganisms to be ingested have usually negative-charged surface and thus they repel each other. In order to establish a bond between bacteria and the cell membrane of phagocytic cell the microorganism gets coated with opsonins, which are naturally occurring factors in the serum.

The two main opsonins present in serum and their corresponding receptors on the surface of phagocytic cells are as under:

1. Immunoglobulin G opsonins and its corresponding receptor on the surface of polymorphs and monocytes is Fc fragment of immunoglobulin.
2. C3b opsonin fragment of complement and its corresponding receptor for C3b on the surface of phagocytic cells.

Engulfment Stage

The opsonised particles binding triggers engulfment. Pseudopods are extended around the object to be engulfed eventually forming a phagocytic vacuole. The lysosome of the cell fused with phagocytic vacuole and form phagolysosome or phagosome.

Secretion (Degranulation) Stage

The preformed granules stored products of PMNs are discharged or secreted into the phagosome and extracellular environment.

The ultimate step in phagocytosis of microbes is killing and degradation.

The microorganisms after being killed by antibacterial substances are degraded by hydrolytic enzymes. However, the mechanism fails to kill and degrade same bacteria like tubercle bacilli.

The antimicrobial agents act by either of following mechanism:

- ❑ Oxygen-dependent bactericidal mechanism.
- ❑ Oxygen-independent bactericidal mechanism.
- ❑ Nitric oxide (NO) mechanism.

Oxygen-dependent Mechanism

Phagocytosis stimulates an oxidative burst characterised by a sudden increase in oxygen consumption, glycogen catabolism (glycogenolysis), increased glucose oxidation and production of reactive oxygen metabolites. The generation of the oxygen metabolites is due to rapid activation of leukocyte NADH oxidase, which oxidizes reduced NADPH and in the process reduces oxygen to superoxide ion (O_2^-).

$$2O_2 + NADPH \longrightarrow 2O_2^- + NADP^+ + H^+$$

Superoxide is then converted mostly by spontaneous dismutation into hydrogen peroxide.

$$O^{2-} + 2H^+ \longrightarrow H_2O_2$$

This type of bacterial activity is carried out either via enzymes myeloperoxidase (MPO) present in granules of neutrophils or independent of enzyme MPO.

MPO-dependent Killing: (H_2O_2-MPO-halide system)

In this mechanism the enzyme MPO acts on H_2O_2 in the presence of halides (Cl^-, Br^-, I^-) to form hypohalous acid (HOCl, HOI, HOBr), which is more potent antibacterial agent than H_2O_2.

$$H_2O_2 \xrightarrow[Cl^-, Br^-, I^-]{MPO} HOCl + H_2O \text{ (Hypochlorous acid)}$$

MPO-dependent Killing

Mature macrophages lack the enzyme MPO and they carry OH^- ions and superoxide singlet oxygen (O') from H_2O_2 in presence of O_2' (Haber-Weiss reaction) or in Fe^{++} (Fenton reaction).

Fenton's Reaction

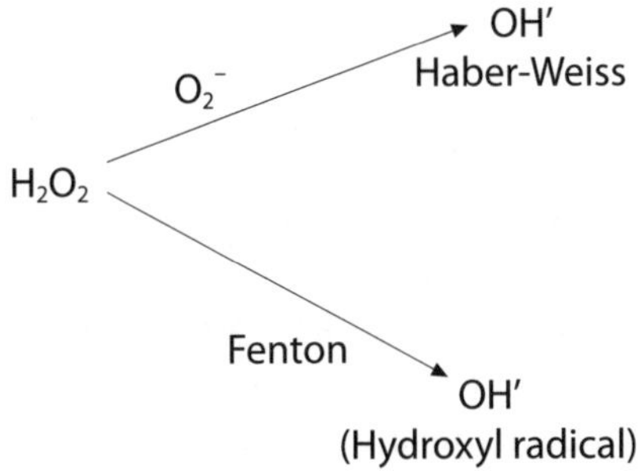

Reactive oxygen metabolites are particularly useful in eliminating microbial organism that grows within phagocytosis, e.g. *M. tuberculosis, H. capsulatum*.

Oxygen-independent Bacterial Mechanism

Some agents released from granules of phagocytic cell do not need oxygen for bactericidal activity. These include lysosomal hydrolases, permeability increasing factors defensins and cationic.

Nitric Oxide Mechanism

in addition to others, the nitric oxide is produced by endothelial cells as well as by activated macrophages. In experimental animals, nitric oxide has been shown to have fungicidal and anti-parasitic action but its role is bactericidal activity in human being is yet not clear.

Question 3

What are the cells of inflammation and immunity?

Answer

Various cells of immunity and inflammation are as follows:

- ❑ Mast cells.
- ❑ Dermal dendrocytes.
- ❑ Peripheral dendritic cells.
- ❑ Neutrophils and monocytes/macrophages.
- ❑ Lymphocytes.
- ❑ T-cells.
- ❑ B-cells.
- ❑ Natural killer cells (NK cells) **(Fig. 10.4)**.

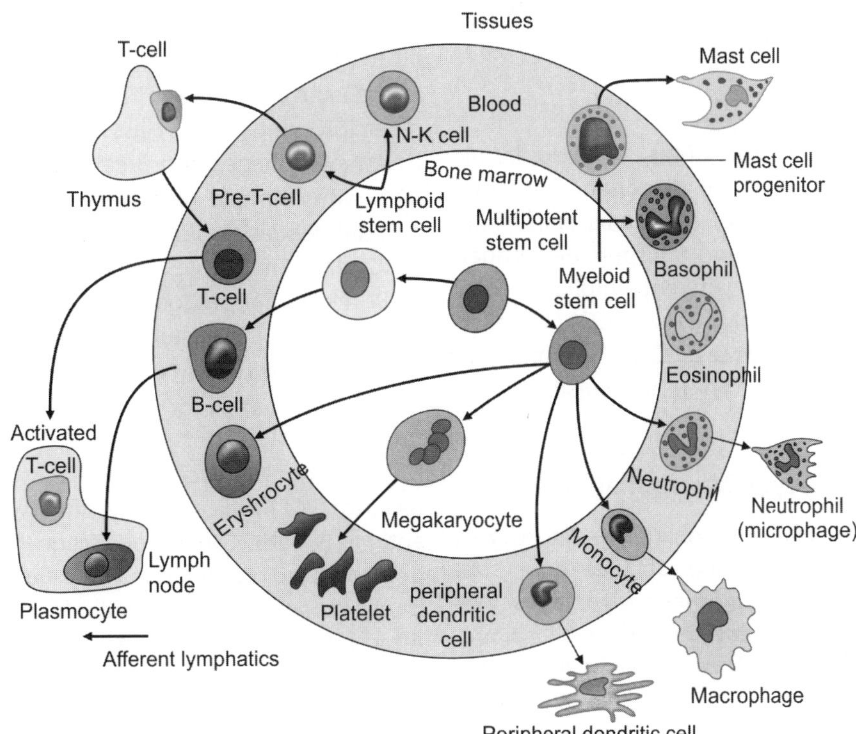

Fig. 10.4: Various cells of inflammation.

Mast Cells

Mast cells are mainly present in the connective tissue around the blood vessels and also in the junctional epithelium. Their most prominent feature is that there is a presence of cytoplasmic granule known as lysosomes, eosinophil chemotactic factor, neutrophil chemotactic factor and heparin. They also contain receptors for IgE antibodies which are found in the gingiva. These cells can synthesise inflammatory mediators like the slow-reacting substances of anaphylaxis (SRS-A), TNF α, IL-6 and leukotriene C4.

Mast cells are important in mediating inflammatory process and they also possess toll like receptors, which allow the innate immune system to adapt which is transitory. Stimulation of these receptors can lead to activation and secretion of vasoactive substances that increase the vascular permeability and dilation.

Dermal Dendrocytes

They are also known as histiocytes and are widely distributed and form a large system of collagen associated dendritic cells (DCs) of myeloid origin. These cells are distributed near the blood vessels and possess receptors for the complement C3a by which they participate in immediate inflammation. They express the major histocompatibility complex (MHC) class II molecules. They can express the matrix metalloproteinases (MMPs) in response to the bacterial challenge and help in periodontal tissue destruction.

Peripheral Dendritic Cells

They are leukocytes with dendrites or cytoplasmic projections, Langerhans cells are dendritic Cells that reside in suprabasilar portions of squamous epithelium. They ingest the antigen locally and transport the antigen to the lymph nodes through the afferent lymphatics. They express high levels of MHC II molecules and CD1, as well as intercellular adhesion molecules (e.g. ICAM-1, lymphocyte function-associated antigen 3 (LFA-3) and co-stimulatory factors.

Neutrophils and Monocyte/Macrophages

Neutrophils are closely related to phagocytic leukocytes neutrophils and macrophages are of the same size. Neutrophils, also known as polymorphonuclear leukocytes (PMNLs), are the predominant leukocyte in blood, accounting for about two-thirds of all blood leukocytes (1,000–8,000 cells/mm^3).

Neutrophils possess receptors for metabolites of the complement molecule C3, designated complement receptors 1, 3 and 4 (CR1, CR3, CR4) and C5 (C5aR). They also possess receptors for IgG antibody (fcy R).

These receptors enable:

- Neutrophils to be recruited from the blood.
- Locate offending agents and.
- Ingest (phagocytose) and kill the offending agents.

Monocytes: When macrophages leave the blood, they form monocytes. They complete their differentiation in local tissues and may become greater than 22 µm in diameter because macrophages differentiate and live in the local tissues; they suited for communicating with lymphocytes and other surrounding cells. Macrophages live along enough to present antigen to T cells. Monocytes and macrophages possess CR1, CR3, CR4, C5aR receptors several classes of Fcy receptors (FcyRI, FcyRII, FcyRIII) and molecules important in antigen presentation (MHC class II receptor CD1).

Lymphocytes

Three main types of lymphocytes are distinguished on the basis of their receptors for antigens: T lymphocytes, B-lymphocytes, and NK cells.

T cells

T cells recognise diverse antigens using a low affinity trans-membranous complex, the T cell antigen receptor (TCR). T cells are subdivided based on whether they possess the co-receptors CD4 or CD8. The CD4 co-receptor reversibly binds MHC class II molecules that are found DCs, macrophages and B cells. CD4+ T cells initiate and help with immune responses by providing proliferation and differentiation signals. The CD8 co-receptor scans for MHC, class I molecules, which are found on all cells. The CD8+ T cells are predominantly cytotoxic T cells involved in controlling intracellular antigens (e.g. certain bacteria, hyphal fungi, viruses).

B cells

B cells recognise diverse antigens using the B cell antigen receptor (BCR), which is a high affinity antigen receptor. The antigen is tightly bound not scanned. Ingested antigen is degraded and presented to T cells. Before antigen exposure, B cells express immunoglobulin M (IgM) as part of the BCR. After antigen exposure, some B cells differentiate to form plasma cells dedicated to the production and secretion of antibodies of IgM isotype. Memory B cells give rise to plasma cells on secondary exposure to antigen and produce high affinity antibodies of the appropriate isotype.

Natural Killer Cells

Natural killer cells (NK cells) recognise and kill certain tumour and virally-infected cells possess several classes of antigen receptors including killer inhibitory receptors (KIRs) and killer activating receptor (KAR). Normal cells possess MHC class I molecules that present antigens recognised as self; these interact with KIRs and protect the cells from NK cell mediated killing. Alterations in antigens presented by the MHC class I molecules, occurring in tumour-infected and virally-infected cells, may result in NK cell activation because the KIRs do not detect sufficient self-antigens. KAR activation can override KIR inhibition and cause the NK cells to kill the target cell.

Question 4

Write short notes on mast cells.

Answer

Mast cells are mainly present in the connective tissue around the blood vessels and also in the junctional epithelium. Their most prominent feature is that there is a presence of cytoplasmic granule known as lysosomes, eosinophil chemotactic factor, neutrophil chemotactic factor and heparin. They also contain receptors for IgE antibodies which are found in the gingiva. These cells can synthesise inflammatory mediators like the SRS-A, TNF α, IL-6, and leukotriene C4.

Mast cells are important in mediating inflammatory process and they also possess toll like receptors, which allow the innate immune system to adapt which is transitory. Stimulation of these receptors can lead to activation and secretion of vasoactive substances that increase the vascular permeability and dilation.

Question 5

What are the various outcomes of acute inflammation?

Answer

Various outcomes of acute inflammation are mentioned below:

Complete Resolution

When the injury is limited or short lived, when there has been little tissue destruction, and when tissue is capable of regeneration, the most usual outcome is restoration to histological and functional normalcy.

This resolution involves neutralisation or removal of chemical mediators, with subsequent normalisation of vascular permeability and halting of leukocyte emigration.

Eventually, the combined efforts of lymphatic drainage and macrophages lead to clearance of the oedema fluid, inflamed cells and necrotic debris from the battlefield.

Scarring or Fibrosis

This results when inflammation occurs in tissues that do not regenerate or after substantial tissue destruction.

In addition, extensive fibrous exudates that cannot be completely absorbed are organised by ingrowth of connective elements, resulting in the formation of a mass of fibrous tissue.

Abscess Formation

It may occur in the setting of certain bacterial or fungal infections (pyogenic).

Progression to Chronic Inflammation

This may follow acute inflammation.

Question 6

What are cytokines? What are their roles in inflammation?

Answer

Cytokines are the peptides or protein mediators or intercellular messengers which regulate immunological, inflammatory and reparative host responses.

They are released by wide variety of cells like lymphocytes, macrophages, platelets, and fibroblasts.

Cytokines can include interleukins, growth factors, chemokines and interferons. They act on various cells like macrophages, fibroblasts, keratinocytes, PMNLs.

Various roles of cytokines are as follows:

- To initiate and maintain immune and inflammatory response.
- Interleukins forms a link between leukocytes, endothelial cells, fibroblasts and epithelial cells.
- Interleukin-6, IL-1 and TNF α are important for periodontal destruction.
- Cytokines mainly associated with periodontal diseases are IL-1, IL-2, IL-4, IL5, IL-6, IL-8, IL-10, TNF, PGE_2.

Question 7

What are the functions of various cytokines?

Answer

Functions of various cytokines are as follows:

- **Interleukin-1:** It is produced mainly by macrophages and lymphocytes. Fibroblasts, platelets, keratinocytes and endothelial cells may also produce IL-1. IL-1, triggers the release of PGE2 in large quantities. It also stimulates the secretion of MMPs.

- **Interleukin-2:** Monocytes and T lymphocytes produce IL-2. It stimulates T cells and enhances clonal expansion of beta cells into plasma cells.
- **Interleukin-4, IL-5, and IL-10:** They all are produced by TH2 cells and also help in the activation of beta cells into plasma cells and downregulate monocytic response.
- **Interleukin-6:** It is produced by lymphocytes, fibroblasts and monocytes. It is responsible for conversion of blood monocytes into osteoclasts.
- **Interleukin-8:** Monocytes, keratinocytes and fibroblasts are responsible for releasing IL-8. It is a strong chemo-attractant of PMNLs at low concentrations.
- **Tomour necrosis factor:** It is produced by macrophages and release lymphotoxins. It stimulates the proliferation of osteoclast precursor cells and also activates the mature osteoclasts to resorb bone.
- **Prostaglandin E_2:** PGE_2 is produced by macrophages and fibroblasts, but IL-1 also induces its production. It is a responsible for osteoclastic resorption.

Question 8

What are immunoglobulins?

Answer

- Immunoglobulins are gamma globulins produced by plasma cells in response to antigens with which they can react in a specific way.
- They can be found in blood, tissues, secretions, and are effectors of the humoral response.
- These molecules are composed of two light chains (λ, κ) and one of the five types of heavy chains (γ, α, δ, μ, ε). The class of the Ig molecules is donated by the heavy chain.
- Basic structure of this molecule resembles the letter Y, where the tail of the Y contains the ends of the heavy-chains Fc fragments and complement-binding site. The remaining area is the heavy chains antibody binding site.
- Functions of immunoglobulins:
  - Immunoglobulin G.
    - › Complement fixation.
    - › Delayed antibody response.
    - › Opsonisation.
    - › Cross placental barrier.
    - › Increased concentration in gingival crevicular fluid.
  - Immunoglobulin A.
    There are two types of IgA: serum IgA and secretory IgA.
    - › Serum IgA helps in complement fixation by alternate pathway.
    - › Secretory IgA has increased concentrations in saliva.
    - › Secretory IgA protects mucosal surfaces and prevents adhesion of bacteria to tissue surfaces especially in the early stages of periodontal diseases.
  - Immunoglobulin M
    - › Responsible for early antibody response and complement fixation.
  - Immunoglobulin E
    - › It causes immediate hypersensitivity reactions.
  - Immunoglobulin D
    - › The functions of IgD are not known.

Question 9

What is transendothelial migration?

Answer

Trans-endothelial migration is selective interaction between leukocytes and endothelium that result in the leukocyte pushing its way between endothelial cells to exit the blood and enter the tissues.

In a local inflammatory response, trans-endothelial migration occurs in the following sequential phases:

- Step 1: Rolling.
- Step 2: An insult to local tissue.
- Step 3: Signalling the endothelium.
- Step 4: Increased rolling.
- Step 5: Signal for rolling arrest.
- Step 6: Strong adhesion.
- Step 7: The zipper phase.

Leukocytes use the lectin (a non-enzymatic carbohydrate binding protein) designated L-selectin to interact with carbohydrate molecules known as vascular adhesion (CD 34) on the luminal surface of endothelial cells. This brief interaction manifests itself as the rolling of the leukocyte along the luminal surface of the endothelium.

A local insult triggers the release of a variety of inflammatory signals (e.g. IL-1, IL-1β, TNF α) from cells in the tissue, especially from resident leukocytes such a mast cells. Mast cells are crucial in initiating neutrophil recruitment against bacteria and responding to anaphylatoxins such as C3a and C5a.

Interleukin-1β, TNF α, C5 and lipopolysaccharides can stimulate endothelial cells to express P-selectin and E-selectin in their luminal surfaces.

The stimulated endothelium also releases chemokines which small peptide cytokines, first recognised for their chemo-attractant activities.

Chemokines function as a signal for rolling arrest. The interaction of a chemokine, IL-8, with the leukocyte receptor CXCR2 causes the leukocyte to shed L-selectin and upregulate the integrins leukocyte function–associated antigen-1(LFA-1). Integrins are transmembrane adhesions, some of which have been adapted for use by the immune system. LFA-1 binds intercellular adhesion molecule-2 (ICAM-2), which is expressed constitutively by endothelium.

Because leukocytes differ with respect to their chemokine receptors, the chemokines dictate which leukocytes (e.g. neutrophils, macrophages, lymphocytes, eosinophils, and basophils) dominate the leukocyte infiltrates. Different stimuli (e.g. cytokines, tissue injury, viral or microbial insults) can lead to expression of different chemokines.

Chronic inflammatory leukocytes (monocytes and lymphocytes) possess integrins that are not expressed by neutrophils. One such integrin, very late antigen-4 (VLA-4), binds endothelial vascular cell adhesion molecule-1 (VCAM-1). Endothelium expresses VCAM-1 after prolonged inflammation, thus providing a mechanism for the selection of chronic inflammatory cells.

CD31 (platelet-endothelium cell adhesion molecule-1) is a 130-kD trans-membrane glycoprotein present at the intercellular borders of endothelial cells facing into lumen and on all leukocytes. CD31 is a homophilic adhesion molecule because CD31 molecules bind to one another.

Once the leukocyte locates the inter-endothelial junction, it uses its own CD31 as a zipper effect has been proposed as a mechanism of minimizing the leakage of fluid. As the endothelium unzips its CD31, the leukocyte rapidly "zips" between the endothelial cells.

Leukocytes possess several proteases including urokinase plasminogen activator receptor (μPAR). The μPAR leads to the activation of collagenase which then may degrade the basement membrane and enable the leukocyte to enter the connective tissues.

Defects in trans-endothelial migration are associated with aggressive periodontitis reflecting are importance in periodontal diseases.

Question 10

What is chemotaxis?

Answer

Chemotaxis is leukocyte's ability to sense a chemical gradient across its cell body and migrates in the direction of increasing concentration.

The phagocyte senses only a limited number of chemicals: chemotaxins for which it has receptors and chemotaxis receptors.

The receptors for chemotaxis belong to a family called the G-protein coupled family. This family of receptors also includes the various light receptors in our retains; thus in some ways, leukocytes "see" a chemotactic gradient much as we see light. The only class of chemotaxins derived directly from bacteria are formyl-methionyl peptides.

To migrate toward a target leukocyte, assume an asymmetric or polarized shape rather than the rounded morphology evident in blood.

Question 11

What are the various defects in leukocyte function?

Answer

Various defects in leukocyte function are mentioned in **(Table 10.1)**:

Table 10.1: Various defects in leukocyte function

Disease	Defect
Genetic Leukocyte adhesion	Beta chain of CD11/CD18 integrins
Deficiency 1 Leukocyte adhesion	Sialyl-Lewis X (selectin receptor)
Deficiency 2 Neutrophil-specific	Absence of neutrophil-specific granules
Granule deficiency Chronic granulomatous disease	Defective chemotaxis decrease oxidative burst NADPH oxidase (Membrane component)
X-linked Autosomal recessive	NADPH oxides (cytoplasmic component)
Myeloperoxidase deficiency	Absent MPO-H_2O_2 system
Chediak-Higashi syndrome	Membrane protein involved in organelle trafficking
Acquired 1. Thermal injury, diabetes, sepsis, etc.	Chemotaxis
2. Hemodialysis, diabetes	Adhesion
3. Sepsis, diabetes, malnutrition, etc.	Phagocytosis and microbicidal activity

CHAPTER 11

Microbial Interactions with the Host in Periodontal Diseases

Question 1

Explain in detail host microbial interactions.

Answer

There are two aspects of host microbial interaction:

1. Microbiologic aspect.
2. Immunologic aspect.

Microbiologic Aspect

- Bacterial colonisation and the survival in the periodontal region.

  - **Bacterial adherence in the periodontal environment:** The bacteria get attached to tooth or root surfaces, tissue surfaces and pre-existing plaque mass.

  - **Host tissue invasion:** Many bacterial species have been recognised which are capable of tissue invasion. These species are responsible for producing periodontal diseases. There localisation into the tissues provide a position from where they can release toxic substance into the host tissue which further lead to tissue destruction.

  - **Bacterial evasion of host defence mechanisms:** Bacteria produce substances which help them in evading the host defence mechanisms for its survival, e.g. bacteria produce immunoglobulin degrading proteases which counteract the effect of immunoglobulins which forms an important host defence constituent.

- Microbial mechanisms of host tissue damage.

There is a number of bacterial products which can retard the growth and alter the metabolism of host tissue cells. For example, ammonia, fatty acids, volatile sulphur, collagenase and matrix metalloproteinases, etc.

Bacterial byproducts can disturb the host system which may lead to tissue destruction. These products can also lead to bone resorption and inhibit other host immune cells.

Immunologic Aspects

Bacteria are responsible for causing periodontal disease and can directly interact with the host tissues leading to tissue destruction. If the destruction exceeds the reconstruction rate, it leads to periodontal disease.

There is a major role of immune system in periodontal pathogenesis.

There are three important paradigms involved in this process.

1. Innate factors like complement system, resident leucocytes like mast cells play an important role in initiating inflammation.

2. Neutrophils which are the acute inflammatory cells protect the tissue by controlling the periodontal microorganisms.

3. Macrophages and lymphocytes which are the chronic inflammatory cells protect the entire host from within the subjacent connective tissues and do all that is necessary to prevent local infection into a systemic one, including the sacrifice of local tissues.

Question 2

Which are the various mediators of inflammation?

Answer

The various mediators of inflammation are:

1. **Proteinases:** Primary proteinases are the matrix metalloproteinases (MMPs) which are responsible for tissue destruction.

These are produced by neutrophils, macrophages, fibroblasts, osteoblasts, osteoclasts and epithelial cells.

Other proteinases which are associated with periodontitis are elastase, cathepsin G, and neutrophil serine proteinases.

2. **Cytokines:** There are three important pro-inflammatory cytokines which play an important role in tissue destruction viz. interleukin 1 (IL-1), interleukin 6 (IL-6) and tissue necrotic factor (TNF).

   ○ Interleukin: 1 is produced by macrophages and lymphocytes.
   ○ TNF-α is also produced by macrophages.

The effect of IL-1 and TNF-α include:

○ Stimulation of endothelial cells to express selectins, which facilitate recruitment of leucocytes.
○ Activation of macrophage IL-1 production.
○ Induction of prostaglandin E2 (PGE2) by macrophages and gingival fibroblasts.

3. **Prostaglandins:**

   ○ They are arachidonic acid metabolites which are released by cyclooxygenases.
   ○ Macrophages and fibroblasts are primarily responsible for production of prostaglandins.
   ○ PGE2 is responsible for bone resorption.

CHAPTER 12

Smoking and Periodontal Diseases

LONG ESSAYS

Question 1

Explain the association of smoking and periodontal disease?

Answer

Smoking has a widespread effect on health of gingival and periodontal tissues like:

- **Physiological effects:**
  - There is decreased flow of gingival crevicular fluid (GCF).
  - Altered bleeding on probing.
  - There is a decrease in sub-gingival temperatures.
- **Microbiological effects:** It has been seen that smoking is closely associated with increased levels of periodontal pathogens specially in deep pockets.
- **Immunological effects:**
  - There is an alteration of the processes of neutrophil chemotaxis, oxidative bursts and phagocytosis.
  - There is an increase in the concentration of tumour necrosis factor alpha (TNF-α), and prostaglandin E2 (PGE2).
  - There is an increase in the enzymes collagenase and elastase.

Impact of smoking on periodontal diseases are as follows:

- **Gingivitis:** There is a decreased gingival inflammation and bleeding on probing.
- **Periodontitis:**
  - Smoking is associated with increased incidence of pocket depth, attachment loss and bone loss.
  - Rate of periodontal destruction is hastened.
  - The prevalence on severity of periodontal destruction is increased.
  - Chances of prevalence of severe periodontitis are seen in smokers as compared to non-smokers.
  - Chances of tooth loss are commonly associated with smoking.
  - The frequency of cigarette smoking per day is directly proportional to the all the above-mentioned points.
  - Patients who have stopped smoking show decrease in the prevalence and severity of periodontal diseases.

CHAPTER 13

Host Modulation and Host Modulation Agents

Question 1

What is the modulatory therapy? Discuss various host modulating agents?

Answer

According to carranza host is defined as the organism from which a parasite obtains its nourishment and modulation is defined as the alteration of function or status of something in response to a stimulus or an altered chemical or physical environment.

Host modulatory therapy (HMT) is a treatment concept that aims to reduce tissue destruction and stabilize or regenerate periodontics by modifying or down-regulating destructive aspects of the host response and up-regulating protective or regenerative response and is used for treating the host side of the host-bacteria interaction.

A variety of agents acts as host modulating agents. They are mentioned below.

Systemically Administrered Agents

❑ Non-steroidal anti-inflammatory drugs (NSAIDs).
❑ Bisphosphonates.
❑ Sub-antimicrobial dose doxycycline (SDD).

Locally Administered Agent

1. Non-steroidal anti-inflammation drugs.
2. Enamel matrix proteins.
3. Growth factors, and bone morphogenic proteins.

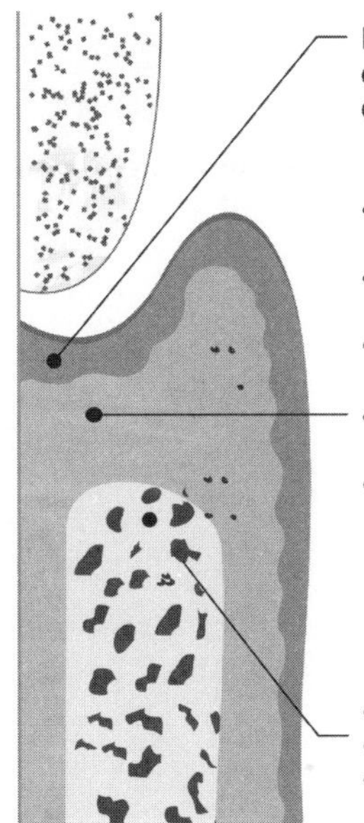

Fig. 13.1: Diagram showing how doxycycline inhibits connective tissue break down.

Non-steroidal Anti-inflammatory Drugs

- They inhibit the formation of prostaglandins, released by neutrophils, macrophages, fibroblasts, and gingival epithelial cells.
- Inflammation is reduced by administering NSAIDS, as it inhibits the production of prostaglandin.
- NSAIDs are given for the treatment of pain, acute inflammation and a variety of chronic inflammatory conditions.

Bisphosphonates

- These drugs inhibit osteoclastic activity, there by inhibiting bone resorption.
- They also have anti-collagenous properties.

Sub-antimicrobial Dose Doxycycline

- It is a 20 mg dose of doxycycline (periostat) that is indicated as an adjacent to SRP for the treatment of chronic periodontitis.
- It is taken for 3 months, twice only.
- It can be taken maximum for 9 months continuously.
- It acts by inhibiting the action of enzyme, cytokines and osteoclasts, rather than by exerting any antibiotic effect.

The rationale for using Sub Antimicrobial dose doxycycline (SDD) as an Host modulatory therapy (HMT) in the treatment of periodontitis is that doxycycline inhibits the activity of MMP's by a variety of mechanisms including reduction in cytokine levels and by stimulating osteoblastic activity and new bone formation by promoting collagen production (**Fig. 13.1**).

Locally Administered Agents

1. **NSAIDs:** Topical Mouthrinse containing NSAIDs for eg ketorolac have been found very effective in reducing the GCF leves of PGE2.
2. **Enamel matrix proteins, growth factor, and bone morphogenic proteins:** These have been shown to be very effective as HMTs.

SHORT ESSAYS

Question 1

What is best comprehensive periodontal management?

Answer

The best clinical improvement can be achieved by combination of various treat more treatment (**Fig. 13.2**).

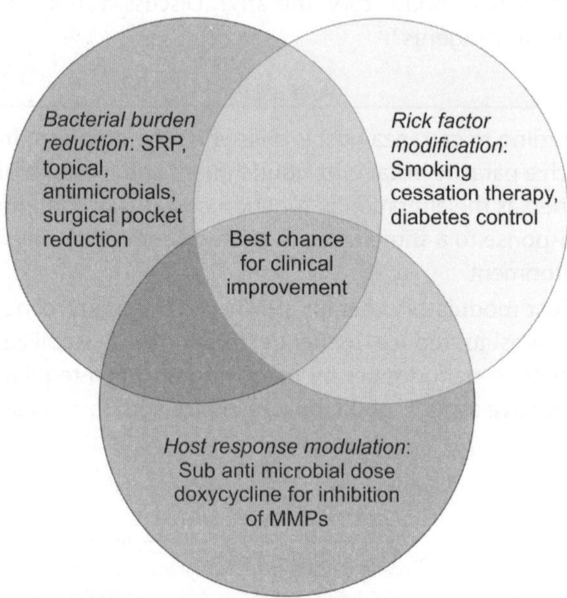

Fig. 13.2: Diagram showing best clinical improvement.

CHAPTER 14

Influence of Systemic Disorders and Stress on the Periodontium

LONG ESSAYS

Question 1

Describe the relationship between diabetes and periodontal diseases. Discuss the management of a diabetic patient having periodontitis.

Answer

Diabetes is defined as clinically and genetically heterogeneous group of metabolic disorders manifested by high levels of glucose in blood.

It can be classified into two types:

1. **Type I:** It is also known as insulin-dependent diabetes.
2. **Type II:** It is also known as non-insulin dependent diabetes.

The most common clinical signs of diabetes are:

- Polydipsia which means excessive thirst
- Polyuria which means excessive urination
- Polyphagia which means excessive hunger, which can be associated with loss in weight.

Various oral manifestations of diabetes mellitus are as follows:

- Cheilosis
- Mucosal drying and cracking
- Burning mouth and tongue
- Decreased salivary flow
- Abscess formation
- Change in the oral flora with predominance of *Candida albicans*, haemolytic streptococci and staphylococci.

Complications of Diabetes Mellitus

There are five classic complications of diabetes mellitus:

1. Retinopathy.
2. Nephropathy.
3. Neuropathy.
4. Altered wound healing.
5. Macrovascular disease.

Periodontal disease is more severe in persons having diabetes. Indeed the periodontal signs and symptoms are now recognized as the "sixth complication".

Relationship between Diabetes and Periodontitis

Pathogenesis

The various factors which lead to increased prevalence of periodontitis in diabetic patients are as follows:

- Vascular changes.
- Functions of polymorphonuclear neutrophils (PMNs).
- Biochemistry of crevicular fluid.
- Changes in plaque microflora.

Vascular Changes

There are certain vascular changes observed in diabetic patients such as:

- Thickening and hyalinization of vascular walls.
- Diastase resistant thickening of capillary basement membranes.
- Swelling and occasional proliferation of the endothelial cells.
- Splitting of capillary basement membrane.

All these diabetes induced vascular changes can lead to inhibitory effect on the transport of oxygen, white blood cells, immune factors and waste product, which further leads to impaired tissue repair and regeneration. This results in greater chances of having periodontitis.

Functions of PMNs

Functional impairment of PMNs is a classic feature of periodontitis.

There are various disorders of PMNs which can be observed in diabetic patients. They are:

- Reduced phagocytosis and intracellular killing.
- Impaired adherence.
- Impaired chemotaxis.

There is also inhibition of the glycolytic pathway with PMNs, abnormal cyclic nucleotide metabolism, which can lead to a disturbance in the organization of microtubules and microfilaments, and also a decrease in leukocyte membrane receptors.

All these factors cause increased prevalence of periodontitis.

Biochemistry of Crevicular Fluid

There has been observed a change in the composition of gingival crevicular fluid (GCF) in patients having diabetes.

This change favours the growth of periodontogenic bacteria which leads to increase rate of periodontitis.

Also levels of cyclic AMP also reduce in patients having diabetes.

Changes in Plaque Microflora

In the plaque of diabetic patients, there is a decreased activity of hyaluronidase.

There is a shift in the flora, with a greater prevalence of *Candida albicans*, haemolytic streptococci, and staphylococci.

Because of the earlier reasons, it has been concluded that patients having diabetes are more susceptible to periodontitis, which is mainly characterized by widening of periodontal ligament, increase in tooth mobility, suppuration, abscess formation, and bone loss.

Laboratory Diagnosis of Diabetes

Diabetes can be diagnosed by any of the laboratory methods:

- **Random blood glucose:** Less than 200 mg/dL.
- **Fasting plasma glucose:** Normal fasting glucose is 70–100 mg/dL.
- **2-hours post-prandial glucose:** Normal 2-hours post-prandial glucose is Less than 140 mg/dL.
- **Glycosylated haemoglobin assay (HbA1c):** Normal is 4–6%; Less than 7% good diabetes control; 7–8% suggests moderate diabetes control; >8% action suggested to improve diabetes control.

Treatment

If the patient is suspected to be diabetic, following procedures should be performed:

- Patients physician should be consulted.
- Laboratory tests should be analysed like fasting blood glucose, post-prandial blood glucose, HbA1c and urinary glucose.

- In the patients having uncontrolled diabetes, periodontal treatment is contraindicated.
- Diabetic patients with periodontitis, should receive oral hygiene instructions, mechanical debridement to remove the local factors and regular maintenance.
- In case of periodontal conditions, which require immediate care, prophylactic antibiotics should be given.
- If there is a patient of brittle diabetes, optimal periodontal health is necessary. Glucose levels should be monitored continuously and periodontal treatment should be performed, when the disease is in a well-controlled state.
- Prophylactic antibiotic treatment should be started and penicillin is the drug of choice.

Guidelines for a Diabetic Patient Receiving Periodontal Therapy

- Early morning appointments should be scheduled because of less stress and insulin levels are optimal.
- Post-operative dose of insulin should be altered, after any surgical procedure.
- Tissues should be handled as minimally and as a traumatically as possible.
- Preoperative sedation is necessary if the patient is anxious.
- Not more than 1:100,000 concentrations of epinephrine should be used.
- In case of extensive therapy, antibiotics are recommended.
- Recall appointments and meticulous home oral care should be prescribed.

Question 2

What is the role of vitamin C/ascorbic acid in aetiology of periodontal diseases. Discuss the oral manifestations of scurvy?

Answer

- Scurvy is caused due to the severe deficiency of vitamin C, which is characterised by haemorrhagic diathesis and delayed wound healing.
- It may be seen both in infants and adults.
- It may be seen in infants in their first year of life if the formulate are not fortified with vitamins and in adults because of malnutrition.
- Malnutrition associated with alcoholism may predispose an individual to scurvy.

Role of Vitamin C in Aetiology of Periodontal Disease

- Vitamin C plays an important role in periodontal diseases through—for the maintenance of epithelial barrier, function to bacterial products, optimal level of vitamin C are required. Vitamin C is also required to maintain the integrity of periodontal vasculature, also the vascular response to bacterial plaque and wound healing.

❑ Metabolism is affected with low levels of vitamin C due to which there is deficient ability of the tissue to regenerate and repair itself.

❑ Bone formation is also impaired leading to periodontal support in the deficiency of ascorbic acid. In the deficient state of vitamin C, there is a failure of osteoblasts to form osteoid.

❑ In the presence of vitamin C, both the chemotactic and the migratory action of are enhanced without influencing their phagocytic activity.

❑ There is an increase in the pathogenicity of the bacterial plaque because of the interference of the ecologic equilibrium because of the decreased vitamin C

❑ Deficiency of vitamin C results in scurvy which further leads to defective formation and maintenance of collagen, impaired osteoid formation and osteoblastic function.

❑ There is an increased capillary permeability, traumatic haemorrhages susceptibility, hyporeactivity of the contractile elements of the peripheral blood vessels, and sluggishness of blood flow in the deficient state of vitamin C.

Clinical Manifestation of Scurvy

❑ Bleeding, swollen gingiva and loosened teeth.
❑ Haemorrhagic lesions into the muscles of extremities, joints, nail beds and sometimes hair follicles.
❑ Petechial haemorrhages can also be seen.
❑ There is impaired wound healing.
❑ There is increased susceptibility to infections.

Gingivitis

❑ There is enlarged haemorrhagic bluish-red gingiva seen in deficiency of Vitamin C.
❑ Patients having Vitamin C deficiency do not always have gingivitis.
❑ Vitamin C deficiency does not cause gingivitis, but it can increase its severity.
❑ Deficiency of Vitamin C can aggravate the gingival response to plaque and can increase enlargement and bleeding.
❑ If the levels of Vitamin C become normal then there would be reduction in the severity of the disorder but gingivitis will remain as long as the bacterial plaque persists.

Periodontitis

❑ Deficiency of Vitamin C can result in swelling and haemorrhage in the periodontal ligament.
❑ Vitamin C deficiency can cause osteoporosis in the alveolar bone which can cause increase in the tooth mobility.
❑ Deficiency of Vitamin C alone does not cause periodontitis since it requires bacterial factors are required for attachment loss to occur.
❑ Decrease in Vitamin C can aggravate the pre-existing periodontitis.

Question 3

Discuss the pathogenesis of diabetes and periodontal disease.

Answer

The various factors which lead to increased prevalence of periodontitis in diabetic patients are as follows:

❑ Vascular changes.
❑ Functions of PMNs.
❑ Biochemistry of crevicular fluid.
❑ Changes in plaque microflora.

Vascular Changes

There are certain vascular changes observed in diabetic patients such as

❑ Thickening and hyalinization of vascular walls.
❑ Diastase resistant thickening of capillary basement membranes.
❑ Swelling and occasional proliferation of the endothelial cells.
❑ Splitting of capillary basement membrane.

All these diabetes induced vascular changes can lead to inhibitory effect on the transport of oxygen, white blood cells, immune factors and waste product, which further leads to impaired tissue repair and regeneration. This results in greater chances of having periodontitis.

Functions of Polymorphonuclear Neutrophils

Functional Impairment of PMNs is a classic feature of periodontitis.

There are various disorders of PMNs which can be observed in diabetic patients. They are:

❑ Reduced phagocytosis and intracellular killing.
❑ Impaired adherence.
❑ Impaired chemotaxis.

There is also inhibition of the glycolytic pathway with PMNs, abnormal cyclic nucleotide metabolism, which can lead to a disturbance in the organization of microtubules and microfilaments, and also a decrease in leukocyte membrane receptors.

All these factors cause increased prevalence of periodontitis.

Biochemistry of Crevicular Fluid

There has been observed a change in the composition of GCF in patients having diabetes

This change favours the growth of periodontogenic bacteria which leads to increase rate of periodontitis.

Also levels of cyclic AMP also reduce in patients having diabetes.

Changes in Plaque Microflora

In the plaque of diabetic patients, there is a decreased activity of hyaluronidase

There is a shift in the flora, with a greater prevalence of *Candida albicans*, haemolytic streptococci, and staphylococci.

Because of the above reasons, it has been concluded that patients having diabetes are more susceptible to periodontitis, which is mainly characterized by widening of periodontal ligament, increase in tooth mobility, suppuration, abscess formation, and bone loss.

SHORT ESSAYS

Question 1

What is the treatment of diabetic patients having periodontitis and what are the treatment guidelines?

Answer

Treatment

If the patient is suspected to be diabetic, following procedures should be performed:

- Patients' physician should be consulted.
- Laboratory tests should be analysed like fasting blood glucose, post-prandial blood glucose, glycated haemoglobin and urinary glucose.
- In the patients having uncontrolled diabetes, periodontal treatment is contraindicated.
- Diabetic patients with periodontitis should receive oral hygiene instructions, mechanical debridement to remove the local factors and regular maintenance.
- In case of periodontal conditions, which require immediate care, prophylactic antibiotics should be given.
- If there is a patient of brittle diabetes, optimal periodontal health is necessary. Glucose levels should be monitored continuously and periodontal treatment should be performed, when the disease is in a well-controlled state.
- Prophylactic antibiotic treatment should be started and penicillin is the drug of choice.

Guidelines for a Diabetic Patient Receiving Periodontal Therapy

- Early morning appointments should be scheduled because of less stress and insulin levels are optimal.

- Post-operative dose of insulin should be altered, after any surgical procedure.
- Tissues should be handled as minimally and as a traumatically as possible.
- Pre-operative sedation is necessary if the patient is anxious.
- Not more than 1:100,000 concentrations of epinephrine should be used.
- In case of extensive therapy, antibiotics are recommended.
- Recall appointments and meticulous home oral care should be prescribed.

Question 2

What is the management of periodontal diseases in pregnant patients?

Answer

Periodontal therapy aims to minimise the potential exaggerated inflammatory response related to pregnancy-associated hormonal alterations, in pregnant females.

- The second trimester of pregnancy is considered as the most safest period for performing dental procedures. But still long, stressful appointments and surgical procedures should be delayed until the period of post-partum.
- The non-emergency periodontal procedures performed in pregnant patients are meticulous plaque control, scaling, root planning and polishing.
- Appointments should be short and patient should be allowed to change positions frequently.
- In an ideal condition no medicines should be prescribed but based on the needs of the pregnant female they

should be reviewed for the potential adverse effects on the foetus before prescribing drugs such as analgesics, antibiotics, local anaesthetics and other drugs.

❑ Dental radiographs should be avoided during pregnancy. The American Dental Association has stated that normal radiographic guidelines do not need to be altered during pregnancy, use of a properly positioned lead apron is an absolute requirement.

Question 3

What are the periodontal manifestations of HIV infection?

Answer

Periodontal manifestations of an HIV infection are as follows:

❑ Linear gingival erythema
❑ Necrotising ulcerative gingivitis
❑ Necrotising ulcerative periodontitis.

Linear Gingival Erythema

❑ It is characterised by reddish to bluish-red, oedematous gingival tissue.
❑ There is usually presence of swollen interdental papilla and tendency to bleeding in increased.
❑ There are significantly more bleeding sites and destruction of interdental papilla is seen.

Necrotising Ulcerative Gingivitis

❑ It is characterised by red and swollen gingiva with a yellowish-grey marginal areas of necrosis.
❑ Loss of interdental papilla is also seen.
❑ It has an extremely rapid progression and there is increased destruction of the periodontal ligament and alveolar bone which is usually accompanied by severe pain.

Necrotising Ulcerative Periodontitis

❑ It is characterised by severe attachment loss and bone loss with increased tooth mobility.
❑ There is severe gingival bleeding.
❑ There is also deep seated along with tooth mobility and halitosis.

Question 4

What is necrotising gingivostomatitis?

Answer

The three conditions, i.e. linear gingival erythema, necrotizing ulcerative gingivitis and necrotizing ulcerative periodontitis, all these conditions may be collectively referred to as necrotizing gingivostomatitis.

Staging of Necrotizing Gingivostomatitis

Staging of necrotizing infections was proposed by Pindborg, who described four stages:

1. Only the tip of the interdental papilla is affected.
2. Marginal gingiva was affected, with punched out papilla.
3. Attached gingiva is also affected.
4. Exposure of bone.

Question 5

What are the periodontal findings of AIDS?

Answer

All HIV infected patients may not know that they are infected when they report for dental treatment. Individuals with known HIV infection may not admit their status on the medical history.

❑ Thus, every patient receiving dental treatment should be managed as a potentially infected person, using universal precautions for all therapy.
❑ Extensive periodontal treatment plans must be considered in regard to the patients' systemic health, prognosis, and survival time.
❑ Large variations in progression of HIV disease exist among individuals, and selection of an appropriate treatment plan depends on the state of the patients overall health.
❑ Although there appears to be few contraindications to routine dental treatment for many HIV infected patients, the periodontal treatment plan is influenced by the patients overall systemic health and coincident oral infections or diseases.
❑ An awareness of oral disorders associated with HIV infection allows the clinician to recognise previously undiagnosed disease or to modify treatment protocols appropriately.

Question 6

Describe in detail the periodontal manifestations of leukaemia

Answer

The leukaemias are the malignant neoplasias of WBC precursors characterised by:

❑ Diffuse replacement of the bone marrow with proliferating leukaemic cells.
❑ Abnormal numbers and forms of immature WBCs in the circulating blood.

❑ Widespread infiltrates in the liver, spleen, lymph nodes, and other body sites.

Periodontal Manifestations in Leukaemic Patients

Oral and periodontal manifestations of leukaemia consist of leukaemic infiltration, bleeding, oral ulcerations and infections.

❑ Gingival enlargements:
- ○ The enlargements are primarily the result of a massive leukemic cell infiltration into the gingival connective tissue. When present, it is usually a feature of acute monocytic leukaemia, although it has been reported as a feature of other forms, including chronic lymphocytic leukaemia.
- ○ The enlarged gingiva hinders mechanical plaque removal, and hence there is an inflammatory component enhancing this enlargement.

❑ Gingival bleeding:
- ○ Gingival bleeding can be seen as an early sign of leukaemia and is secondary to thrombocytopenia that accompanies the leukaemia.
- ○ It is specially marked when the platelet count drops below 10,000/mL and is compounded by poor oral hygiene.
- ○ Gingival haemorrhage is a common finding in leukaemic patients, even in the absence of clinically detectable gingivitis.
- ○ Bleeding tendency can also manifest in the skin and throughout the oral mucosa, where the petechiae are often found, with or without leukaemic infiltrates. More diffuse submucosal bleeding manifests as ecchymosis.
- ○ Bleeding can also be a side effect of the drugs used to treat leukaemia.

❑ Periodontal infections:
- ○ Infections of the periodontal tissues secondary to leukaemia can be of two types:
  - ➤ An exacerbation of an existing periodontal disease.
  - ➤ Through an increased susceptibility of the periodontium to fungal, viral or bacterial infections.

❑ Oral ulcerations and infections :
- ○ The response to bacterial plaque and other local irritation is altered, the cellular component of the inflammatory exudates differs both quantitatively and qualitatively from that in non-leukaemic individuals.
- ○ Granulocytopenia results from the displacement of normal bone marrow cells by leukaemic cell, which increases the host susceptibility to opportunistic microorganisms and leads to ulcerations and infections.
- ○ These lesions occur in sites of trauma such as buccal mucosa in relation to the line of occlusion or on the palate.
- ○ Discrete, punched-out ulcers penetrating deeply into the sub-mucosa and covered by a firmly-attached white slough can be found on the oral mucosa.
- ○ The gingival appearance is peculiar bluish-red. It is sponge-like and friable and bleeds persistently on slightest provocation or even spontaneously.
- ○ There are a variety of changes seen in the epithelium. It may be thinned or hyperplastic. Common findings include degeneration associated with intercellular and intracellular oedema and leukocytic infiltration with diminished surface keratinisation.
- ○ A gingival bacterial infection can be seen as a result of an exogenous bacterial infection.

CHAPTER 15

Periodontal Medicine

Question 1

Which are the various systemic diseases which can be effected by periodontitis? Explain in detail.

Answer

Various systemic diseases which can be effected by periodontitis are as follows:

- Cardiovascular system (CVS) and Cerebrovascular system:
  - Atherosclerosis.
  - Coronary artery disease (CAD) and stroke.
  - Myocardial infarction.
- Endocrine system:
  - Diabetes mellitus.
- Reproductive system:
  - Pre-term low birth weight (PLBW).
  - Pre-eclampsia.
- Respiratory system:
  - Chronic obstructive pulmonary disease.
  - Acute bacterial pneumonia.

Cardiovascular and Cerebrovascular System

- Daily oral-hygiene activity, e.g. mastication/tooth brushing creates greater bacteremia than from dental procedures.
- Periodontal disease predisposes the patient to bacteremia via the virulent Gram-negative periopathogens.
- 8% of infective endocarditis cases are associated with periodontal disease even in absence of dental procedures.
- American Heart Association (AHA) recommendations: Importance of establishing and maintaining best possible oral health to reduce potential sources of bacterial seeding.
- Thrombogenesis: Platelet aggregation is the primary cause for, periopathogens involved in coronary thrombogenesis especially platelets selectively bind with *Streptococcus sanguinis (plaque)*, *Porphyromonas gingivalis* with help of platelet aggregation-associated protein (PAAP) resulting formation of thromboemboli.
- Atherosclerosis: Focal thickening of arterial intima and media of the vessel.

Pathological Changes

- Circulating monocytes adhere to endothelium via adhesion molecules. Intercellular adhesion molecule-1, endothelial leukocyte adhesion molecule-1, vascular cell adhesion molecule-1, that are triggered by prostaglandins, bacterial LPS, cytokines. Complex penetrates the endothelium, ingests LDL and form foam cells significant of atheromas.
- Monocytes, macrophages liberating pro-inflammatory cytokines (IL-1, TNF, PGE2) that proliferate lesion.
- FGF, PDGF mitogenic factors stimulate collagen formation, arterial thickening, narrow lumen and less blood supply.

Systemic inflammatory markers, i.e. acute phase reactant proteins (CRP and fibrinogen) serve as a proven risk assessment tool for cardiovascular disease. Serum CRP and fibrinogen is elevated in periodontitis.

Periodontal disease has two-fold effects systemically:

1. Direct effects on Blood vessels (atheroma formation).
2. Indirect effects stimulating CVS changes (elevation of systemic inflammatory responses) (**Figs 15.1 to 15.6**).

Stroke and Periodontal Disease

- Studies reveal that poor dental health is a significant risk factor for stroke (25%).
- Periodontitis is a severe risk factor than smoking.
- Longitudinal study states that the periodontal patients with more than 20% bone loss at baseline were three times more likely to develop stroke versus those with less than 20% bone loss (**Fig 15.7**).

❑ Periodontitis increases individual's risk factor by threefold to develop stroke.

Diabetes and Periodontal Disease

Complications of diabetes mellitus are as follows:
❑ Retinopathy.
❑ Nephropathy.
❑ Neuropathy.
❑ Macrovascular disease.

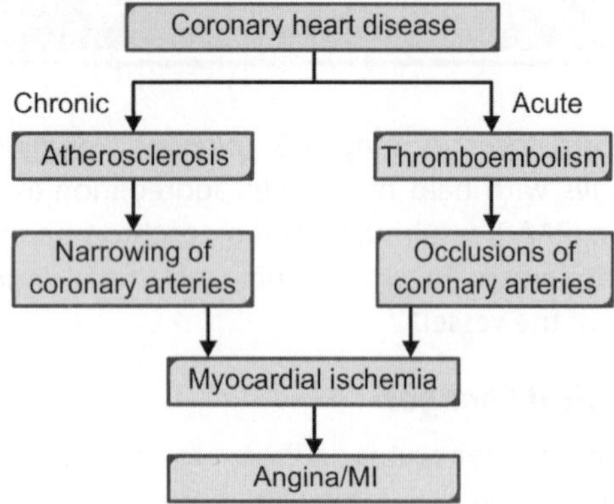

Fig. 15.1: Acute and chronic pathways to ischemic heart disease.

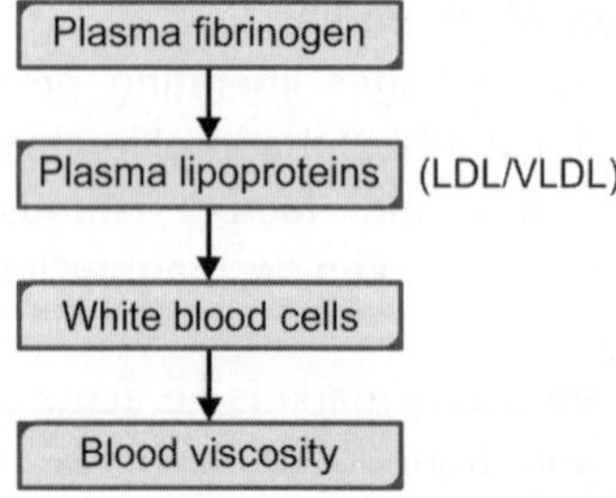

Fig. 15.2: Factors affecting blood viscosity in health.

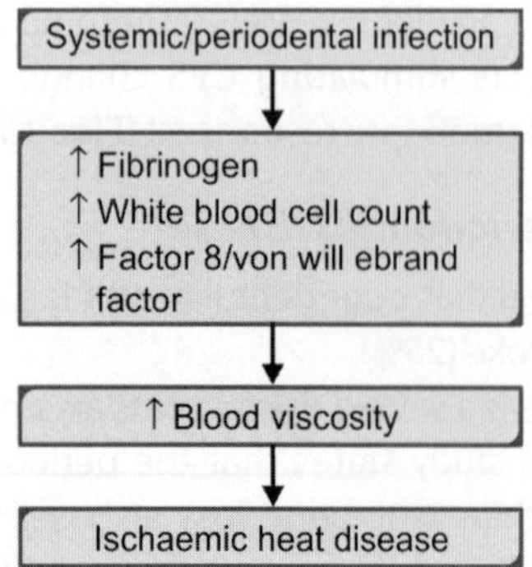

Fig. 15.3: Effect of infection on blood viscosity.

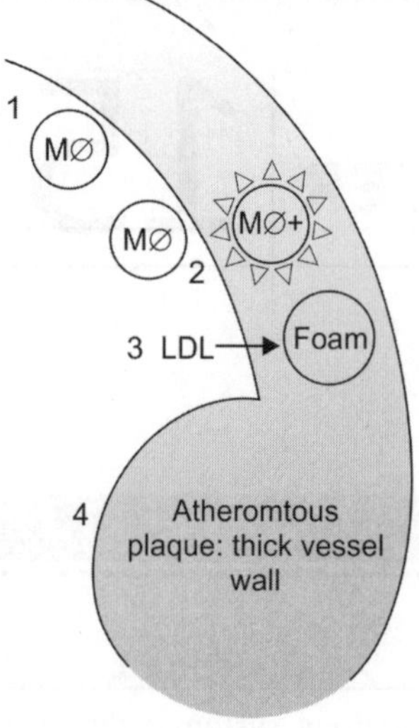

Fig. 15.4: Pathogenesis of atherosclerosis.

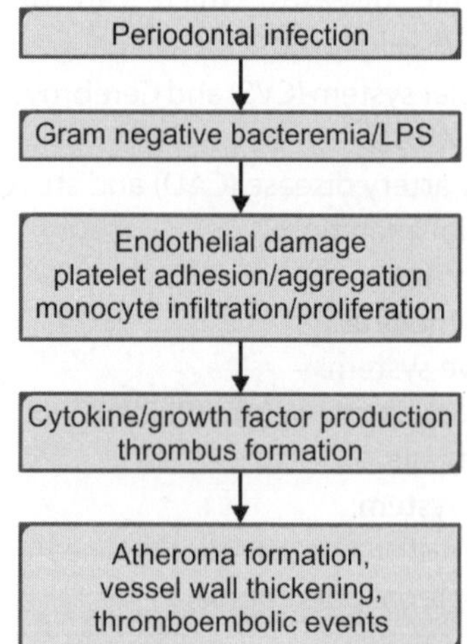

Fig. 15.5: Influence of periodontal infection on atherosclerosis.

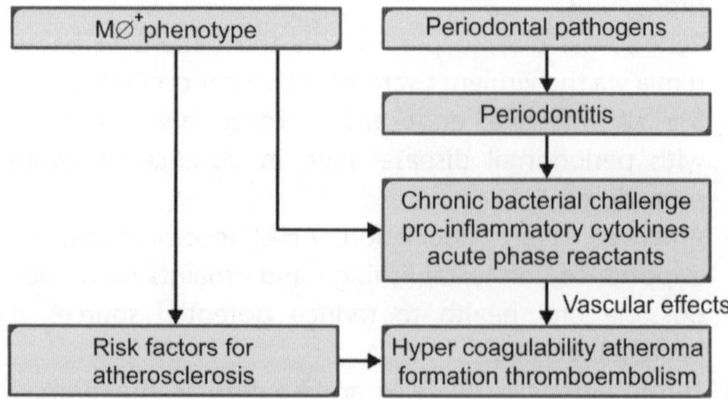

Fig. 15.6: Cardiovascular and periodontal consequences of hyper-responsive monocyte/macrophage phenotype.

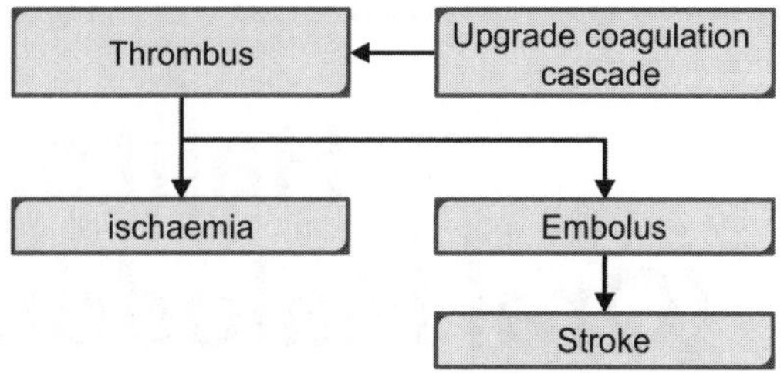

Fig. 15.7: Mechanism of stroke.

❏ Altered wound healing.
❏ Periodontal disease.
❏ Diabetes mellitus type 2 and severe periodontitis at baseline resulted in worsened glycemic control over time.
❏ Periodontal therapy along with systemic antibiotics significantly improves glycemic levels in cases with severe periodontitis with poor metabolic control.
❏ Antibiotics act as adjunct to periomechanical therapy.
❏ Mode of action of doxycycline 20 mg (tetracycline).
❏ Eliminates residual microorganisms.
❏ Anticollagenase property reduces the MMP's activity and protein glycation henceforth suppressing the AGE complex formation and improving metabolic control **(Fig 15.8)**.

Periodontitis and Pregnancy

Low birth weight infants less than 2,500 g at birth have high risk for death in neonatal period or on survival increased risk for congenital defects, respiratory disorders, etc.

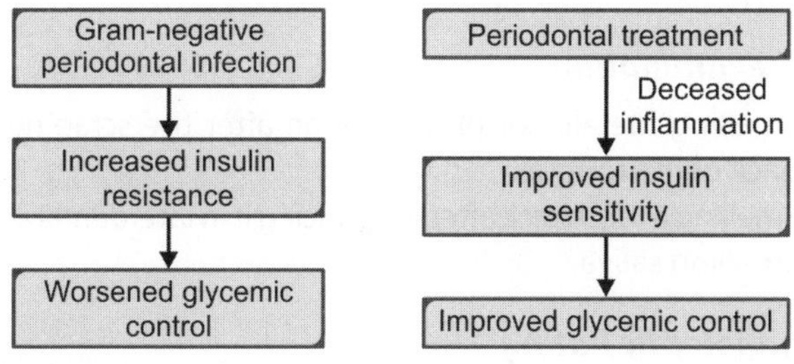

Fig. 15.8: Potential effects of periodontal infection and periodontal therapy on glycemic control in patients with diabetes

Aetiology for Low Birth Weight

In Pre-term labour, premature rupture of membrane. Risk factors are smoking, drug use, hypertension, diabetes, low socioeconomic status, genitourinary tract infections (bacterial vaginosis), etc.

❏ Periodontitis primarily a Gram negative infection, plays a role in low birth weight (LBW) infants chiefly by stimulation of host cytokine production.
❏ Studies state high levels of *Tannerella forsythia, P. gingivalis* found in subgingival plaque of women with LBW infants.
❏ Women with higher PGE2 and IL-1 levels in gingival crevicular fluid (GCF) are more prone to pre-mature births.
❏ Pre-eclampsia (hypertensive disorder) acts as risk in presence/severity of periodontal disease (2.5%).
❏ Maternal infection raises prematurely the pro-inflammatory cytokines and prostaglandin levels in amniotic fluid premature labour **(Fig 15.9)**.

Periodontal Disease and COPD

❏ COPD is characterized by airflow obstruction resulting from chronic bronchitis/emphysema.
❏ Pathogenic mechanisms are similar to periodontal disease, i.e. host response aggravated by bacteria in periodontal disease and smoking in COPD.
❏ Correlation is still in an infancy stage.

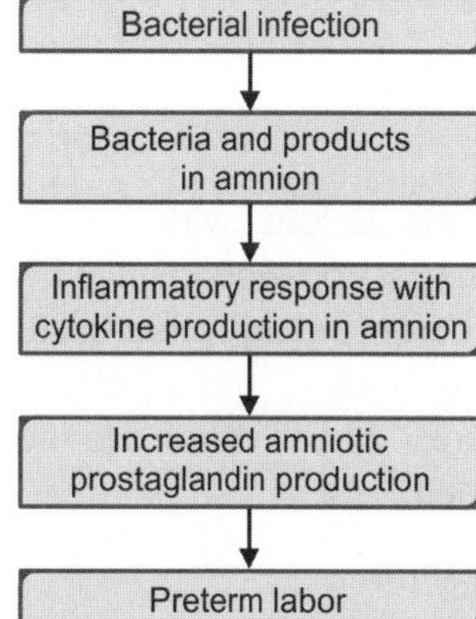

Fig. 15.9: Mechanisms by which infection may induce preterm labor

CHAPTER 16

Halitosis (Oral Malodour)

Question 1

Define oral malodour/halitosis/breath malodour. Give its aetiology, diagnosis and management.

Answer

Breath malodour can be defined as the unpleasant subjective perception after smelling someones breath due to some pathological cause.

Breath malodour should not be confused momentarily disturbing odour caused by food intake or smoking.

Aetiology

The unpleasant smell of breath is due to the presence of volatile sulphide compound (VSC) specially hydrogen sulphide, methyl mercaptan and dimethyl sulphide.

Intra-oral Causes

Dentition

- In deep carious lesions with food impaction and putrefaction, extraction wounds filled with blood clots, purulent discharge or any other factor causing food impaction.
- Acrylic dentures when worn overnight or are not regularly cleaned.

Periodontal Infections

- Bacterias associated with gingivitis or periodontitis like *porphyromonas gingivalis, prevotella intermedia, prevotella nigrescens, Campylobacter rectus, fusobacterium nucleatum, peptostreptococcus micros, tannerella forsythia, spirochetes*, etc. produce VSC, thus causing breath malodour.
- Anaerobic conditions, deep periodontal pockets help in the decarboxylation of lysine and ornithine to cadaverine and putrescine which are malodourous in nature.

Dry Mouth

- In patients with xerostomia, large amount of plaque are found on teeth, prosthesis and tongue surface.
- This plaque causes increase in the microbial load thus producing a lot of VSC and thus breath malodour.

Extra-oral Causes (Ear-Nose-Throat)

- In patients with acute pharyngitis, purulent sinusitis, chronic sinusitis or regurgitation oesophagitis, strong breath malodour is commonly seen.
- **Bronchi and lungs:** Breath malodour is commonly seen in cases of chronic bronchitis, bronchiectasis, and bronchial carcinoma.

Diabetes

Accumulation of ketone bodies in type 1 diabetes causes alteration of breath malodour and may prove useful in diagnosis.

Diagnosis

Self-examination

- Smelling metallic or plastic spoon after the scraping of back of the tongue.
- Smelling a tooth pick after introducing it in interdental area.
- Smelling saliva.

Organoleptic Rating

- It is considered gold-standard.
- In this, a trained judge sniffs the expired air and rates the intensity from 0 to 5:
  - 0—no odour present.
  - 1—barely noticeable odour.
  - 2—slight but clearly noticeable odour.
  - 3—moderate odour.
  - 4—strong offensive odour.
  - 5—extremely foul odour.

- The judge smells a series of different air samples:
  - 1—oral cavity odour: Judge places his or her nose close to the mouth opening while the patient refrains from breathing and counts from 1 to 20.
  - 2—breath odour: The subject expires through the mouth, while the judge smells both at the beginning and at the end.
  - 3—tongue coating: The judge smells the tongue scraping.
  - 4—nasal breath odour: The judge places his nose near the nostrils while the patient expires through the nose keeping the mouth closed.

Specific Characteristics of Breath Malodour

- Rotten-egg smell indicates the presence of VSC.
- A dead mice smell is associated with liver insufficiency, VSC, aliphatic acids.
- Rotten-apple smell indicated type I diabetes.
- Fish odour indicates kidney insufficiency.

Technology to Detect Oral Malodour

- Portable volatile sulphide monitor.
- Gas chromatography.
- Dark-field or phase-contrast microscopy.
- Saliva intubation test.
- Electronic nose.

Treatment

- **Mechanical reduction of intra-oral nutrients and microorganisms:** Tongue cleaning, tooth-brushing, interdental cleaning, scaling.
- **Chemical reduction of oral microbial load:** Chlorhexidine, triclosan-based mouthwashes, chlorine dioxide, two-phase oil water rinses, Listerine rinses, amino fluoride/stannous fluoride, 3% hydrogen peroxide rinses, oxidizing lozenges.
- **Conversion of malodourous gases into non-volatile compounds:** Metal salt solutions metal salts like zinc ions, combined with sulphur making volatile sulphide compound into non-volatile sulphide compounds.
- **Toothpastes:** Baking soda based dentifrices have been shown to be effective by reducing VSC levels.
- **Masking the malodour:** Mouth rinses, mouth sprays, and lozenges contain pleasant odour which mask the breath malodour for a short duration.

CHAPTER 17

Defence Mechanism of Gingiva

Question 1

Describe in detail defence mechanism of gingiva?

Answer

Sulcular Fluid or Gingival Crevicular Fluid

- Gingival crevicular fluid (GCF) is an inflamtmatory exudate and not a continuous transudate.
- In normal gingiva little or no fluid can be collected.
- **Methods of collection of GCF:**
  - **Brill Technique:** In this a filter-paper strip is inserted into the pocket till resistance is encountered.

    This method introduces irritation of sulcular epithelium which can trigger the low of fluid, therefore this gives an inaccurate picture.
  - **Loe and Holm-Pedersen technique:** In this method they place the filter-paper strip at the entrance of the pocket to minimise the irritation.

    In this method fluid seeping out of the pocket is picked up by the strip but sulcular epithelium does not come in contact with the paper.
  - **Weinstein method:** In this method they use pre-weighed twisted threads which are placed in the gingival crevice along the tooth and the amount of fluid collected is estimated by re-weighing the thread.
  - **Micropipette:** In this method micropipettes are used, which are placed in the pocket.

    These collect the fluid by the capillary action.
- **Composition of GCF:**
  - **Cellular elements:** Bacteria, desquamated epithelial cells, leucocytes [polymorphonuclear neutrophils (PMNs)], lymphocytes, monocytes/ macrophages.
  - **Electrolytes:** Potassium, sodium and calcium ions are seen in GCF.
  - **Organic compounds:** Glucose hexose amine and hexuronic acid are commonly seen.
- Glucose concentration in GCF is three to four times than serum.
- Metabolic and bacterial products commonly seen in GCF are lactic acid, urea, hydroxyproline, endotoxins, hydrogen sulphide and antibacterial factors.
- Many enzymes are also seen.
- **Clinical Significance of GCF:**
  - GCF is an inflammatory exudate whose presence in sulci gives an indication of inflammation even in the sulcus which appears normal to naked eye.
  - The amount of GCF is proportional to the severity of inflammation.
- **Factors that influence the amount of GCF are:**
  - **Circadian periodicity:** Between 6 am to 10 pm a gradual increase in GCF amount is seen which decreases post 10 pm.
  - **Sex hormones:** Females sex hormones enhance vascular permeability thus enhancing GCF flow.
  - **Mechanical stimulation:** Chewing and vigorous gingival brushing stimulates the increases of GCF flow.
  - **Smoking:** Smoking produces an immediate but transient increase in GCF flow.
  - **Periodontal therapy:** GCF production is increased during the healing period after periodontal surgery.

Leucocytes in Dentogingival Area

- Leucocytes which are predominantly polymorphonuclear neutrophils (PMNs) are found in clinically healthy gingival sulci.
- These appear in small numbers extravacularly in connective tissue adjacent to the bottom of the sulcus.

- From here these travel across the epithelium into the gingival sulcus.
- 91.2–91.5% PMNs and 8.5–8.8% mononuclear cells together form the leucocyte population.
- Mononuclear cells are composed of 58% B lymphocytes, 18% mononuclear phagocytes and 24% T lymphocytes.
- Leucocytes form a major protective mechanism against plaque in the gingival sulcus.

Saliva

- Saliva in oral cavity performs following functions:
  - Lubrication with the help of glycoproteins and muccoids.
  - Physical protection with glycoprotein and muccoids.
  - Cleansing with the physical flow.
  - Buffering action with the help of bicarbonate and phosphate action.
  - Anti-bacterial action.

Anti-bacterial Factors

- **Inorganic Factors:**
  - Ions and gases, bicarbonate , sodium, potassium, phosphates, calcium, fluorides, ammonium and carbon dioxide.

- **Organic Factors:**
  - **Lyzozyme:** It is a hydrolytic enzyme which works on both Gram-negative and Gram-positive organisms.
  - *Lacto peroxidase-thiocyanate system:* It is bactericidal to some strains of Lactobacillus and Streptococcus.
  - *Lactoferrin:* It is effective against Actinobacillus species.
  - *Myeloperoxidase:* This enzyme is released by leucocytes and is bactericidal towards Actinobacillus and also inhibits attachment of actinomyces to hydroxyapatite.

- **Salivary Antibodies:**
  - Saliva contains IgG, IgM and IgA immunoglobulins.
  - However out of these, IgA has the highest concentration in the saliva while IgG is seen more in GCF.

- **Salivary Enzymes:**
  - Most common enzyme is parotid amylase; however, in periodontal diseases, following enzymes are also seen: hyaluronidase, lipase, beta glucuronidase, chondroitin sulphatase, amino acid decarboxylase, catalase, peroxidase and collagenase.
  - Saliva also contains anti-proteinases, which inhibit cysteine proteinases like cathepsin and anti-leucoproteases which inhibit elastase.
  - Tissue inhibitor of matrix metalloproteinase (TIMP) inhibits the activity of collagen degrading enzymes.

CHAPTER 18

Gingival Inflammation

Question 1

What are the various stages of gingivitis? Explain in detail with histopathology.

Answer

There are four stage of gingivitis:

1. Stage I gingivitis: The initial lesion.
2. Stage II gingivitis: The early lesion.
3. Stage III gingivitis: The established lesion.
4. Stage IV Gingivitis: The advanced lesion.

Stage I Gingivitis: The Initial Lesion

- Clinically, this initial response to bacterial plaque is not apparent and therefore referred to as subclinical gingivitis.
- It is the first manifestation of gingival inflammation.
- There are vascular changes in this stage consisting of dilated capillaries and an increase in blood flow.
- If the host respose is good, the initial lesion would resolve rapidly, leaving the tissue to the normal state.
- But if the host does not responds well, then the lesion might take up a chronic form and there might be infiltration of macrophages and lymphoid cells.

Histologically

- There is increase in the number of leucocytes.
- There is increase in the gingival crevicular fluid (GCF) flow, due to increased accumulation of leucocytes within the gingival sulcus.
- Leucocytes increase within the junctional epithelium and the connective tissue.
- There is widening of the blood vessels.

Stage II Gingivitis: The Early Lesion

- Early lesion evolves form the initial lesion.
- This process starts in about one week after the beginning of plaque accumulation.
- This stage shows erythema due to the proliferation of capillaries and increase formation of capillary loops between rete pegs or ridges.
- Bleeding on probing also becomes evident.
- Between 6 and 12 days after the onset of clinical gingivitis, the gingival fluid flow and the number of leucocytes reach to the maximum level.
- About 70% of collagen is destroyed around the cellular infiltrate.
- The polymorphonuclear leukocytes (PMNs) are now evident in the gingival epithelium, since they leave the blood vessels and through chemotactic stimuli from plaque, migrate to the epithelium.
- Process of phagocytosis occurs, in which the PMNs engulf the bacteria.
- There is a decreased capacity of collagen production, and fibroblast shows cytotoxic alterations.

Histologically

- Seventy-five percent lymphocytes, mainly T lymphocytes are found in the connective tissue, just beneath the junctional epithelium.
- Neutrophils, macrophages and some amount of plasma cells and mast cells are also seen within the connective tissue.
- Rete pegs may be seen in the Junctional epithelium.
- The features of initial lesion aggravate in early lesions.

Stage III Gingivitis: The Established Lesion

- This lesion is predominated by plasma cells and B lymphocytes.
- B lymphocytes are mainly of immunoglobulin G1 (IgG1) and G3 (IgG3) subclasses.
- This stage occurs around 2–3 weeks of plaque accumulation.

- There is presence of localised gingival anoxemia which is due to engorged and congested blood vessels, impaired venous return and sluggish blood flow.
- Anoxemia leads to bluish hue on the reddened gingiva.
- Colour of the gingiva can deepen due to extravasation of erythrocytes and into the connective tissue and break down of haemoglobin into its component pigments.
- Collagenase is an enzyme which is normally present in gingival tissue it is produced by PMNs and also by some bacteria.
- The activity of this collagenase is increased in inflamed gingival tissue which causes destruction of the gingival connective tissue.
- In the chronically inflamed gingiva there is also increased levels of acid phosphatase, alkaline phosphatase, β-glucuronidase, β-glucosidase, β-galactosidase, esterases, aminopeptidase and cytochrome oxidase.

Histologically

- There is presence of a chronic inflammatory reaction.
- There is increase in the number of plasma cells and B lymphocytes.
- Intercellular spaces within the Junctional epithelium widens.

- Intercellular spaces are filled with granular debris, along with lysosomes derived from disrupted neutrophils, lymphocytes and monocytes.
- Tissue components can be destroyed, because of acid hydrolases released by lysosomes.
- Rets ridges can be seen in the Junctional epithelium that protrude into the connective tissue.
- Collagen fibres are also destroyed within the connective tissue, around, the infiltrate disrupted plasma cells, neutrophils, lymphocytes, monocytes and mast cells.

Stage 4 Gingivitis: The Advanced Lesion

- These lesion evolves from stage three gingivitis.
- It is characterised by extension of inflammation into the alveolar bone.
- Therefore, it is referred to as phase of periodontal break down.

Histologically

- Extensive inflammation and immunopathologic tissue damage is seen.
- Plasma cells continue to dominate the connective tissue.
- PMNs dominate the Junctional epithelium and crevice.
- Gingiva becomes fibrotic.

C H A P T E R **19**

Clinical Features of Gingivitis

LONG ESSAYS

Question 1

What is gingivitis? Describe gingivitis. Discuss clinical features of gingivitis in detail.

Answer

Inflammation of gingiva is refrred to as gingivitis.

- It can occur as a sudden onset for short duration can be painful.
- Gingivitis which reappears even after having been eliminated by treatment is referred to as recurrent gingivitis.
- Gingivitis which is slow in onset and is for longer duration is inferred to as chronic gingivitis. It is most commonly found.
- Gingivitis which is confined to the gingiva of a single tooth or group of teeth is referred to as localised gingivitis.
- Gingivitis, involving the margin of the gingiva and may include a portion of the contiguous attached gingiva is referred to as marginal gingivitis.
- Gingivitis involving the interdental papillae and may extend to the gingival margin, is referred to as papillary gingivitis.
- Gingivitis affecting the gingival margin, the attached gingiva and the interdental papillae is referred to as. Diffuse gingivitis.
- Gingival disease can be described as follows:
  - *Localised marginal gingivitis:* It is confined to one or more areas of the marginal gingiva.
  - *Localised diffuse gingivitis:* It extends from margin to the mucobucccal fold in a small area.
  - *Localised papillary gingivitis:* It is seen in one or more interdental regions in a small area.
  - *Generalised marginal gingivitis:* It is seen in the gingival margin in relation to all the teeth.
  - *Generalised diffuse gingivitis:* It involves the complete gingiva that includes the interdental, marginal and the attached gingiva.

- **Clinical features of gingivitis are as follows:**
  - A. Gingival bleeding on probing.
  - B. Colour changes in the gingiva.
  - C. Changes in consistency of gingiva.
  - D. Changes in surface texture of gingiva.
  - E. Changes in position of the gingiva.
  - F. Changes in gingival contour.

A. Gingival Bleeding on Probing

- Bleeding on probing is one of the clearest signs of gingival inflammation seen before the gingivitis is established, other being the increase in gingival crevicular fluid production rate.
- It may vary in severity duration and case of provocation.
- It has been seen that bleeding on pooling appears before visual signs of inflammation, thus it is a more objective sign that requires less subjective estimation by the examiner.
- Presence of bleeding is not a definite indicator of clinical attachment loss, but its absence definitely indicates an excellent negative predictor of future attachment loss.

Factors causing gingival bleeding could be local or systemic

- **Local factors causing gingival bleeding:**
  - Other than plaque, there are various other contributing factors for gingivitis. They can be anatomic and developmental tooth variations, caries, frenum pull, iatrogenic factors, malposition of teeth, mouth breathing, overhangs, partial dentures, lack of attached gingiva and recession.
- **Chronic and recurrent bleeding:**
  - Chronic inflammation is the most common cause of abnormal gingival bleeding
  - Mechanical trauma can provoke gingival bleeding, either chronic or recurrent

- Mechanical trauma could be from tooth brushing tooth picks, food impactions or biting into solid foods for example apples
- The severity of bleeding and the ease of its provocation depends upon the intensity of inflammation
- Once the vessels are ruptured and damaged, mechanism of hemostasis starts, which include contraction of the vessel wall, decrease in blood flow, platelets adhere to the edges of the tissue forming a fibrous clot which contracts, resulting in approximation of the edges of the injured area
- But when this area is irritated, bleeding starts again
- Bleeding on probing is a sign of active tissue destruction
- Injury can lead to active episodes of gingival inflammation
- Injury could be laceration of gingiva during tooth brushing or by sharp pieces of hard food, gingival burns from hot foods or chemicals
- Spontaneous bleeding is also seen in acute necrotising ulcerative gingivitis as the inflamed connective tissue consists of engaged blood vessels, which get enrobed by ulceration due to necrotic surface epithelium.

❑ **Systemic factors causing bleeding:**
- Certain conditions have common feature of a haemostatic mechanism failure which result in abnormal bleeding in the skin, internal organ and other tissues including oral mucosa.
- In such condition, the bleeding is spontaneous.
- Haemorrhagic disorders, in which there is abnormal gingival bleeding is seen are as follows: Vascular abnormalities like vitamin C deficiency or allergy like Schonlein-Henoch purpura, platelet disorders like thrombocytopenic purpura, hypoprothrombinemia like vitamin K deficiency, other coagulation defects such as haemophilia, leukaemia or Christmas disease, deficient platelet thromboplastic factor (PF3) resulting from uraemia, multiple myeloma and post rubella purpura.
- There are certain other . They can be effects of hormonal replacement therapy, oral contraceptives, pregnancy and the menstrual cycle.
- Fluctuation in certain hormones such as androgonic hormones have been associated in modifying gingivitis, especially during puberty.
- Certain medications also alter the gingivitis like, anticonvulsants antihypertensive calcium-channel blockers and the immunosuppressant drugs, cause gingival enlargements, which cause gingival bleeding, secondarily.

B. Colour Changes in Gingiva

❑ Colour of the gingiva is dependent on three factors vascularity, degree of keratinisation and pigments within the epithelium.
❑ Colour change is a very important clinical sign of gingivitis.
❑ The normal colour of gingiva is coral pink, and is because of vascularity and overlying epithelial layers.
❑ If the vascularity increase, the colour changes to reddish pink.
❑ Thus, in chronic periodontitis, the colour changes to reddish pink due to increased proliferation of blood vessels and reduced keratinisation. Bluish hue may be seen in later stages due to venous.
❑ The colour change starts from the interdental and the marginal gingiva and may extend to the attached gingiva.
❑ Colour changes in acute gingivitis differs in both distribution and nature from those in chronic gingivitis.
❑ The colour change may be marginal, diffuse or patch like, depending upon the acute condition.
❑ For example in acute necrotising ulcerative gingivitis, the marginal gingiva is involved. In herpetic gingivostomatitis the involvement is diffuse and in acute reaction to chemical irritation can be diffuse or patch like.
❑ If the condition does not worsen, the colour remains red and may revert back but if the condition worsens in acute inflammation, then the colour changes to dull, whitish grey.

Metallic Pigmentation

❑ Systematic absorption of heavy metals like bismuth, arsenic, mercury, lead and, from therapeutic was or occupational or household environment might discolour the gingiva and other areas of the oral mucosa.
❑ A black or bluish line is present in the gingiva due to these metals.

Colour Changes Associated with Systemic Factors

❑ There are certain systemic factors which may influence the colour of the gingiva.
❑ There could be endogenous or endogenous source of pigments.
❑ Endogenous oral pigments are melanin, bilirubin and iron which can cause oral pigmentation.
❑ Melanin pigmentation is a normal physiologic process which is found in highly-pigmented ethnic groups.

- Following are the diseases in which there is increase in melanin pigmentation:
  - **Addison's disease:** Isolated patches of discolouration are seen in this disease, which is of varying degree from bluish-black to brown.
    - ➢ It is basically caused due to adrenal dysfunction.
  - **Peutz- syndrome:** This disease causes intestinal polyposis.
    - ➢ Melanin pigmentation is seen in oral mucosa and lips.
  - **Albright syndrome:** (fibrous dysplasia) and von reckling hausen's disease (neurofibronatosis) produces areas of oral melanin pigmentation.
    - ➢ Bile pigments can also stain the skin and the mucous membrane.
    - ➢ Iron deposition seen in case of haemochro-matosis also produces a blue-grey pigmentation of the oral mucosa.
    - ➢ Disorders related to blood can produce colour changes of the oral mucosa such as anaemia, polycythaemia or leukaemia.
    - ➢ Disorders related to endocrine system and metabolic disturbance can also produce colour change such as diabetes and pregnancy.
    - ➢ Exogenous factors which are responsible for colour changes in gingiva are as follows:
      - » Irritants such as coal, metal dust and colouring agents in food and lozenges.
      - » Tobacco leads to increase in melanin pigmentation and hyperkeratosis of the gingiva.
      - » Amalgam implantation in the mucosa can lead to localised bluish black areas of pigmentation.
- If a patient wants to get his gingiva depigmented because of aesthetic concern, procedure known as gingival depigmentation can be performed.
- There are various ways of gingival depigmentation such and with the help of scalpels, chemicals, electrocautery and lasers.

C. Changes in Consistency of Gingiva

- Both the acute and chronic form of gingiva produces changes in the consistency of gingiva.
- In chronic gingivitis, both the forms, i.e. destructive which is oedematous and reparative which is fibrotic, coexists and the form which is predominated, will define the consistency of gingiva.
- The various clinical and histopathological changes seen in the gingival consistency in chronic and acute form of gingivitis are as follows:

Chronic Gingivitis

Clinical Changes	Microscopic Features
Saggy and puffiness that pits on pressure.	It is because of infiltration by fluid and cells of inflammatory exudate.
Highly soft and friable gingiva which readily gets fragmented on exploration with a probe and pinpoint surface areas of redness and desquamation are seen.	Degeneration of the connective tissue and epithelium associated with injurious substances that provoke the inflammation and inflammatory exudate. There is a change in the connective tissue and epithelium relationship, with inflamed, engorged connective tissue expanding to within a few epithelial cells of surface. Thinning of the epithelium and degeneration is associated with oedema and leucocyte invasion, separated by areas in which rets pegs are elongated.
Firm Leathery Consistency	It is because of fibrosis and due to epithelial proliferation associated with long-standing chronic inflammation.

Acute Gingivitis

Clinical Changes	Microscopic Features
Diffuse puffiness and softening.	It is because of diffuse oedema of acute inflammatory origin.
Sloughing with greyish flake like particles of debris adhering to eroded surface.	There is necrosis with formation of pseudo membrane which can be composed of bacteria, PMNs and degenerated epithelial cells in a fibrous meshwork.
Vesicle formation	There is intercellular and intracellular oedema with degeneration of nucleus and cytoplasm and rupture of cell wall.

D. Changes in Surface Texture of the Gingiva

- The normal surface of gingiva is usually stippled.
- Stippling, basically refers to an orange peel appearance of gingiva which is caused by numerous small depressions and elevations.
- It is seen in interdental gingiva and attached gingiva.
- Surface of gingiva can be either smooth and shiny or firm and nodular depending whether the changes are exudative or fibrotic.
- Nodular texture is seen in cases of drug-induced gingival overgrowth.

E. Changes in Position Gingiva

- Normal position of gingiva is usually at cementoenamel junction (CEJ)
- In cases of inflammation the gingiva can be above CEJ, due to increase in the size of gingiva
- Also in cases of gingival enlargement, the gingiva will be above CEJ, most of the times covering the clinical crowns as well
- In case of attachment loss, there can be shift in the position of gingiva apical to CEJ
- This is referred to as gingival recession
- Recession is exposure of the root surface by the apical shift in the position of gingiva
- There can be two positions of gingiva in recession
- First is the actual position, which is the level of the epithelial attachment on the tooth
- Second is the apparent position which is the level of the crest of the gingival margin
- Actual position of the gingiva would determine the severity of the recession and not the apparent position (Fig. 19.1).
- Causes of recession are as follows:
  - Faulty tooth brushing techniques (gingival abrasion)
  - Tooth malposition
  - Friction from soft tissues (gingival ablation)
  - Gingival inflammation
  - Abnormal frenum attachment
  - Iatrogenic dentistry
  - Trauma from occlusion
  - Orthodontic treatment

Clinical Significance of Recession

Gingival recession can lead to:

- Root caries
- Recession can causes abrasion or erosion of the cementum leading to hypersensitivity of dentin

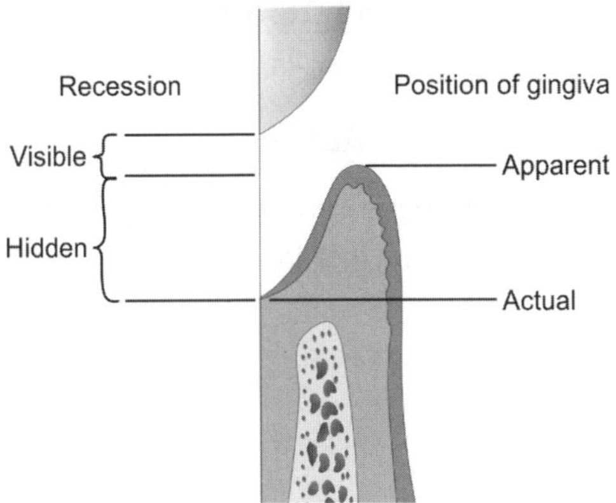

Fig. 19.1: Diagram showing apparent and actual position of the Gingiva along with visible and hidden recession.

- It can cause hyperaemia of pulp and associated symptoms may result from excessive exposure of the root surface
- Oral hygiene can be a problem in cases of interproximal recession, resulting in plaque accumulation.

F. Changes in Gingival Contour

- Change in the contour of gingiva is mainly seen in cases of gingival enlargement
- Normal contour of the gingiva is scalloped
- In cases of disease, the contour of gingiva becomes scalloped
- Inflammatory changes is in the marginal gingiva can lead to formation of and clefts
- Some suggest they occur because of traumatic occlusion and the treatment would be occlusal adjustments clefts and narrow, triangular shaped gingival recession
- As the recession progression apically, the cleft becomes broader, causing exposure of the root cementum
- McCall festoons are rolled, thickened band of gingiva which is generally seen along the canines, when the recession approaches the muco gingival junction.

SHORT ESSAYS

Question 1

What is the effect of tooth brushing on the consistency of the gingiva?

Answer

There are various effects of tooth brushing on the consistency of gingiva such as:

- It promotes keratinisation of oral epithelium.
- Capillary gingival circulation is enhanced.
- Thickening of alveolar bone.
- It has been seen in various studies that tooth brushing increases the proliferative capacity of the functional epithelium.
- Therefore, it means that the tooth brushing can increase the turnover rate and desquamation of junctional epithelial surfaces.
- This process holds an important clinical significance as it prevents direct access to the underlying tissue by periodontal pathogens and may repair small breaks in the junctional epithelium.

Question 2

What is the significance of calcified masses in gingiva?

Answer

Calcified masses in gingiva can be found as alone or in groups.

❑ They may vary in size, location, shape and structure.

❑ These calcified masses are removed from the tooth and displaced into the gingiva during scaling root remnants, cementum fragments or cementicles.

❑ These masses leads to chronic inflammation and fibrosis and sometimes foreign body giant cell activity.

❑ Sometime they can be enclosed within an osteoid like matrix.

CHAPTER 20

Gingival Enlargement

Question 1

What is gingival enlargement and its classification and grades? Discuss in detail about drug-induced gingival enlargement?

Answer

Gingival enlargement is the increase in the size of gingiva.

It is also referred to as gingival over growth.

Classification of gingival enlargements are as follows: (According to Carranza)

I. Inflammatory enlargement
  A. Chronic
  B. Acute
II. Drug induced enlargement
III. Enlargements associated with systemic disease or conditions
  A. Conditioned enlargements
    › Pregnancy
    › Puberty
    › Vitamin C deficiency
    › Plasma cell gingivitis
    › Non-specific conditioned enlargements (pyogenic granuloma)
  B. Systemic diseases causing gingival enlargements
    › Leukaemia
    › Granulomatous diseases (e.g. Wegener's granulomatosis, sarcoidosis)
IV. Neoplastic enlargement (gingival tumors)
  A. Benign tumors
  B. Malignant tumors
V. False enlargements.

- Depending upon the location and distribution, gingival enlargement can be given the following designations:
  - Localized: Limited to gingiva adjacent to a single tooth or group of teeth.
  - Generalised: Involving the gingiva throughout the mouth.
  - Marginal: Confined to the marginal gingiva.
  - Papillary: Confined to the interdental papilla.
  - Diffuse: It involves the marginal, attached gingiva and papilla.
  - Discrete: It an isolated sessile or pedunculated tumor like enlargement.

Degree of gingival enlargement are as follows:

- **Grade 0:** No signs of gingival enlargement
- **Grade I:** Enlargement confined to interdental papilla.
- **Grade II:** Enlargement involving papilla and marginal gingiva.
- **Grade III:** Enlargement covering three quarters or more of the crown.

Drug-induced Gingival Enlargement

- Few drugs are responsible for causing clinical enlargements.
- These include anti-consultants, immuno suppressants and calcium-channel blockers.
- Enlargement can creates problem in speech, mastication, tooth eruption and problems with esthetics.
- Clinical and microscopic features of different drugs are almost similar.

Clinical Features

- Enlargement starts as a painless, beadlike enlargement of the interdental papilla and extends to the facial and lingual gingival margins.
- As the enlargement progresses the growth from the marginal and papillary gingiva unites and converts into a massive tissue fold covering a considerable portion of crowns, which may interfere with occlusion.

- The enlargement appears as pale pink, firm, resilient and resembles the shape of a mulberry with a small lobulated surface with no bleeding.
- The enlargement appears beneath the gingival margin, from which it is separated by a linear groove.
- Because of the enlargement, the plaque control becomes difficult.
- Because of poor plaque control, a secondary inflammatory process starts, which complicates the gingival enlargement caused due to drug.
- Because of the above reasons, the enlargement becomes a combination of overgrowth due to drugs and inflammation caused by bacteria.
- Secondary inflammatory changes produce a red or a bluish-red discoloration, increases the bleeding tendency and obliterates the lobulated surface demarcations.
- Enlargement can be generalized in the mouth, but is more commonly seen in the maxillary and mandibular anterior regions.
- Enlargement is not seen in edentulous areas. It is always seen in areas, where teeth are present.
- Enlargement gets disappeared from the area where the teeth are extracted.
- In very few cases, hyperplasia of edentulous sites have been reported.
- Drug induced gingival enlargements, may be absent in mouths with excessive plaque and calculus and it may be present in mouth with little or no plaque.
- Maintaining the oral hygiene using toothpaste, toothbrush, floss or mouthwash can reduce the inflammation, but not the overgrowth.
- It can recur, even after it is surgically excised.
- Enlargement is chronic and increases slowly in size.
- If the causative drug is discontinued, there is a spontaneous disappearance within a few months.
- Enlargement begins as a hyperplasia of the connective tissue core of the marginal gingiva.
- It increases by its expansion and proliferation beyond the crest of the gingival margin.
- There is presence of an inflammatory infiltrate at the bottom of sulcus or the pocket.

Histopathology

- There is a pronounced hyperplasia of the connective tissue and the epithelium within the enlargement.
- Rete pegs become elongated and go deep inside the connective tissue.
- There are densely arranged collagen bundles within the connective tissue, with an increase in the number of fibroblasts and new blood vessels.

- Epithelium shows acanthosis.
- There is presence of enough amount of ground substance.
- Enlargement starts as a hyperplasia of the connective tissue core of the marginal gingiva and is increased due to proliferation and expansion beyond the crest of the gingival margin.
- Enlargements which reoccur, appears as granulation tissue, composed of several new capillaries and fibroblasts and irregularly arranged collagen fibrils with few lymphocytes.
- Sometimes, the connective tissue is more vascularized along with chronic inflammatory cells at the foci, specially plasma cells in case of cyclosporine enlargements.
- In a phenytoin enlargement, there is an equal ratio of fibroblast to collagen, which is seen in a normal gingiva of normal individuals. This shows that at some point, the development of the lesion must have abnormal high fibroblastic proliferation.
- There are numerous oxytalan fibres seen beneath the epithelium and in the areas of inflammation.
- Along the sulcular surfaces of the gingiva, inflammation is common.

1. Anti-convulsants

- Anti-convulsants are the drugs used to treat epilepsy.
- Phenytoin (Dilantin) is the first drug inducing gingival enlargement.
- Phenytoin is a hydantoin introduced by Merritt and Putman is the year 1938.

Clinical Features

- Fifty percent of the patients receiving the drug, suffer from gingival enlargement.
- It is more commonly seen in young patients.
- After a threshold level has been exceeded, the occurrence and severity of the enlargement are then not related to the dosage.

Pathogenesis

- Proliferation of fibroblast like cells and epithelium are proliferated by phenytoin.
- There are two analogues of phenytoin the have similar effect on fibroblast like cells and two analogues are:
  1. 1-allyl-5-phenylhydantoinate.
  2. 5-methyl-5-phenylhydantoinate.
- There is an increased synthesis of glycosaminoglycan by fibroblast from a phenytoin induced gingival overgrowth.

❑ There is also a reduction in collagen degradation because of phenytoin. It is due to production of an inactive fibroblastic collagenase.

❑ Gingival enlargement may result from the genetically determined ability or inability of the host to deal effectively with prolonged administration of this drug.

❑ It has been seen that fibroblasts in a non inflamed gingiva, are less active and do not respond to phenytoin.

❑ But fibroblasts in an inflamed tissue are active and respond to phenytoin.

❑ Therefore it can be concluded, that the pathogenesis of phenytoin-induced gingival enlargement is not very specific and clear but three factors, i.e.,
1. Specific genetically predetermined subpopulations of fibroblast.
2. Inactivation of collagenase and
3. Plaque induced gingival inflammation are thought to be important in causing and accelerating the phenytoin-induced gingival enlargement.

2. Immunosuppressants

❑ Immunosuppressants are the drugs which are given to several autoimmune diseases and to prevent organ transplant rejections.

❑ Most commonly used drugs are immunosuppressants.

❑ These drugs inhibit the function of helps T cells, which play an important role in cellular and humoral immune responses.

❑ Dosage of greater than 500 mg/day have been reported to induced gingival overgrowth.

❑ Vascularisation is more in cyclosporine induced gingival enlargement as compared to phenytoin enlargement.

❑ Microscopic examination reveals that the enlargement is a hypersensitivity response to cyclosporine as there is presence of abundant amorphous extracellular substance.

❑ It is more commonly seen in children.

❑ Patients who are medicated both with cyclosporine and calcium-channel blockers, are more like to have greater gingival enlargement.

❑ Cyclosporine has other side effects also, other than gingival enlargement, they are nephrotoxicity, hypertension and hypertrichosis.

❑ Tacrolimus, is another immunosuppressive drug that can be used as an substitute for cyclosporine and has very less side effects as compared to cyclosporine.

3. Calcium-Channel Blockers

❑ These drugs are given to treat cardiovascular problems such as angina pectoris, hypertension, coronary artery spasms, and cardiac arrhythmias.

❑ They act by blocking the intracellular mobilization of calcium, by inhibiting the calcium ion influx across the cell membrane of heart and smooth muscle.

❑ Because of this the coronary arteries and arterioles are dilated, due to which the oxygen supply to the heart muscle gets improved.

❑ It also dilates the peripheral vasculature due to which the hypertension is reduced.

❑ Examples of some of these drugs are amlodipine, feladipine, nifedipine, verapamil, cardizem.

❑ Nifedipine is the most common drug which induces gingival enlargement.

❑ Isradipidine is a dihydropyridine derivative which can act as a substitute for nifedipine and would not cause gingival enlargement.

❑ Nifedipine along with cyclosporine is given in kidney transplant recipients.

❑ This combination of drugs causes more gingival enlargement.

Question 2

What are conditioned gingival enlargements?

Answer

Conditioned gingival enlargements are the enlargements that occurs when there is exaggerated systemic condition of the patient or when it distorts the usual gingival response to dental plaque.

❑ Initiation of this type of enlargement requires dental plaque, but dental plaque is not the sole determinant of the nature of the clinical features.

❑ There can be three kinds of conditioned gingival enlargements:
1. Hormonal that include pregnancy and puberty.
2. Nutritional that include vitamin C deficiency.
3. Allergic.

Non-specific conditioned enlargement can also be seen.

1. Enlargements in Pregnancy

❑ These enlargements can be marginal or generalised or can occur as single or multiple tumor like masses.

❑ There is an increase in the level of progesterone and estrogen at the time of pregnancy, which reaches up to 10 and 30 times the levels during menstrual cycle during the end of third trimester respectively.

❑ There is a change in the vascular permeability due to the change in the hormonal levels, because of which there is gingival edema and an increased inflammatory response to the dental plaque.

- There is also a shift in the subgingival microbiota. There is an increase in prevotella intermedia.

Marginal enlargement: This enlargement does not occur without the presence of dental plaque.

- This enlargement results from aggravation of the previous inflammation.
- It is more prominent on the interproximal surfaces, than on the facial or lingual surface.
- The enlargement is generally generalised.
- It appears as bright red in color, friable, soft and has a shiny, smooth surface.
- Bleeding or slight provocation is seen.

Tumour-Like Gingival Enlargement

- It is usually seen after the 3rd month of pregnancy, though earlier incidences have also been reported.
- This is an inflammatory response to the plaque and is modified by the patients condition.
- Enlargement is mushroom like, discrete, flattened spherical mass that protrudes from the gingival margin.
- It can be attached to sessile or a pedunculated base.
- It is magenta or dusky red in colour.
- It has a tendency to expand laterally, its flattened appearance is perpetuated by pressure from the tongue and cheeks.
- It has a smooth, shiny surface and often exhibits numerous deep red, pinpoint markings.
- It does not invade the bone, as it is a superficial lesion.
- The consistency is semi-firm and may have various degrees of softness and friability.
- It is painless.
- If its size and shape foster accumulation of debris under its margins or interferes which occlusion, in which, painful ulceration may occur.
- If proper plaque control is performed, many gingival diseases during pregnancy can be avoided.

Histopathology

- Angiogranuloma is the term given to gingival enlargement during pregnancy.
- There is presence of central mass of connective tissue, with numerous diffusely arranged, newly formed, and engorged capillaries which are lined by cuboidal endothelial cells.
- There is a moderately fibrous stroma, with varying degrees of oedema, and chronic inflammatory infiltrates.
- There is thickening of stratified squamous epithelium.
- Rete pegs become prominent.
- There is some amount of intra-cellular and extra-cellular oedema, prominent intercellular bridges, and leucocyte infiltration.

2. Enlargement in Puberty

- It is seen both in male and female adolescents at the time of puberty.
- It is generally seen in plaque retentive areas.
- It is seen on the marginal and interdental gingiva mainly, which peculiar bulbous interdental papilla.
- The size of the enlargement far exceeds the enlargement caused by local factors.
- Because of the mechanical action of the tongue and the excursion of food, the enlargement is less on lingual side as compared to labial or buccal, since this action prevents a heavy accumulation of local irritants on the lingual surface.
- The clinical features of puberty enlargement are almost similar to that of chronic inflammatory gingival disease.
- There is a spontaneous reduction in the enlargement after puberty, but does not disappear completely until the local causative factors are removed.
- Microscopically, there is presence of chronic inflammation with prominent oedema and associated degenerative changes.

3. Enlargement Due to Vitamin C Deficiency

- Gingival enlargement due to vitamin C deficiency in referred to as scurvy.
- Vitamin C deficiency itself does not cause inflammation, it also requires bacterial plaque.
- Acute vitamin C deficiency causes haemorrhage, collagen destruction and oedema of the connective tissue, all of which modify the response of gingiva to dental plaque to an extent that the normal defensive reaction of gingiva is limited.
- Because of this inflammation also exaggerates.
- Massive gingival enlargement is produced as a combined effect of acute vitamin C deficiency and the inflammation.

Clinical Features

- Marginal gingiva is most commonly involved
- Gingiva is bluish red in color.
- It is soft, friable and has a shiny, smooth surface.
- There is haemorrhage on spontaneous or on slight provocation.
- Surface necrosis is seen, with pseudomembrane formation.

Histopathology

- Gingiva consists of chronic inflammatory cellular infiltration with a superficial acute response.
- Scattered areas of haemorrhage is seen, with engorged capillaries.
- There is collagen degeneration, marked diffuse oedema of scarcity of collagen fibrils or fibroblasts.

4. Plasma Cell Gingivitis

- It can also be referred as Atypical Gingivitis or Plasma Cell Gingivostomatitis.
- Enlargements starts from the marginal gingiva and extends up to the attached gingiva.
- Plasma cell Granuloma– It is a small lesion which is localised can also be present.

Clinical Features

- Gingiva is red, friable, and sometimes granular and can bleed easily.
- There is generally no loss of attachment.
- This is located in the oral aspect of the attached gingiva and thus differs from plaque induced gingivitis.
- Cheilitis and glossitis can be seen.
- Aetiology of plasma cell gingivitis is usually allergic specially to substances like churning gum, dentifrices and various other diet components.

Histopathology

- There is spongiosis and infiltration with inflammatory cells in the oral epithelium.
- Spinous layers and basal layers are damaged.
- There is a dense infiltrate of plasma cells in the connective tissue which can extend into the epithelium.
- It there is cessation of the allergen, the condition would be normal.
- In a very few cases, rapidly progressive periodontitis can be seen due to presence of marked inflammatory gingival enlargements with a predominance of plasma cells.

5. Non-specific Conditioned Enlargement (Pyogenic Granuloma)

- It is a tumour-like enlargement.
- It is an exaggerated conditioned response to minor trauma.

Clinical Features

- The lesion varies from a discrete spherical, tumor like mass with a pedunculated attachment to a flattened, keloid like enlargement having a broad base.
- It colour ranges from red to purple, can be either friable or firm.
- In most of the cases, if presents with surface ulceration and purulent exudation.
- The lesion can convert into a fibro-epithelial papilloma or may remain unchanged.
- Removal of the lesion and elimination of local irritating factors is the treatment option for pyogenic granuloma.
- Fifteen percent is the recurrence rate.
- Clinical and microscopic features of pyogenic granuloma is similar to that of enlargement seen during pregnancy.

Histopathology

- It appears as a mass of granulation tissue, with chronic inflammatory cellular infiltration.
- Prominent features of pyogenic granuloma are endothelial proliferation and the formation of numerous vascular spaces.
- Atrophic surface epithelium can be seen in some areas and hyperplastic in others.
- Surface ulceration and exudation are common features.

SHORT ESSAYS

Question 1

What is gingival abscess?

Answer

It is a localised, painful and rapidly expanding lesion that is generally of sudden onset.

- It is usually limited to marginal gingiva and the interdental papilla.
- Appears as a red swelling with a smooth, shiny surface.
- The lesion becomes fluctuant and pointed with a surface orifice from which a purulent exudate is expressed, within 24-48 hours.
- If the lesion continues to expand, it can rupture spontaneously.
- The adjacent teeth are generally sensitive to percussion.

Aetiology

- It is caused because of bacteria carried deep into tissues when any foreign substance such as toothbrush bristle, piece of apple, or a lobster shell, fragment, etc are forcefully embedded into the gingiva.
- The lesion is confined to gingiva and does not extend to the periodontal ligament.

Histopathology

- Gingival absence consists of purulent focus in connective tissue.
- It is surrounded by a diffuse infiltration of PMNs oedematous tissue and vascular engorgement.

- There is varying degrees of intracellular and extracellular oedema and invasion by leucocytes over the surface epithelium.
- Surface epithelium sometimes shows ulceration.

Question 2

What are false enlargements?

Answer

- These enlargements are not the true enlargements of the gingival tissue.
- They appear because of increase in the size of underlying bony of dental tissue.
- There are no abnormal clinical features seen over the gingiva, except the massive increase in size of the area.

Underlying Osseous Lesions

- Tori and exostosis are the most common bony enlargements, subjacent to the gingival area.
- It can also be seen in Paget's disease, fibrous dysplasia, central giant cell granuloma, cherubism, ameloblastoma, osteoma and osteosarcoma.
- The gingival tissues appear normal.
- They might have unrelated inflammatory changes.

Underlying Dental Tissue

- At the time of eruption, especially the primary dentition, the labial gingiva may show a bulbous marginal distortion caused by superimposition of the bulk of the gingiva on the normal prominence of the enamel in the gingival half of the crown.
- This kind of enlargement has been termed as development enlargement.
- If often persists until the junctional epithelium has migrated from the enamel to the cemento-enamel junction.

- The enlargement are physiologic and does not causes any problem.
- When such enlargements have inflammation then it looks like an extensive gingival enlargement.
- Treatment of inflammation is the treatment of choice in such cases.

Question 3

What is a gingival cyst?

Answer

- It is benign tumour of gingiva.
- When they reach a clinically significant size, they appear as localised enlargements, which involve the marginal and the attached gingiva.
- They are most commonly seen in the lingual areas of mandibular canine and premolar area.
- They are generally painless, but if they expand, they might cause erosion of the surface of alveolar bone.
- Gingival cyst can be differentiated from a lateral periodontal cyst as it arises within the alveolar bone, adjacent to the root and is developmental in origin.
- Gingival cyst develops from odontogenic epithelium or from surface or sulcular epithelium traumatically implanted in the area.
- Its treatment include its removal which is followed by uneventful recovery.

Histopathology

- Gingival cyst cavity is lined by a thin flattened epithelium with or without localised areas of thickening.
- Epithelium like unkeratinised stratified squamous epithelium, keratinised stratified squamous epithelium and parakeratinized epithelium with palisading basal cells can be found.

CHAPTER 21

Acute Gingival Infections

LONG ESSAYS

Question 1

Discuss in detail about the aetiology, clinical features, differential diagnosis and treatment options for acute necrotising ulcerative gingivitis.

Answer

It is also referred to as Vincent's infection.

- Acute necrotising ulcerative gingivitis (ANUG) is rapid in onset, painful microbial disease of the gingiva.
- Its main causative microorganism is fusobacterium species, along with spirochaetes.
- ANUG has been renamed as necrotising ulcerative gingivitis (NUG)
- It is also referred to as trench mouth, because of its prevalence in the soldiers working in trenches during World War I.
- The disease is known as Vincents angina because this disease was first described by Vincent.

Aetiology

- It is mainly caused by fusobacterium and spirochaetes, therefore it is a fusospirochaetal infection.
- The complex of microorganisms consists of following bacteria– Treponema microdentium, intermediate spirochaetes, vibrios, fusiform bacilli and filamentous organism- Borrelia species.

Predisposing Factors

It can be divided into three factors:

1. Local factors.
2. Systemic factors.
3. Psychosomatic factor.

Local Factors

- Smoking and use of tobacco

- Pre-existing gingivitis, deep periodontal pockets, and pericoronal flaps which favour the proliferation of anaerobic fusiform bacilli and spirochaetes.

Systemic Factors

- Immunodeficient patients
- Nutritional deficiencies like vitamin C and B2 deficiencies
- Chronic sleep deficiency leading to fatigue
- Habits like alcohol or drug above
- Systemic diseases like diabetes
- Other debilitating diseases like syphilis, cancer, severe gastrointestinal tract disorders, anaemia, leukaemia and acquired immune deficiency syndrome.

Psychosomatic Factor

This disease is related to stressful situations like patients with depression or any emotional disturbances, patients feeling inadequate at handling life situations.

Clinical Features

- It presents as an acute disease and symptoms are sudden in onset.
- In some cases, it can resolve on its own, and shows milder symptoms which lead to subacute stage.
- Some common predisposing factor could be debilitating disease or acute respiratory tract infection, psychological stress, nutritional deficiencies use of tobacco, smoking and continuous work without rest.

Characteristics Clinical Signs are as follows

- This infection shows punched out, crater like depressions at the crest of the interdental papillae and it might involve the marginal gingiva. Attached gingiva and oral mucosa are rarely involved
- A slough which is grey in colour and pseudomembranous in nature, cover the gingival craters.

- It can be demarcated from the healthy gingiva by a pronounced linear erythema.
- In some cases lesions may be denuded of the pseudomembrane, exposing red, shiny and haemorrhagic gingival surface.
- Lesion bleeds even on slightest provocation.
- Fetid odour.
- Increased salivation.
- Pasty saliva.
- Metallic foul taset.
- Generally patient complains off a constant radiating, gnawing pain that is aggravated upon taking hot and spicy food and upon chewing.
- Extraoral and systemic sign and symptoms are local lymphadenopathy and mild fever.
- In very severe cases following signs can be seen: High fever, increased pulse rates, leukocytosis, loss of appetite, and general lassitude.
- These signs and symptoms are more severe in children.

Clinical Courses

If NUG is untreatued, it may progress to necrotising ulcerative periodontitis.

The staging of NUG given by Horning and Cohen is as follows:

- **Stage 1:** Necrosis of the tip of the interdental papilla (NUG).
- **Stage 2:** Necrosis of the inertia papilla (either NUG or NUP).
- **Stage 3:** Necrosis of the marginal gingiva (NUP).
- **Stage 4:** Necrosis extending to the marginal gingiva (NUP).
- **Stage 5:** Necrosis involving the buccal and labial mucosa (necrotising stomatitis).
- **Stage 6:** Necrosis exposing alveolar bone (necrotising stomatitis).
- **Stage 7:** Necrosis perforating skin of check (NOMA).

Various Zones of the Lesion

Various zones in the lesion, described by Listgarten, may overlap one another, and all zones may not be present at the same time.

Zone 1 (Bacterial Zone)

- This is the most superficial zone.
- It consists of various bacterias and few spirochaetes which can be of small, medium and large types.

Zone 2 (Neutrophil Rich Zone)

- This zone contains numerous leukocytes, mainly leukocyte with bacteria, including spirochaetes of various types interspersed in between the leukocytes.

Zone 3 (Necrotic Zone)

- It consists of disintegrated tissue cells, fibrillar material, remnants of collagen fibres, and many intermediate and large types of spirochaetes with few other bacteria.

Zone 4 (Zone of Spirochaetes Infiltration)

- This zone contains well preserved tissues infiltrated with intermediate and large spirochaetes without other organisms.

Diagnosis

- Diagnosis can be made by clinical picture of the patient which include gingival pain, bleeding and ulceration.
- Biopsy specimen, or a microscopic examination of a bacterial smear, would not give a clear diagnosis.
- Necrotising ulcerative gingivitis can be differentiated from other infections such as tuberculosis through a biopsy specimen.

Treatment for Necrotising Ulcerative Gingivitis

Treatment objectives of NUG are as follows:

- Resolution of acute phase.
- Treatment of chronic disease either underlying the acute involvement or elsewhere in the oral cavity.
- Alleviation of generalized symptoms such as fever and malaria.
- Correction of systemic aetiological factors such as smoking and stress.
- Necrotising ulcerative gingivitis can be treated in thee clinical visits:

First Visit

- Primary goal of this visit is the treatment of acute lesion.
- Complete medical history and history of present illness should be recorded.
- Dietary history and smoking history should be taken.
- Human immunodeficiency virus risk factor and psychological factors should be evaluated.
- Vitals signs should be recorded, along with palpation of lymph nodes, mainly submaxillary and segmental lymph nodes.
- Any skin lesion present, should be evaluated.
- After all these basic evaluations and recordings, the pseudomembrane and surface debris should be gently removed with a moist cotton and a topical anaesthetic should be applied over the affected area.
- Supra-gingival scaling, using an ultrasonic instrument should be done.
- Sub-gingival scaling and curettage are contraindicated at this stage, since it can lead to extension of the infection and bacteremia.

❑ Any kind of periodontal surgery or extractions are postponed, until the patient becomes symptom free. And it usually takes about 4 weeks for a patient to become symptom free.
❑ Patient should be prescribed the following antibiotics:
  ○ Amoxicillin 500 mg orally every 6 hours for 10 days.
  ○ If patient is allergic to penicillin, then in that case, erythromycin 500 mg every 6 hours, or metronidazole 500 mg twice daily for 7 days.

Analgesics such as non-steroidal anti-inflammatory drugs (NSAIDs) can be prescribed to the patient, so as to get relief from pain.

Instructions to be given to the patient on first visit are as follows:

❑ Patient should avoid habits such as tobacco, smoking, alcohol and condiments.
❑ Patients are advised to rinse with 3% hydrogen peroxide mixed with equal amount of warm water every 2 hours, or twice daily with 0.2% chlorhexidine mouth wash.
❑ Overzealous tooth brushing and interdental cleaning device should be avoided.
❑ For tooth brushing, an ultra-soft toothbrush should be used.
❑ Adequate rest should be taken by the patient.

Second Visit

❑ One to two days after the first visit, the second visit should be scheduled.
❑ All the systemic signs and symptoms should be checked if they have resolved or not.
❑ The lesion would be still erythematous but with marked reduction of necrotic tissue.
❑ Scaling can be performed during their visit.
❑ All the instructions given during the first visit, should be followed by the patient.

Third Visit

❑ The patient is recalled after a prised of 5 days, after the second visit, to check for resolution of the symptoms.
❑ Complete protocol for the periodontal management is planned, during this visit.
❑ Patient advised to discontinue the hydrogen peroxide rinse and continue with chlorhexidine mouth wash for 2 or 3 weeks.
❑ Scaling and root planning can be repeated if required.
❑ Patient should be reinforced to follow proper plaque control measurements.
❑ The patients is counselled on nutrition, smoking cessation and other associated habits, to prevent further possible recurrence.

❑ All the local irritants like faulty restorations etc should be removed.
❑ Chronic gingivitis, periodontal pockets should be treated well.
❑ After a period of 1 month, the patient is re-evaluated for oral hygiene maintenance, habits, psychosocial factors and determination of the need for reconstructive or aesthetic surgery.
❑ Other than this treatment, some additional treatment should also be given to the patient such as:
  ○ Contouring of gingival margin (gingivoplasty).
  ○ Nutritional supplements.

Contouring of gingival margin (gingivoplasty)

The normal gingival architecture is spoiled in cases of NUG because there is severe loss of interdental gingiva and bone.

This can be restored by a procedure known as gingivoplasty or gingivectomy in which the normal gingival architecture is obtained.

Nutritional supplements

❑ Patient is unable to take food because of pain, therefore nutritional supplements should be indicated with the local treatment.
❑ A standard multivitamin preparation should be given to the patient, along with therapeutic dose of vitamins B and C.

Question 2

Describe in detail about the aetiology, clinical features, histopathology and differential diagnosis of acute herpetic gingivostomatitis.

Answer

❑ Acute herpetic gingivostomatitis mostly affects infants and children younger than 6 years of age
❑ The causative organisms is herpes simplex virus type-1 (HSV-1)

Clinical Features

❑ This infection is mostly seen in children and young adult.
❑ Males and females are equally affected.
❑ There are vesicular lesions which are painful and develop on all mucosal surfaces and rupture to produce foul smelling ulcers.
❑ Patient is usually febrile, drools and has significant malaise and will have tender cervical lymphadenopathy.
❑ Acute illness and lesions lasts about 10 days and resolve with scar formation.
❑ Herpes simplex virus type-1 has access to the patient through direct or airborne water droplet transmission from an infected individual.

- The mucous membrane lesions represent direct viral infection at the site of inoculation.
- After primary infection, the virus ascends through sensory and autonomic nerves and persists as latent HSV in the neuronal ganglia that innervates the sites.
- Herpes simplex virus type-1 mostly resides in the trigeminal ganglion.
- Various stimuli such as sunlight, trauma, fever and stress can result in secondary manifestation.

Oral Signs

- Gingiva and oral mucosa, both are involved.
- In the initial stage, the characteristic feature is the presence of discrete, spherical grey vesicles on the gingiva, labial and buccal mucosa, soft palate, pharynx, lingual mucosa and the tongue.
- The vesicles rupture after 24 hours and form painful, small ulcers with a red, elevated, halo like margin and a depressed, yellowish or greyish white central portion.
- The ulcers may occur in dust as or can be widely separated.
- In a few cases, the lesion may be diffuse, erythematous, shiny discoloration and oedematous enlargement of the gingiva with a tendency to bleed.
- The lesion wound resolve by 7–10 days, or its own.
- It heals without scarring.

Symptoms

- Soreness of the mouth associated with difficulty in drinking and chewing food.
- Lesions are painful and sensitive to touch.

Constitutional signs and symptoms are as follows:

- High grade fever.
- Generalized malaise.
- Cervical adenitis.

Diagnosis

- Diagnosis is made mainly by taking a detailed history and performing a proper clinical examination
- Virus culture and immunologic tests should be performed using monoclonal antibodies or deoxyribonucleic acid hybridization techniques to confirm the diagnosis.

Differential Diagnosis

- Necrotising ulcerative gingivitis
- Recurrent aphthous stomatitis
- Erythema multiforme
- Stevens Johnson syndrome
- Bullous lichen planus.

Treatment

- Earlier the treatment only consisted of supportive care but recently an antiviral therapy with 15 mg/ kg of an acyclovir suspension is given 5 times daily for 7 days. But this therapy is effective only if the patient reports or is being diagnosed within 3 days of onset.
- Patients reporting after 3 days of onset should be given a palliative care which includes removal of plaque and food debris, administrations of NSAIDs and nutritional supplements.
- Periodontal therapy should be postponed until the acute symptoms subsides.

SHORT ESSAYS

Question 1

What is pericoronitis? What are its types and clinical features? Explain in detail about the management of pericoronitis.

Answer

- Pericoronitis is an acute infection in which there is inflammation of gingiva and surrounding soft tissues of an incompletely erupted tooth.
- It is most common in lower third molars.

Types of Pericoronitis

- Acute.
- Subacute.
- Chronic.

Clinical Features

- The pericoronal flap or the operculum is markedly swollen and red along with presence of exudate.
- Patient complains of pain radiating to the ear, throat and floor of the mouth.
- Because of inability to open the jaws, the patient is extremely uncomfortable.
- Patient would complain of foul taste.
- Swelling of the cheek may also be seen in the region of the angle of the jaw.
- There may be presence of lymphadenitis.
- Fever, malaise and leukocytosis are also present.

Complications of pericoronitis are as follows:

❑ Pericoronal abscess.
❑ Peritonsillar abscess, cellulitis and ludwig's angina, are the potential sequelae of acute pericoronitis.

Treatment

Treatment of pericoronitis is dependent on three factors.

They are as follows:

1. Severity of inflammation
2. Systemic involvement
3. Possibility of retaining the tooth
❑ Treatment can take more than one visit:

First Visit

❑ Debris, irritants and exudate should be removed with gentle irrigation of area with warm saline.
❑ Occlusion has to be evaluated. One should check for the occlusion of the opposing tooth with the pericoronal flap.
❑ Occlusal adjustment should be done in case of opposing tooth traumatizing the flap.
❑ In cases with lymph node involvement, antibiotics are prescribed.
❑ A 15 no. blade can be used for drainage for a fluctuant swelling, if present.
❑ Patient should be prescribed hourly warm saline rinses.

Second Visit

❑ After the resolution of acute symptoms the pericoronal flap should be surgically excised using the periodontal knives.
❑ The surgical produce which is done for removal of operculum is referred to as operculectomy.
❑ It can be performed using scalpel, knives, cautery or lasers.
❑ An easily maintainable site should be created for the patient which can be achieved by removing the flap.

Question 2

What are differences between primary herpetic gingivo stomatitis and necrotising ulcerative gingivitis?

Answer

Table 21.1: Differences between primary herpetic gingivo stomatitis and necrotising ulcerative gingivitis.

	Primary herpetic gingivo stomatitis	Necrotising ulcerative gingivitis
Aetiology	Caused by virus herpes simplex virus type-1.	Fusospirochaetal complex.
Clinical features	Diffuse erythema and vesicular lesion which rupture leaving slightly depressed area of ulcer. Diffuse involvement of the gingiva.	A necrotising condition with punched out gingival margins covered by a pseudomembrane. Only marginal gingiva involved.
Age	Children and adolescents.	In children it is rare.
Course	Course of 7–10 days.	No definite duration.
Contagion	Contagious.	Non contagious.

Question 3

What is gingival abscess?

Answer

Gingival abscess is a localised, acute inflammatory lesion that can arise due to various number of sources such as microbial, trauma, foreign body impactions.

Aetiology

It can be caused due to impingement by any foreign body like dental floss, food particle or impression material in previously healthy sites.

Clinical Findings

❑ Gingival is red, swollen and painful.
❑ Impacted foreign object may still be embedded into the gingiva.

Treatment

❑ Scaling and root planing are completed to establish drainage and any foreign body present is removed. Scaling can be done with or without local anaesthetic.
❑ The area is irrigated with warm water and covered with moist gauze under light pressure.
❑ Once bleeding is arrested, the patient is dismissed with instructions to rinse with warm saline and gargle every 2 hours for the rest of the day.
❑ After 24 hours the area is re-evaluated.

Question 4

Enumerate various acute lesions of gingiva.

Answer

According to Manson, acute gingival lesions can be classified as follows:

❑ Traumatic lesions of gingiva
  ○ Physical injury
  ○ Chemical injury

- ❑ Viral infections
    - ○ Acute herpetic gingivostomatitis
    - ○ Herpangina
    - ○ Measles
    - ○ Herpes varicella/zoster virus infections
    - ○ Glandular fever
- ❑ Bacterial infections
    - ○ Acute necrotising ulcerative gingivitis
    - ○ Tuberculosis
    - ○ Syphilis
- ❑ Fungal disease
    - ○ Candidiasis
- ❑ Gingival abscess
- ❑ Aphthous ulcers
- ❑ Erythema multiform
- ❑ Drug allergy and contact hypersensitivity.

CHAPTER 22

Gingival Diseases in Childhood

Question 1

What are the changes seen in gingiva during tooth eruption?

Answer

During the transition phase of dentition, gingival changes are seen. It is important to differentiate between these physiological changes from gingival diseases.

Various changes seen during tooth eruption are:

- **Pre-eruption bulge:** A gingival bulge is seen at the site of crown eruption. The gingiva in this bulge is firm, slightly blanched and is in confirmation with the underlying shape of crown.
- **Formation of gingival margin:** As the crown erupts into the oral cavity penetrating through the oral mucosa, development of marginal gingiva and sulcus is seen.
  - During eruption, the marginal gingiva appears oedematous, rounded and erythematous.
- **Normal prominence of gingival margin:** During mixed dentition stage, the gingiva around the newly erupted teeth, specially in the anterior region appears quite prominent.

This prominence is due to the fact, that gingiva is still attached to crown due to which it gets superimposed on the bulk of underlying enamel.

Question 2

What are the types of gingival diseases seen in childhood?

Answer

Types of gingival diseases seen in childhood are:

- Chronic marginal diseases.
- Localised gingival recession.
- Acute gingival infections.

Chronic Marginal Diseases

It is the most common type of gingival change seen in childhood.

Changes in colour, size, texture and consistency resembling chronic inflammation are seen.

In some cases fiery red discolouration may also be noticed.

These changes in children are commonly caused due to gingivitis and should not be associated with bleeding and increase in pocket depth.

Aetiology

- Plaque.
- Materia alba.
- Poor oral hygiene.
- Calculus is mainly seen in age group of 7–15 years.
- Tooth eruption associated gingivitis due to accumulation of plaque around erupting tooth.

Partially exfoliated deciduous teeth are a common site of plaque accumulation and thus cause gingivitis.

Gingivitis occurs more commonly in children with increased over bite and over jet, nasal obstruction and mouth-breathing habits.

High prevalence and intensity of gingivitis is seen in patients who are in circumpubertal period and this type of gingivitis is termed as pubertal gingivitis. Bleeding from interdental sites is commonly seen and this condition autoresolves after puberty.

Localised Gingival Recession

- Gingival recession in childhood is generally seen in teeth, which are labially placed in the arch.
- It is also seen in teeth that are excessively tipped, rotated due to which there roots project labially, thus making them prone to gingival recession.

- Local irritants may also cause gingival recession.
- Gingival recession is also seen in teeth which are near highly attached fraenum.
- The gingival recession due to positioning of teeth may autocorrect with growth of the arches or may have to be treated orthodontically.

Acute Gingival Infections

- **Primary herpetic gingivostomatitis:** Most common acute gingival infection in childhood and generally occurs as a sequela to upper respiratory tract infection.
- **Candidiasis:** Fungal infection caused by *Candida albicans*.
- **Necrotising ulcerative gingivitis (NUG):** Incidence is generally low in children.

Seen more commonly in malnourished children and children with Down syndrome.

Primary herpetic gingivostomatitis can be sometimes erroneously diagnosed as NUG.

CHAPTER 23

Desquamative Gingivitis

Question 1

Define desquamative gingivitis. Discuss about its aetiology, clinical features, pathogenesis and management.

Answer

Desquamative gingivitis is a clinical term to describe red, painful, glazed and friable gingiva, which may be a manifestation of some mucocutaneous conditions such as lichen planus or the vesiculobullous disorders.

❑ It is characterised by intense redness and desquamation of the surface epithelium of the attached gingiva.
❑ Initially, it was referred to as "gingivosis" as it was considered to be degenerative condition.
❑ In 1960, McCarethy et al. said that desquamative gingivitis is not a specific entity, instead it is a non-specific gingival manifestations of many systemic disturbances.

Clinical Features

❑ It is an oral manifestation of dermatosis like lichen planus, mucous membrane pemphigoid, bullous pemphigoid or pemphigus.
❑ Based upon clinical manifestation, it can be mild, moderate or severe.
  ○ Mild form:
    ➢ It is usually seen in females between the age of 17 years and 24 years.
    ➢ Characterised by diffuse erythema of the marginal, interdental and attached gingiva.
    ➢ It is generally painless.
    ➢ Patient would generally complain of discolouration of gingiva.
  ○ Moderate form:
    ➢ Individuals between 30 years and 40 years are mainly affected.

➢ This form present as a patchy distribution of bright, red and grey areas involving the marginal and attached gingiva.
➢ Gingival surface exhibits pitting on pressure and appears soft, smooth and shiny.
➢ Epithelium not firmly attached to the underlying connective tissue. It pulls off on massaging with finger, which leads to exposure of the connective tissue.
➢ Patients complain of burning sensation in the mouth.
➢ Tooth brushing may lead to denudation of the gingival surface, which can cause pain. Because of this, patient is not able to brush properly, which leads to deposition on the teeth, which in turn causes the gingival inflammation.
  ○ Severe form:
    ➢ It is characterised by irregularly-shaped areas which are denuded from the gingiva.
    ➢ The area is bright-red in colour and scattered all over the gingival surface.
    ➢ This form is very painful and it is constantly dry and there is burning sensation.
    ➢ There is presence of Nikolskys sign in which the epithelium can be easily peeled off.
    ➢ Oral mucosa is smooth and shiny.
    ➢ Patients having severe form, cannot tolerate coarse food, condiments or changes in temperature.

Histopathology

❑ The lesions may be of lichenoid or bullous types.
❑ The lichenoid type resembles lichen planus, whereas bullous type has the features of mucous membrane pemphigoid.
❑ There is separation of collagen fibres because of which there is a separation of epithelium from underlying connective tissue.

- There is also a decrease in number of anchoring fibrils.
- Epithelium is atrophic, keratinisation is reduced.
- There is infiltration of the connective tissue with inflammatory cells.

Diagnosis

- Diagnosis is very important to form a line of treatment.
- Oral cavity should be inspected carefully for any lesions.
- In case of lichen planus, gingiva as well as other parts of the oral mucosa may be affected.
- Papular skin lesions are present on wrist and ankles.
- A detailed history should be taken.
- Conjunctivitis, burning sensation on urination, vaginal irritation, etc. are suggestive of mucous membrane pemphigoid.
- Hormonal aetiology has also been suggested specially in cases of menopause or hysterectomy.
- Biopsy helps in confirmation of diagnosis of lichen planus, mucosa membrane pemphigoid and rare bacterial conditions, such as candidiasis.

Management

- It is essential to reduce the gingival inflammation, which can be achieved by improvement in oral hygiene.
- Soft tooth brushes should be prescribed to patients, for routine plaque control. Care should be taken not to injure the gingival tissues.
- Hydrogen peroxide (3%) diluted with two part of warm water can be used as mouth wash, twice daily.
- Topical corticosteroid ointment can be used many times in a day. Before application, gingiva should be gently dried with sterile sponge.
- Triamcinolone acetonide (0.1%), fluocinonide (0.05%), or desonides (0.05%) may be used for topical application.
- Systemic corticosteroids can also be given. It should be given only after complete evaluation of the general health of the patient and the physicians consent.
- Mucous membrane pemphigoid responds favourably to systemic steroid therapy. Prednisone 30–40 mg daily or on alternate days to begin and gradually should be reduced to 5–10 mg daily or on alternate days as maintenance dose may be used.
- Nutritional supplements should also be given.
- The patient should have patience, since the lesion takes long time to heal. And also patient should not discontinue the treatment before the lesion heals and to patiently wait for the results.

Explain in detail about mucous membrane pemphigoid.

Mucous membrane pemphigoid is also referred to as cicatricial pemphigoid, which is a group of putative autoimmune, chronic inflammatory, subepithelial blistering disease predominantly affecting mucous membrane, with or without clinically observable scarring.

- It is most commonly seen in women in their 5th decade of life.
- Young children are rarely affected.
- It is characterised by an auto immune reaction involving auto-antibodies, directed against basement membrane zone, followed by complement activation and subsequent leucocyte recruitment.
- Proteolytic enzyme release and dissolve the basement membrane zone.
- Cicatricial pemphigoid involves the oral cavity, conjunctiva and mucosa of the nose, vagina, rectum, oesophagus and urethra.

Clinical Features of Oral Lesions

- Oral lesions are characterised by erosive or desquamative gingivitis.
- Vesicles and ulceration may be seen on the gingiva.
- Attached gingiva is erythematous.
- Bullae rupture in about 2–3 days forming irregular shaped ulcers.
- Healing of the ulcers is generally delayed and takes up to 3 weeks.

Histopathology

- Lesion shows sub-epithelial vesiculation.
- Epithelium is separated from the connective tissue.
- Basement membrane shows a split, under electron microscope.

Treatment

- It is generally treated with systemic corticosteroids.
- Oral hygiene should be maintained.
- Use of hydrogen peroxide mouthwash should be recommended.
- Soft brush should be used.

SHORT ESSAYS

Question 1

What is the classification of desquamative gingivitis lesions?

Answer

Classification of disease that clinically present at desquamative gingivitis is as follows:

Dermatological:

- ❑ Lichen planus.
- ❑ Mucous membrane pemphigoid.
- ❑ Bullous pemphigoid.
- ❑ Pemphigus vulgaris.
- ❑ Chronic ulcerative stomatitis.
- ❑ Linear IgA disease.
- ❑ Lupus erythematosus.

CHAPTER 24

Periodontal Pocket

Question 1

Define periodontal pocket. What are its classifications and clinical features? Discuss the pathogenesis in detail.

Answer

According to Carranza, periodontal pocket is defined as a pathologically deepened gingival sulcus. It is a very important feature of periodontal disease.

Classification

It can be classified as:

- Based on morphology and their relationship to adjacent structures:
  - ○ **Gingival pocket:** It is also referred as false or relative pocket. It is formed by gingival enlargement without destruction of the supporting tissues of the periodontium.
  - ○ **Periodontal pocket:** It is also referred to as true pocket. It is formed by pathologic deepening of the gingival sulcus due to apical proliferation of epithelial attachment. It can be further classified as:
    - ➢ Suprabony pocket: Also referred to as supracrestal/supra-alveolar pocket. It is present above the crest of alveolar bone, i.e. the bottom of the pocket is coronal to the underlying alveolar bone.
    - ➢ Infrabony pocket: Also referred to as intrabony/subcrestal pocket **(Fig. 24.1)**. It is present below the crest of alveolar bone, i.e. the bottom of the pocket is apical to the level of adjacent alveolar bone. The lateral pocket wall lies between .the tooth surface and the alveolar bone **(Fig. 24.2)**.
- Based on the number of surfaces involved:
  - ○ **Simple pocket:** In this pocket involves one tooth surface.
  - ○ **Compound pocket:** In this pocket, two tooth surfaces are involved.
  - ○ **Complex pocket:** It is spiral pocket which originates on one tooth surface and on some other tooth surface of the same tooth. These types of pockets are most commonly seen in furcation areas **(Fig. 24.3)**.

Clinical Features

Clinical features are as follows:

- Bluish-red, thickened marginal gingiva.

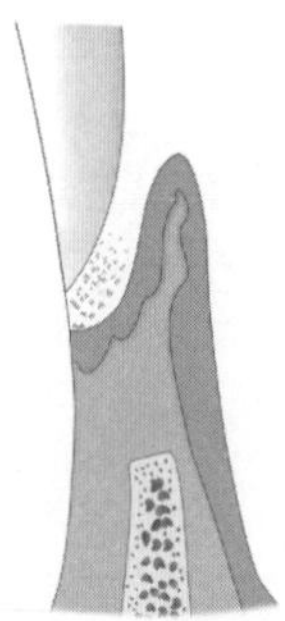

Fig. 24.1: Diagram showing Gingival pocket and Periodontal pocket.

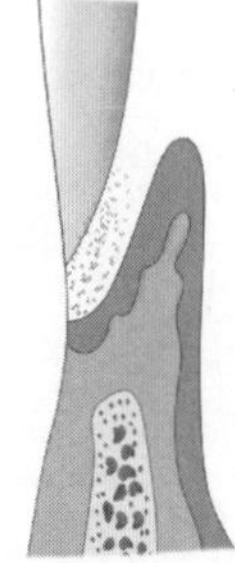
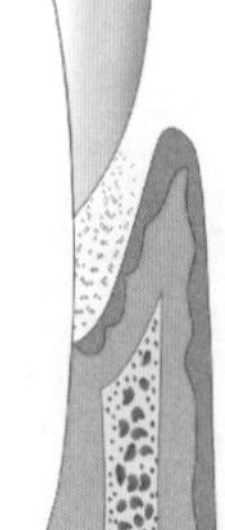

Fig. 24.2: Diagram showing Subrabony pocket and Intra bony pocket.

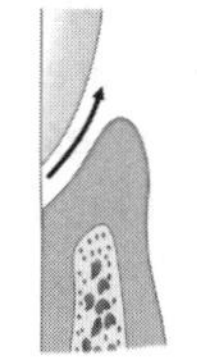 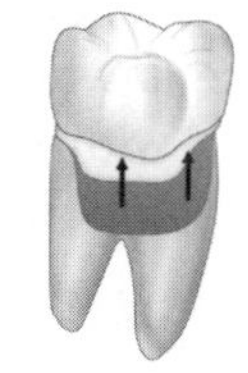 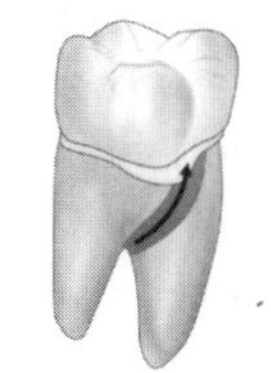

Simple pocket   Compound pocket   Complex pocket

Fig. 24.3:

- A bluish-red, vertical zone from the gingival margin to the alveolar mucosa.
- Gingival bleeding and suppuration.
- Tooth mobility.
- Diastema.
- Localised pain or deep pain in pockets.

Pathogenesis of periodontal pocket:

- periodontal pockets occur because of the micro-organism and their by-products that produce pathologic changes which lead to deepening of the gingival sulcus.
- Deepening of gingival sulcus may be because of either migration of the junctional epithelium apically and its separation from the tooth surface, or because of movement of the gingival margin in the direction of the crown resulting in a pocket or it could be due to both the reasons.
- Changes which are involved in the transition from the gingival sulcus to the pocket are due to increase in number of spirochetes and motile rods.
- This transition involves several zones of inflammatory changes, along with destruction of connective tissue attachments in the connective tissue wall of the sulcus.
- Apical to the junctional epithelium an area of destroyed collagen fibres develops and is occupied by inflammatory cells and oedema.

- Immediately apical to this, is a zone of partial destruction and then an area of normal attachment. There are two mechanisms involved for collagen destruction:
    1. Collagenases and other lysosomal enzymes from polymorphonuclear leukocytes (PMNLs) and macrophages become extracellular and destroy collagen.
    2. Fibroblasts phagocytize collagen fibres by extending cytoplasmic process to the ligament interface and by resorbing the inserted collagen fibrils and fibrils of the cementum matrix.
- Because of the loss of collagen, the apical portion of the junctional epithelium proliferates along the root. Extension of junctional epithelium along the root requires the presence of healthy epithelial cells.
- Marked degeneration or necrosis of the junctional epithelium retards rather than accelerates pocket formation because of lack of healthy epithelial cells.
- As the apical portion migrates, the coronal portion of the junctional epithelium detaches from the root. It occurs because of cohesiveness of the junctional epithelium as a result of rapidly proliferating bacteria, bacterial enzymes and the relative volume of PMNs.
- Therefore, the gingival sulcus shifts in an apical direction from the base and the sulcular epithelium is replaced by pocket epithelium.
- Because of this transformation from the gingival sulcus to a periodontal pocket, the plaque accumulation increases and becomes even more difficult to clean, increasing the severity of disease.
- Therefore, with continued inflammation, crest of the gingival margin extends coronally and junctional epithelium extends apically along the root, separating from it.

SHORT ESSAYS

Question 1

Describe the histopathology of pocket formation.

Answer

- The connective tissue is oedematous and densely infiltrated with plasma cells and lymphocytes and scattered PMNLs.
- Blood vessels are increased in number, they become dilated and engorged, single or multiple necrotic foci are occasionally present.

- Connective tissue also shows proliferation of the endothelial cells with newly formed capillaries, fibroblasts and collagen fibres.
- The junctional epithelium at the base of the pocket is usually much shorter than that of a normal sulcus.
- The corono-apical length of the junctional epithelium is 50–100 μm.
- The most severe degenerative changes in the periodontal pocket occur along the lateral wall.
- Epithelial buds or interlacing cords of epithelial cells project from the lateral wall into the adjacent inflamed

connective tissue and frequently extend further apically than the junctional epithelium.

❑ Progressive degeneration and necrosis of the epithelium leads to ulceration of the lateral wall, exposure of the underlying marked inflamed connective tissue and suppuration.

❑ The epithelium at the gingival crest of a periodontal pocket is generally intact and thickened with prominent rete pegs.

❑ Filaments, rods and coccoids organisms with predominant gram-negative cell walls have been found in the intercellular space initially under exfoliating epithelial cells, but they are also found between deeper epithelial cells and accumulating on the basement lamina.

❑ Few bacteria can traverse the basement lamina and involve the sub-epithelial connective tissue.

Question 2

What are the contents of a pocket?

Answer

Periodontal pockets consists of debris, mainly containing microorganisms and their products, for example, enzymes, endotoxins and other metabolic products, dental plaque, gingival fluid, food remnants, salivary mucin, desquamated epithelial cells and leukocytes.

In the exudate, living, degenerated and necrotic PMNLs, living and dead bacteria, serum and some amount of fibrin is seen.

Question 3

Describe the microtopography of the gingival wall of the pocket.

Answer

Soft tissue wall in the periodontal pockets in scanning electron microscopy (SEM), shows following areas:

❑ Areas of relative quiescence.
❑ Areas of bacterial accumulation.
❑ Areas of emergence of leukocytes.
❑ Areas of leukocytes-bacterial interaction.
❑ Areas of intense epithelial desquamation.
❑ Areas of ulceration with exposed connective tissue.
❑ Areas of haemorrhage with numerous erythrocytes.

Areas of Relative Quiescence

It is relatively flat surface with minor depression and wounds and occasional shedding of cells.

Areas of Bacterial Accumulation

On the epithelial surface, depressions are seen, along with enough debris and bacterial clumps which penetrate into the intercellular spaces which get enlarged. The main bacteria which are seen are: Cocci, rods and filaments along with few spirochetes. These bacteria are covered with a loose, intercellular, fibrillar substance.

Areas of Emergence of Leukocytes

Holes are located in the intercellular spaces, through which leukocytes appear.

Areas of Leukocytes-bacterial Interaction

Many leukocytes are present which are covered with bacteria, during the process of phagocytosis.

Areas of Intense Epithelial Desquamation

They appear as semi-attached and folded epithelial squames in which one end in generally attached to the pocket wall and the other is free towards the pocket space.

Areas of Ulceration with Exposed Connective Tissue

Haemorrhage is seen occasionally in this area. Bottom of ulcer shows exposed collagen fibres and various connective tissue cells.

Areas of Haemorrhage with Numerous Erythrocytes

Several erythrocytes are seen in this area.

Question 4

What are the differences between suprabony and infrabony pockets?

Answer

Supra-bony pockets	Infra-bony pockets
In this, the base of the pocket is coronal to the alveolar crest.	In this, the base of the pocket is apical to the alveolar crest.
There is a horizontal pattern of bone loss.	There is a vertical or angular pattern of bone loss.
Interproximally, the trans-septal fibres are restored horizontally in the space between the base of the pocket and alveolar bone.	Interproximally, the trans-septal fibres are restored, obliquely, from cementum beneath the base of pocket over the crest of the cementum of adjacent tooth.
On the facial and lingual surfaces, the peridontal ligament fibres beneath the pocket follow their normal course	On the facial and lingual surfaces, the periodontal fibres beneath the pocket follow the angular pattern of adjacent bone.

Question 5

What are the root surface wall changes during pocket formation?

Answer

- ❑ Significant changes are seen in root surface wall of a periodontal pocket.
- ❑ These changes can increase the periodontal infection, cause pain and may complicate the periodontal therapy.
- ❑ Many changes are seen in the root cementum which could be structural, chemical or cytotoxic.
- ❑ New tissues are formed in the continuous effort of repair, but they are degenerative due to cellular exudates released during the changes in the root surface wall.
- ❑ Features, such as colour, consistency and surface texture of the pocket wall are determined by the balance between the destructive and reparative changes.

Question 6

What are the clinical signs and symptoms of the pocket?

Answer

Clinical signs are:
- ❑ Enlarged, bluish red marginal, gingiva with a blunt edge.
- ❑ Shiny, discoloured and puffy gingiva associated with exposed root surface.
- ❑ Break in the continuity of the interdental gingiva.
- ❑ Gingival bleeding, purulent exudate from the gingiva.
- ❑ Extrusion, mobility and migration of teeth
- ❑ Development of diastema.

Symptoms are:
- ❑ Localised pain or a sensation of pressure in the gingiva after eating which diminishes gradually
- ❑ Foul taste
- ❑ Radiating pain deep inside the bone
- ❑ Growing feeling in the gums
- ❑ Sensitivity to hot and cold
- ❑ Pain in the absence of caries
- ❑ Urge to dig a pointed substance like a tooth pick into the gums
- ❑ Patient would generally complain that food sticks to the teeth upon eating.

Question 7

What are the correlation of clinical and histopathological features of periodontal pocket?

Answer

Correlation of clinical and histopathological features of periodontal pocket are as follows:

Clinical features	Histological feature
1. Gingival wall of pocket shows:	
• Various degrees of bluish red discolouration • Flaccidity • Smooth and shiny surface • Pitting on pressure	• This discoloration is caused due to circulatory stagnation • It is because of destruction of gingival fibres and surrounding tissues • It is caused due to atrophy of epithelium and oedema • It is because of oedema and degeneration
2. Gingival wall may be pink and firm	• When fibrotic changes predominate over exudative changes, specially in the outer wall of the pocket, the wall becomes pink and firm. Also degeneration and often ulcerations is seen in the inner wall of the pocket
3. Upon slightest probing, bleeding occurs	• Easy bleeding is because of increase in vascularity, degeneration and thinning of epithelium and proximity of engorged vessels to inner surface
4. Inner part of pocket is generally painful	• It is because of ulceration of inner aspect of pocket wall
5. Upon digital pressure, puss may be expressed	• Pus occurs because of suppurative inflammation of inner wall

Question 8

Write short note on periodontal cyst.

Answer

A periodontal cyst is a localised destruction of the periodontal tissues along a lateral root surface, most commonly mandibular canine premolar area.

Aetiology of periodontal cyst could be:
- ❑ Proliferation of epithelial rests of malassez.
- ❑ Lateral dentigerous cyst retained in this jaw after tooth eruption.
- ❑ Primordial cyst of supernumerary tooth germ.
- ❑ Stimulation of epithelial rests of the periodontal ligament by infection from a periodontal abscess or the pulp through an accessory root canal.

Its clinical features are as follows:
- ❑ Asymptomatic
- ❑ Localised, tender swelling.

Radiographic features would be:
- ❑ Periodontal cyst appears on the interproximal side, on the side of the root.
- ❑ It appears as a radiolucent area bordered by a radiopaque line.
- ❑ Radiographically it is very difficult to differentiate it from a periodontal abscess.

Its microscopic features are as follows:
- The cystic epithelium is non-keratinised, thickened, loosely arranged and proliferating epithelium.

Question 9

Write short note on periodontal abscess.

Answer

Periodontal abscess is a localised purulent inflammation in the periodontal tissues. It is also referred to as lateral abscess or a parietal abscess.

Aetiology

Periodontal abscess may be formed in the following ways:
- Extension of infection from a periodontal pocket deeply into the supporting periodontal tissues and localisation of the suppurative inflammatory process along the lateral aspect of the root.
- When the inflammatory process extends laterally from the inner surface of a periodontal pocket into the connective tissue of the pocket wall and when the drainage into the pocket space is impaired, it result in localisation of abscess.
- A periodontal abscess may form in the cul-de sac, the deep end of which is shut off from the surface.
- Because of incomplete removal of calculus from the periodontal pocket, may result in periodontal abscess.
- Trauma to the tooth or with perforation of the lateral wall of the root during endodontic therapy.

Classification of Periodontal Abscess

Periodontal abscess can be classified as:
- Abscess in the supporting periodontal tissues along the lateral aspect of the root. In this situation generally a sinus is seen in the bone which extends laterally from the abscess to the external surface.
- Abscess in the soft tissue wall of a deep periodontal pocket.

Microscopic Features

- There is accumulation of viable and non-viable PMNLs within the periodontal pocket wall.

- Pus is formed, which is basically formed by the PMNLs which liberate enzymes that digest the cells and other tissue structures, forming the pus.
- The purulent area is surrounded by an acute inflammatory reaction.
- The epithelium overlying it, exhibits extracellular and intracellular oedema and invasion of leukocytes.

Question 10

Describe the surface morphology of tooth wall of periodontal pocket.

Answer

The following zones can be seen on the surface of tooth wall:
- Cementum covered by calculus.
- **Attached plaque:** It covers the calculus and extends apically from it to a variable degree around 100–500 μm.
- **Zone of unattached plaque:** It surrounds attached plaque and extends apically to it.
- **Zone of attachment of junctional epithelium to the tooth:** The extension of this zone, which in normal, sulci is more than 500 μm, is usually reduced in periodontal zocket to less than 100 μm.
- **Zone of semi destroyed connective tissue fibres:** They may be apical to the junctional epithelium.
  - Zones 3, 4, and 5 form the plaque free zone **(Fig. 24.4)**

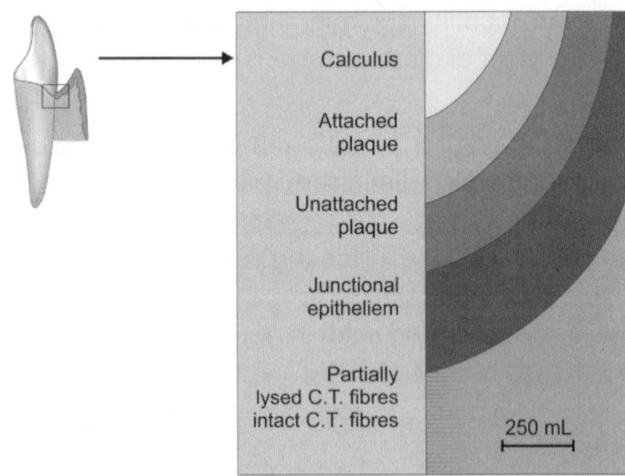

Fig. 24.4: Diagram of the area at the bottom of a pocket; C.T = connective tissue.

CHAPTER 25

Bone Loss and Patterns of Bone Destruction

LONG ESSAYS

Question 1

Explain in detail about mechanism of bone destruction, along with histopathology and diagrams.

Answer

Inflammation has been the most common cause of bone destruction, which spreads from marginal gingiva into the supporting periodontal tissues. "Periodontitis is always caused by gingivitis but not all gingivitis progresses to periodontitis".

The transformation of gingivitis to periodontitis is associated mainly with two changes, i.e.

1. Bacterial composition change.
2. Cellular composition chance.

Other than this, there are various factor associated with bone destruction and they are:

- Local factor
- Systemic factor
  - Bacterial factors
  - Host-mediated factor
  - Trauma from occlusion (TFO)

Bacterial composition change: In cases of gingivitis, more of gram-positive microorganisms are observed, but in case of severe inflammation and destruction, the number of gram-negative microorganisms increase along with motile organisms and spirochete, whereas the number of coccoid rods and straight rod decreases.

Cellular composition change: In the initial stage of gingivitis, fibroblasts and lymphocytes are seen. But as the disease progresses, the cellular composition is changed and more of plasma cells and blast cells are seen.

A fibrin-fibrinolytic system has also been seen in advancing lesion which is been mentioned as "walling off" the advancing lesion.

Various factors for bone destruction are:
- Local
- Systemic.

Local Factors

- Bacterial: Various bacterial products and inflammatory mediators act on osteoblasts or their progenitors, inhibiting their action and reducing their numbers.
- Host factors: Various host factors produced by inflammatory cells are responsible for bone resorption and periodontal destruction. Various host mediator factors which can produce their effect are prostaglandins and their precursors, interleukin-1α (IL-1α), IL-1B and tumour necrosis factor alpha (TNF-α). Non-steroidal anti-inflammatory drugs (NSAIDs) can inhibit PGE2 production thus reducing bone resorption.
- Trauma from occlusion can induce bone destruction in presence as well as absence of inflammation. Bone loss can be seen lateral to the root surface.

Systemic Factors

- Local and systemic factors regulate the physiologic equilibrium of bone.
- When there is a generalised tendency towards bone resorption, bone loss initiated by local inflammatory processes can be magnified.
- A strong relationship exists between periodontal bone loss and osteoporosis. Osteoporosis is a physiologic condition of post-menopausal women, which leads to bone loss and structural bone changes.
- Periodontitis and osteoporosis share a number of risk factors such as ageing, smoking, diseases, medication that interferes with healing.
- Periodontal bone loss may also occur in generalised skeletal disturbances such as hyperparathyroidism, leukaemia, Langerhans cell histiocytosis (LCH).

Histopathology of Bone Destruction

- ❑ Gingival inflammation extends along the collagen fibre bundles and follows the course of the blood vessels through the loosely arranged tissues around them into the alveolar bone **(Fig. 25.1)**
- ❑ Along its course from gingiva to the bone, there is destruction seen in the gingival and transseptal fibres.
- ❑ However there is continuous tendency of transseptal fibres to recreate themselves. Therefore, even in cases of extreme periodontal bone loss, transseptal fibres are present.
- ❑ After reaching to the bone, the inflammation spreads into the marrow spaces.
- ❑ The marrow is replaced with leukocytic and fluid exudate, new blood vessels and proliferating fibroblasts.
- ❑ There is an increase in the number of multinuclear osteoclasts and mononuclear phagocytes and Howship lacunae lines the bone surfaces.

The amount of inflammatory infiltrate correlates with the degree of bone loss but not with the number of osteoclasts.

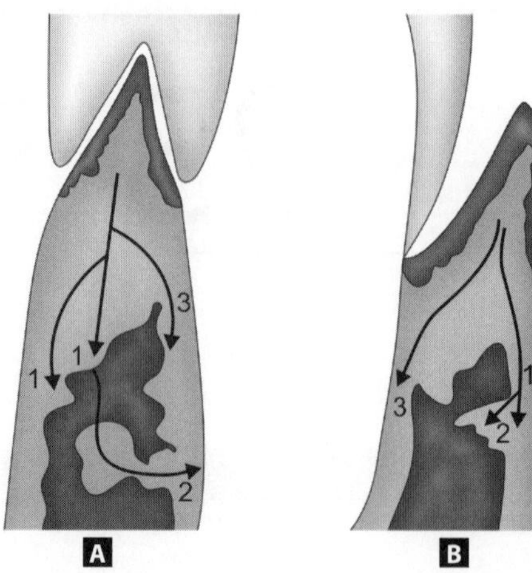

Fig. 25.1: Pathways of inflammation from gingiva into the supporting periodontal tissues in periodontitis [(A) Interproximally, from the gingiva into the bone (1), from the bone into the periodontal ligament (PDL) (2), and from the gingiva into the PDL (3); (B) Facially and lingually, from the gingiva along the outer periosteum (1), from the periosteum into the bone (2), and from the gingiva into the PDL (3)]

SHORT ESSAYS

Question 1

What are the factors determining bone morphology in periodontal disease?

Answer

Various factors that determine bone morphology in periodontal disease are as follows:

- ❑ The thickness, width, and crestal angulation of the interdental septa.
- ❑ The thickness of the facial and lingual alveolar plates.
- ❑ The presence of fenestration and dehiscence.
- ❑ The alignment of the teeth.
- ❑ Root and root trunk anatomy.
- ❑ Root position within the alveolar process.
- ❑ Proximity with another tooth surface.

Question 2

What is radius of action?

Answer

Locally produced bone resorption factors may need to be present in the proximity of bone surface, to produce their effect

- ❑ It has been postulated by Page and Schroeder on the basis of Waerhaug's measurements made on human autopsy specimen, that there is a range of about 1.5–2.5 mm within which bacterial plaque can induce bone loss.
- ❑ Beyond 2.5 mm there is no bone loss.
- ❑ Large defects exceeding a distance of 2.5 mm from the tooth surface (as seen in aggressive types of periodontitis) may be caused by the presence of bacteria in the tissues. {Note to operator: Kindly insert "Discuss the rate of bone loss" from page 6 of Bone loss 1 file.}

Question 3

Explain in detail how bone destruction is caused by trauma from occlusion?

Answer

Bone destruction mechanism from trauma from occlusion (TFO) occurs in following ways:

- ❑ TFO can produce bone destruction in the presence as well as absence of inflammation.
- ❑ In the absence of inflammation the changes caused by TFO varies from increased compression and tension of the PDL and increased osteoclasts of alveolar bone to necrosis of the PDL and bone and resorption of bone and tooth structures.
- ❑ These changes are reversible and can be repaired if the offending forces are removed.

- Continuous TFO, can result in funnel-shaped widening of the crestal portion of the PDL, with resorption of the adjacent bone.
- These changes which may cause the bony crest to have an angular shape represent adaptation of the PDL tissue aimed at cushioning, increased occlusion forces, but the modified bones shape may weaken tooth support and cause tooth mobility.
- In presence of inflammation, TFO aggregates the bone destruction and can lead to bizarre bone patterns.

Question 4

What are periods of destruction?

Answer

Periodontal destruction is not always occurring or is continuous, instead, it occurs in an episodic, intermittent manner. This destructive period results in loss of collagen and alveolar bone with an increase in the depth of periodontal pocket.

Aetiology for onset of destructive periods have been summarised by following four theories:

- Bursts of destructive activity are associated with subgingival ulceration and an acute inflammatory reaction, resulting in rapid loss of alveolar bone.
- Burst of destructive activity coincide with the conversion of a predominantly T-lymphocyte lesion to one with a predominantly B-lymphocyte plasma cell infiltrate.
- Periods of exacerbation are associated with an increase of the loose, unattached, non-motile, gram-negative, anaerobic pocket flora and periods of remission coincide with the formation of dense, unattached, non-motile, gram-positive flora with a tendency to mineralize.
- Tissue invasion by one or several bacterial species is followed by an advanced local host defence that controls the attack.

Question 5

What are the various bone destruction patterns in periodontal disease?

Answer

Various bone destruction patterns in periodontal disease are as follows:

1. Horizontal bone loss
2. Vertical or angular defects
3. Osseous craters
4. Bulbous bone contours
5. Reversed architecture
6. Ledges
7. Furcation involvements.

Horizontal Bone Loss

- It is the most common pattern of bone loss.
- The height of the bone is reduced, but the bone margins remains nearly perpendicular to the surface of the tooth.
- It can occur at different degree around the same tooth.

Vertical Bone Loss

- The bone is lost in an oblique direction leaving a hollowed-out trough in the bone along side the root.
- The base of the defect is apical to the surrounding bone.
- These defects are generally accompanied with infrabony pocket.
- These defects can be classified as one wall two walls or three wall defects on the basis of the number of osseous wall.
    1. **Three wall defect:** This defect has three walls. It has the best prognosis.
    2. **Two wall defect:** This defect has two osseous walls.
    3. **One wall defect:** This defect has one osseous wall (**Fig. 25.2**)
- Sometimes, the numbers of osseous walls are greater in the apical portion of the defect than in its occlusal portion. This type of defect is termed as combined osseous defect.

Surgical exposure of the defect is the only sure way to determine the presence and configuration of vertical osseous defect.

Three wall defects are also referred as intrabony defects, whereas one wall defects are referred as hemiseptum originally.

Osseous Craters

- They are the concavities seen in the crest of the interdental bone, confined within facial and lingual walls.
- Craters form around 35.2% of all defects and occur twice as often in posterior segments as in anterior segments.

Reasons for the high frequency of interdental craters are as follows:

1. The interdental area collects plaque and is difficult to clean.
2. The normal flat or even concave faciolingual shape of the interdental septum in lower molars may favour crater formation.
3. Vascular patterns from the gingiva to the centre of the crest may provide a pathway for inflammation (**Fig. 25.3**).

Bulbous Bone Contours

Bulbous bone contours are bony enlargement caused because of exostosis, adaptation to function, or buttressing

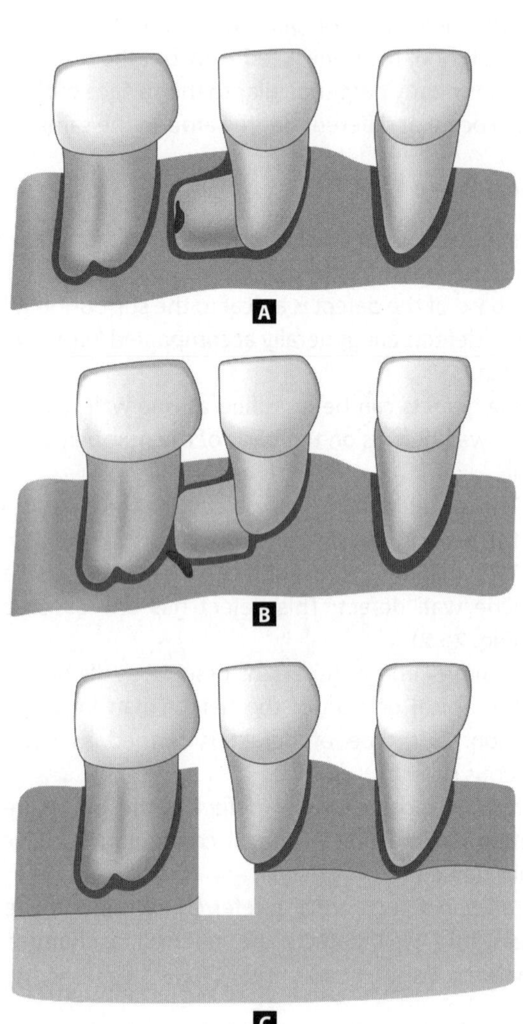

Figs 25.2A to C: (A) Three wall defect, three bony walls present—distal, lingual and facial; (B) Two wall defect, two bony wall present—buccal and lingual; (C) One wall defect, one bony wall present—distal wall only.

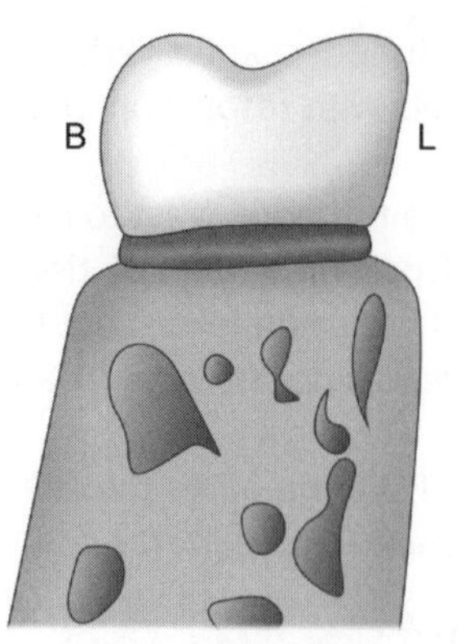

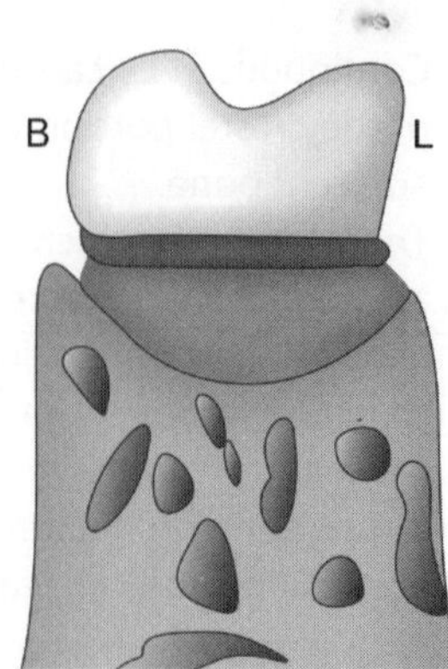

Fig. 25.3: Diagrammatic representation of an osseous crater in a faciolingual section between two lower molars—left, normal bone contour and right, osseous crater

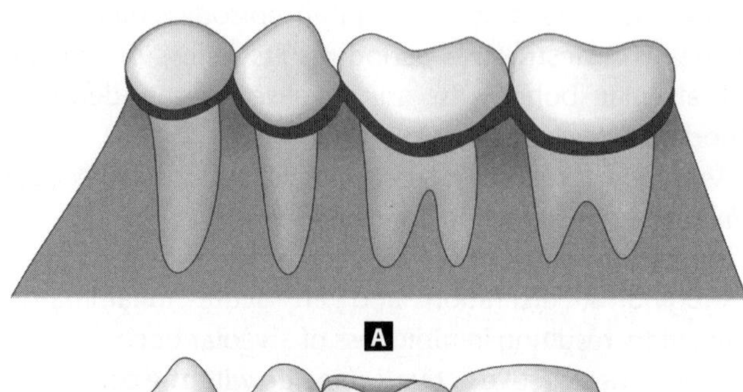

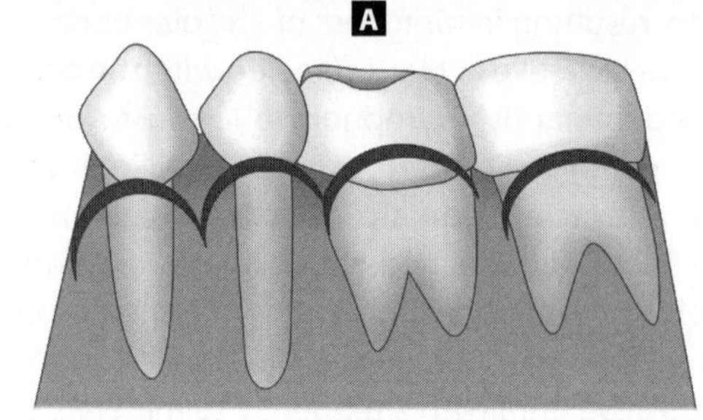

Figs 25.4A and B: (A) Normal architecture, where interdental bone is higher than radicular bone; (B) Reverse architecture where interdental bone is lower than radicular bone

bone formation. They are seen more commonly in the maxilla than in the mandible.

Reversed Architecture

It is found due to loss of interdental bone, both in facial and lingual plates, without the simultaneous loss of radicular bone. Because of this, the normal architecture (i.e. radicular bone at a lower height, than the interproximal bone) is reversed. It is seen more commonly in maxilla (**Fig. 25.4**).

Ledges

They are plateau-like bone margins caused by resorption of thickened bony plates.

Furcation Involvements

- ❑ It refers to invasion of the bifurcation and trifurcation of multirooted teeth by periodontal disease.
- ❑ The furcation can either be visible or may be covered with a pocket wall.
- ❑ There are four grades of furcation:
  - ○ **Grade I:** In this, there is incipient bone loss.
  - ○ **Grade II:** Partial bone loss (cul-de-sac).
  - ○ **Grade III:** Total bone loss, with through-and-through opening of furcation but covered with the pocket wall.
  - ○ **Grade IV:** Complete bone loss (similar to Grade III), but accompanied with gingival recession, exposing the furcation.

Furcation involvement represents progressive periodontal destruction and has the same cause as periodontitis.

Sometimes, plaque removal becomes difficult from the furcation area, which may aggregate the disease process.

Question 6

What are Exostoses?

Answer

Exostoses are outgrowth of bone of varied size and shapes.

- They can be seen as small nodules, large nodules, sharp ridges, spike like projections, or combination of any of these.
- Exostoses have been reported rarely, in areas where free gingival grafts have been placed.

Question 7

What is buttressing bone formation?

Answer

It is also referred to as lipping.

- Sometimes bone formation occurs in an attempt to buttress bony trabeculae, which are weakened by resorption.

- This types of bone formation is referred to as buttressing bone formation.
- It can be of two types: Central and peripheral.
- When it occurs within the jaw it is referred to as central buttressing bone formation.
- When it occurs on the external surface of the jaw, then it is referred to as peripheral buttressing bone formation. It may cause bulging of the bone which can be termed as lipping.

Question 8

What is the role of the food impaction in bone loss?

Answer

Whenever proximal contacts are abnormal or absent, interdental bone defects can be seen. It is generally due to pressure and irritation from food impaction.

- Poor proximal relationship can also result from shift in the position of the teeth, because of which there is food impaction, leading to bone loss.
- Therefore, food impaction is a complicating factor than the cause of bony defects.

CHAPTER 26

Trauma from Occlusion

Question 1

Define trauma from occlusion. What are the various clinical and radiographic features? Discuss in detail the classification of trauma from occlusion. Discuss the treatment of traumatic occlusion.

Answer

Definition

When the forces exceed the adaptive capacity of the tissues, tissue injury results. The resultant injury is termed as trauma from occlusion.

Clinical features are as follows:

- Mobility
- Occlusion
- Fremitus
- Prematurities
- Wear facets
- Tooth migration
- Fractured teeth or tooth
- Thermal sensitivity.

Radiographic indicators of trauma from occlusion (TFO) are as follows:

- Thickening or discontinuity of lamina dura
- Widened periodontal ligament space
- Bone loss
- Root resorption.

Classification

It can be classified as:

- Acute
- Chronic

Acute Trauma from Occlusion

- Acute TFO results from an abrupt occlusal impact which can result from biting over a hard object such as stone or an olive pit
- It can also result from restorations or prosthetic appliances that may interfere with or alter the direction of occlusal force.

Various features of acute TFO are:

- Tooth pain
- Sensitivity to percussion
- Increased tooth mobility
- If this abrupt force can be corrected by shifting the position of the tooth or by wearing away or correction of the restorations, the injury can heal and symptoms can subside. But if this does not happen, then the periodontal injury might worsen and develop into necrosis, which can be accompanied by periodontal abscess formation or persist as a symptom free chronic condition
- Cemental tears can also lead to acute trauma from occlusion.

Chronic Trauma from Occlusion

- Chronic trauma from occlusion is more common than acute trauma from occlusion and has more clinical importance
- It results from gradual changes in occlusion produced by tooth wear, drifting movement and extrusion of teeth combined with a para-functional habit such as bruxism and clenching, rather than as a sequel of acute periodontal trauma
- Chronic trauma from occlusion can be divided into primary and secondary:

Primary Trauma from Occlusion

- Primary trauma from occlusion may be caused by alterations in occlusal forces, reduced capacity of the periodontium to withstand occlusal forces or both
- When TFO results from alteration in occlusal forces, it is referred to as primary TFO.

The main aetiological factors in primary TFO are the local alterations in the occlusion due to the following reasons:

- Because of insertion of a high filling or a prosthetic replacement that creates excessive force on the abutment and antagonist teeth
- The extrusion or the drifting movement of the teeth into spaces created by unreplaced missing teeth or the orthodontic movement of teeth into functionally unacceptable position
- Changes produces by primary trauma do not alter the level of connective tissue attachment and do not initiate pocket formation because supracrestal gingival fibres are not affected and therefore prevent apical migration of the junctional epithelium.

Secondary Trauma from Occlusion

- Secondary TFO occurs when the adaptive capacity of the tissues to withstand occlusal forces is impaired by bone loss resulting from marginal inflammation
- This diminishes the periodontal attachment area and alters the leverage on the remaining tissues
- The periodontium becomes more vulnerable to injury and previously well-tolerated occlusal forces become traumatic (**Fig. 26.1**).

Combined TFO

When the injury results from abnormal occlusal forces applied to teeth or teeth with inadequate periodontal support.

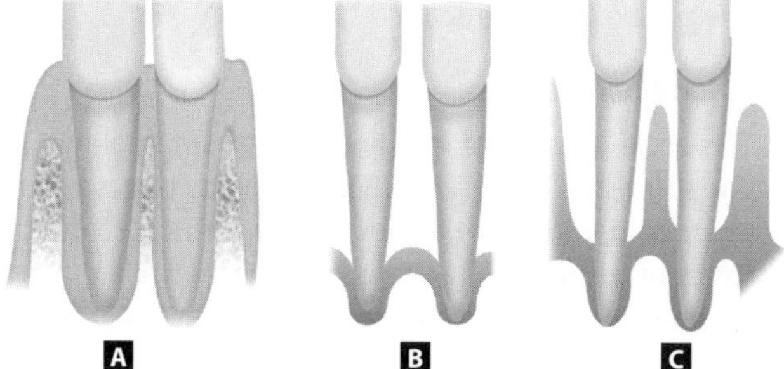

Fig. 26.1: Can occur on; (A) Normal periodontium with normal height of bone (B) Normal periodontium with reduced height of bone (C) Marginal periodontitis with reduced height of bone.

What are the various stages of trauma from occlusion?

Tissue response from trauma can be in three stages. They are as follows:

1. Stage 1: Injury.
2. Stage 2: Repair.
3. Stage 3: Adaptive remodelling of the periodontium.

Stage 1: Injury

- In this stage there is tissue injury resulting from excessive occlusal force
- In this the body attempts to repair the injury and restore the periodontium
- This can occur if the forces are diminished or if the tooth drifts away from them
- If the offending force is chronic, the periodontium is remodelled to cushion its impact. This ligament is widened at the expense of the bone, resulting in an angular bone defects without periodontal pockets and the tooth becomes loose
- Slightly excessive pressure stimulates resorption of the alveolar bone, with a resultant widening of the periodontal ligament space
- Slightly excessive tension can cause elongation of the periodontal ligament fibres and apposition of the alveolar bone
- In the areas of increased pressure there are numerous blood vessels but reduced in size, while in areas of increased tension they become elongated
- A gradation of changes is produced with increase in pressure in the periodontal ligament starting from compression of fibres, which can produce areas of hyalinization
- Fibroblasts and other connective tissue cells get injured subsequently, leading to necrosis of the areas of ligament
- Vascular changes may also be seen
- Within 30 minutes, retardation and stasis of blood flow occurs
- At 2–3 hours, blood vessels appear to be packed with RBCs starts to fragment
- Between 1 and 7 days disintegration of blood vessels walls and release of contents to surrounding tissue
- In addition to this, there is increased resorption of alveolar bone and resorption of tooth surface occur
- Severe tension may cause widening of periodontal ligament, thrombosis, haemorrhage, tearing of the periodontal ligament and resorption of alveolar bone

- Severe pressure can force the root against the bone, which can lead to necrosis of the periodontal ligament and bone
- The bone gets resorbed from the viable periodontal ligament adjacent to necrotic areas and from marrow spaces, and this process is known as undermining resorption
- The areas of periodontium most susceptible to injury from excessive occlusal forces are the furcations
- Injury to the periodontium produces a temporary depression in mitotic activity and rate of proliferation and differentiation of fibroblast, in collagen formation and in bone formation
- This would return to normal levels after dissipation of the forces.

Stage II: Repair

- Repair is a constant phenomenon that is seen normally in the periodontium. TFO further stimulates increased reparative capacity
- The tissue that has been destroyed are removed and new connective tissue cells and fibres, bone and cementum are formed in an attempt to restore the injured periodontium
- When the damage produced, exceeds the reparative capacity of the tissues, till then the forces remain traumatic
- When the bone is resorbed by excessive occlusal forces, the body attempts to replace the thinned bone with new bone. This attempt to compensate for the lost bone is referred to as buttressing bone formation and it is an important feature of the reparative process associated with TFO.

Buttressing bone formation can be of two types:

1. *Central buttressing:* It occurs within the jaws. In this form of buttressing, endosteal cells deposit new bone, which restores the bony trabecula and reduces the size of the marrow spaces.
2. *Peripheral buttressing:* It occurs on the surface of the bone. It can occur on either or facial or lingual surfaces of the alveolar bone. Peripheral buttressing may be seen as a shelf-like thickening of the alveolar margin of the bone, in severe cases, which is referred to as lipping. It basically looks lies a pronounced bulge in the contour of the facial and lingual bone.

Stage III: Adaptive Remodelling of the Periodontium

- If the repair process does not keep pace with the destruction caused by occlusion, the periodontium is remodelled in an effort so as to create a structural relationship in which the forces are no longer injurious to the tissues
- This would result in a thickened periodontal ligament, which is funnel shaped at the crest with vertical defects in the bone, and no formation of pockets
- The affected teeth becomes loose along with increased vascular supply
- The injury phase has increased bone resorption, and decreased bone formation. Repair phase shows increased bone formation and decreased bone resorption. After adaptive remodelling of the periodontium, resorption and formation of bone return to normal.

Explain in detail about the concept of trauma from occlusion in periodontal diseases. Discuss about the physiological and pathological tooth mobility observed in teeth having TFO.

There are various concepts of trauma from occlusion in periodontal disease. They are as follows:

Glickman's Concept

- According this concept, given by Glickman and Smulow in the year 1965 and 1967, if the forces of an abnormal magnitude are acting on teeth harbouring sub-gingival plaque, then the pathway of spread of a plaque associated gingival lesion can be altered
- According to Glickman, instead of an even destruction of the periodontium and alveolar bone, i.e. suprabony pockets and horizontal bone loss, which occurs at the sites with uncomplicated plaque associated lesions, sites which are exposed to abnormal occlusal force will develop angular bony defects and infra bony pockets.

The periodontal structure can be divided into two zones:

1. The zone of irritation and
2. The zone of co-destruction.

The Zone of Irritation

- This zone consists of marginal and interdental gingiva. The soft tissue of this zone is bordered by hard structure on one side, i.e. tooth on one side and is not affected by forces of occlusion. Therefore, it means that inflammation of gingiva cannot be induced by TFO but is because of microbial plaque irritation
- Such plaque associated lesion at a non-traumatised tooth propagates in apical direction firstly by involving the alveolar bone and later the periodontal area.

The advancement of this lesion results in an even or horizontal bone destruction.

The Zone of Co-destruction

❑ This zone includes the periodontal ligament, the root cementum and alveolar bone, and is demarcated coronally by the trans-septal fibres, i.e. interdental and the dentoalveolar collagen
❑ The tissue in this zone might become the seat of lesion caused by TFO
❑ The fibre bundles that separate the zone of co-destruction from the zone of irritation can be affected from two different directions:
   1. From the inflammatory lesion maintained by the plaque in the zone of irritation
   2. From trauma induced changes in the zone of co-destruction.

Because of this exposure from two different directions the fibre bundles become oriented to some other direction which is parallel to the root surface (**Fig. 26.2**).

Waerhaug's Concept

❑ This concept is supported by Prichard in 1965 and Manson in 1976
❑ From his similar studies he came to a conclusion that angular defects and infra bony pockets occur more often at periodontal sites of teeth not affected by TFO
❑ In other words the Glickman's concept/hypothesis that TFO played a role in spread of inflammation into the zone of co-destruction

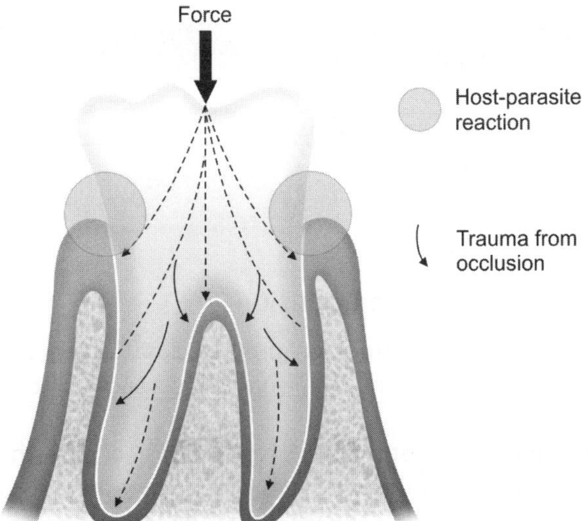

Fig. 26.2: The reaction between dental plaque and the host takes place in the gingival sulcus region. Trauma from occlusion appears in the tissues supporting the tooth.

❑ According to the concept of Waerhaug, because of the inflammatory lesions associated with sub-gingival plaque, the periodontal destruction occurs. He said that the angular or vertical defects occur when the sub-gingival plaque of one tooth has reached more apically, than the microbiota of the neighbouring tooth, also when the volume of the alveolar bone around the roots is comparatively large.

Therefore to conclude, whenever there is gingival inflammation in a tooth, exposed to trauma, four possibilities can be seen:

❑ TFO may alter the pathway of extension of gingival inflammation to the underlying periodontal tissues. Inflammation may proceed into the periodontal ligament rather than to the alveolar bone and the resulting bone loss would be angular with infra bony pockets.
❑ It may favour the environment for the formation and attachment of plaque and calculus and may be responsible for development of deeper lesions.
❑ If the tooth is tilted orthodontically or migrates into an edentulous space, then supra-gingival plaque can become sub-gingival, resulting in formation of a supra bony pocket into an infra bony pocket.
❑ There might be a pumping effect on plaque metabolites increasing their diffusion, due to increased tooth mobility associated with trauma to the periodontium.

Physiologic Adaptive Capacity of the Periodontium to Occlusal Forces

❑ Adaptive capacity is referred to as the dynamics of the periodontium to accommodate the forces exerted on the crown
❑ This can vary in different persons and in the same person at different times. This can be explained by four factors which affect the occlusal forces on the periodontium:
   ○ *Magnitude:* When the magnitude of occlusal forces increases the periodontium shows the following:
     ➤ Thickening of the periodontal ligament
     ➤ An increase in the number and width of periodontal ligament fibres
     ➤ An increase in the density of the alveolar bone.
   ○ *Direction:* Changes in the direction cause a reorientation of the stresses and strains within the periodontium
   ○ *Duration:* Constant pressure on the bone is more injurious than intermittent forces
   ○ *Frequency:* The more frequent the application of an intermittent force, the more injurious to the periodontium.

Pathologic Migration

Pathologic migration refers to tooth displacement that results when the balance among the factors that maintain physiologic tooth position is disturbed.

Pathogenesis

The normal position of the teeth is maintained by two major factors:
1. The health and normal height of the periodontium
2. The forces exerted on the teeth.

Health and Normal Height of the Periodontium

- A tooth with weakened periodontal support is unable to withstand the forces and moves away from the opposing force
- When the periodontal support is reduced, forces that are acceptable to an intact periodontium become injurious. Pathologic migration may continue even after a tooth no longer contacts its antagonist.

Forces Exerted on the Teeth

The changes in the forces may occur as a result of:
- Unreplaced missing teeth
- Failure to replace first molars
- Other causes.

If the periodontium is sufficiently weakened, these forces do not have to be abnormal to cause pathologic migration.

Unreplaced Missing Teeth

- The spaces created by unreplaced missing teeth lead to drifting of adjacent teeth
- Drifting does not result from destruction of the periodontal tissues. But it usually creates conditions that lead to periodontal diseases and thus, the initial tooth movement is aggravated by loss of periodontal support.

Failure to Replace Tirst Molars

- Tilting of the second and the third molars causing a decrease in the vertical dimension
- Movement of premolars distally and the mandibular incisors tilting lingually
- Increased anterior overbite
- Pushing the maxillary incisors labially and laterally
- Extrusion of the anterior teeth due to disappearance of incisal apposition
- Diastema of the anterior teeth.

Other Causes

- Pressure from the tongue may cause drifting of teeth in normal conditions
- When the periodontium is sufficiently weakened, these forces cause pathologic migration
- Pressure from the granulation tissue of the periodontal pocket also causes pathologic migration.

SHORT ESSAYS

Question 1

What is trauma from occlusion and what is traumatic occlusion?

Answer

- When occlusal forces exceed the adaptive capacity of the tissues, tissue injury results. The resultant injury is termed trauma from occlusion
- Therefore, trauma from occlusion refers to the tissue injury, not the occlusal force
- An occlusion that produces such injury is called a traumatic occlusion.

Question 2

What is the classification of trauma from occlusion?

Answer

It can be classified as:
- Acute
- Chronic

Acute Trauma from Occlusion

- Acute TFO results from an abrupt occlusal impact which can result from biting over a hard object such as stone or an olive pip
- It can also result from restorations or prosthetic appliances that may interfere with or alter the direction of occlusal force.

Various features of acute TFO are

- Tooth pain

- Sensitivity to percussion
- Increased tooth mobility
- If this abrupt force can be corrected by shifting the position of the tooth or by wearing away or correction of the restorations, the injury can heal and symptoms can subside. But if this does not happen, then the periodontal injury might worsen and develop into necrosis, which can be accompanied by periodontal abscess formation or persist as a symptom free chronic condition
- Cemental tears can also lead to acute trauma from occlusion.

Chronic Trauma from Occlusion

- Chronic trauma from occlusion is more common than acute trauma from occlusion and has more clinical importance.
- It results from gradual changes in occlusion produced by tooth wear, drifting movement and extrusion of teeth, combined with a para-functional habit such as bruxism and clenching, rather than as a sequel of acute periodontal trauma.
- Chronic trauma from occlusion can be divided into primary and secondary:

Primary Trauma from Occlusion

- Primary trauma from occlusion may be caused by alterations in occlusal forces, reduced capacity of the periodontium to withstand occlusal forces or both
- When TFO results from alteration in occlusal forces, it is referred to as primary TFO
- The main aetiological factors in primary TFO are the local alterations in the occlusion due to the following reasons:
  - Because of insertion of a high filling or a prosthetic replacement that creates excessive force on the abutment and antagonist teeth
  - The extrusion or the drifting movement of the teeth into spaces created by unreplaced missing teeth or the orthodontic movement of teeth into functionally unacceptable position
  - Changes produces by primary trauma do not alter the level of connective tissue attachment and do not initiate pocket formation because supracrestal gingival fibres are not affected and, therefore prevent apical migration of the junctional epithelium.

Secondary Trauma from Occlusion

- Secondary TFO occurs when the adaptive capacity of the tissues to withstand occlusal forces is impaired by bone loss resulting from marginal inflammation
- This diminishes the periodontal attachment area and alters the leverage on the remaining tissues

- The periodontium becomes more vulnerable to injury and previously well-tolerated occlusal forces become traumatic.

Question 3

What are the clinical and radiological signs of trauma from occlusion?

Answer

Clinical features are as follows:
- Mobility
- Occlusion
- Fremitus
- Prematurities
- Wear facets
- Tooth migration
- Fractured teeth or tooth
- Thermal sensitivity.

Radiographic features of TFO are as follows:
- Thickening or discontinuity of lamina dura
- Widened periodontal ligament space
- Bone loss
- Root resorption.

Question 4

What is bone buttressing?

Answer

When the bone is resorbed by excessive occlusal forces, the body attempts to replace the thinned bone with new bone. This attempt to compensate for the lost bone is referred to as buttressing bone formation and it is an important feature of the reparative process associated with TFO.

Buttressing bone formation can be of two types:

1. **Central buttressing:** It occurs within the jaws. In this form of buttressing, endosteal cells deposit new bone, which restores the bony trabecula and reduces the size of the marrow spaces.

2. **Peripheral buttressing:** It occurs on the surface of the bone. It can occur on either or facial or lingual surfaces of the alveolar bone. Peripheral buttressing may be seen as a shelf-like thickening of the alveolar margin of the bone, in severe cases, which is referred to as lipping. It basically looks like a pronounced bulge in the contour of the facial and lingual bone.

Question 5

What is the Glickman's concept of trauma from occlusion?

Answer

- According this concept, given by Glickman and Smulow in the year 1965 and 1967, if the forces of an abnormal magnitude are acting on teeth harbouring sub-gingival plaque, then the pathway of spread of a plaque associated gingival lesion can be altered.
- According to Glickman, instead of an even destruction of the periodontium and alveolar bone, i.e. supra bony pockets and horizontal bone loss, which occurs at the sites with uncomplicated plaque associated lesions, sites which are exposed to abnormal occlusal force will develop angular bony defects and infra bony pockets.
- The periodontal structure can be divided into two zones:
  1. The zone of irritation.
  2. The zone of co-destruction.

The Zone of Irritation

This zone consists of marginal and interdental gingiva. The soft tissue of this zone is bordered by hard structure on one side, i.e. tooth on one side and is not affected by forces of occlusion. Therefore, it means that inflammation of gingiva cannot be induced by TFO but is because of microbial plaque irritation.

Such plaque associated lesion at a non-traumatised tooth propagates in apical direction firstly by involving the alveolar bone and later the periodontal area. The advancement of this lesion results in an even or horizontal bone destruction.

The Zone of Co-Destruction

- This zone includes the periodontal ligament, the root cementum and alveolar bone and is demarcated coronally by the trans-septal fibres, i.e. interdental and the dentoalveolar collagen.
- The tissue in this zone might become the seat of lesion caused by TFO
- The fibre bundles that separate the zone of co-destruction from the zone of irritation can be affected from two different directions:
  1. From the inflammatory lesion maintained by the plaque in the zone of irritation
  2. From trauma induced changes in the zone of co-destruction.

Because of this exposure from two different directions the fibre bundles become oriented to some other direction which is parallel to the root surface.

Question 6

What is Waerhaug's concept of trauma from occlusion?

Answer

- This concept is supported by Prichard in 1965 and Manson in 1976.
- From his similar studies, he came to a conclusion that angular defects and infra bony pockets occur more often at periodontal sites of teeth not affected by TFO
- In other words the Glickman's concept/hypothesis that TFO played a role in spread of inflammation into the zone of co-destruction
- According to the concept of Waerhaug, because of the inflammatory lesions associated with sub-gingival plaque, the periodontal destruction occurs. He said that the angular or vertical defects occur when the sub-gingival plaque of one tooth has reached more apically, than the microbiota of the neighbouring tooth, also when the volume of the alveolar bone around the roots is comparatively large.

Therefore to conclude, whenever there is gingival inflammation in a tooth, exposed to trauma, four possibilities can be seen:

- Trauma from occlusion may alter the pathway of extension of gingival inflammation to the underlying periodontal tissues. Inflammation may proceed into the periodontal ligament rather than to the alveolar bone and the resulting bone loss would be angular with infra bony pockets.
- It may favour the environment for the formation and attachment of plaque and calculus and may be responsible for development of deeper lesions.
- If the tooth is tilted orthodontically or migrates into an edentulous space, then supragingival plaque can become sub-gingival, resulting in formation of a supra bony pocket into an infra bony pocket.
- There might be a pumping effect on plaque metabolites increasing their diffusion, due to increased tooth mobility associated with trauma to the periodontium.

Question 7

What is pathologic migration? Explain with examples.

Answer

Pathologic migration refers to tooth displacement that results when the balance among the factors that maintain physiologic tooth position is disturbed.

Pathogenesis

The normal position of the teeth is maintained by two major factors:
1. The health and normal height of the periodontium.
2. The forces exerted on the teeth.

Health and Normal Height of the Periodontium

- A tooth with weakened periodontal support is unable to withstand the forces and moves away from the opposing force
- When the periodontal support is reduced, forces that are acceptable to an intact periodontium become injurious. Pathologic migration may continue even after a tooth no longer contacts its antagonist.

Forces Exerted on the Teeth

The changes in the forces may occur as a result of:

- Unreplaced missing teeth
- Failure to replace first molars
- Other causes.

If the periodontium is sufficiently weakened, these forces do not have to be abnormal to cause pathologic migration.

Unreplaced Missing Teeth

- The spaces created by unreplaced missing teeth lead to drifting of adjacent teeth.
- Drifting does not result from destruction of the periodontal tissues. But it usually creates conditions that lead to periodontal diseases and thus, the initial tooth movement is aggravated by loss of periodontal support.

Failure to Replace first Molars

- Tilting of the second and the third molars causing a decrease in the vertical dimension
- Movement of premolars distally and the mandibular incisors tilting lingually
- Increased anterior overbite
- Pushing the maxillary incisors labially and laterally
- Extrusion of the anterior teeth due to disappearance of incisal apposition
- Diastema of the anterior teeth.

Other Causes

- Pressure from the tongue may cause drifting of teeth in normal conditions
- When the periodontium is sufficiently weakened, these forces cause pathologic migration
- Pressure from the granulation tissue of the periodontal pocket also causes pathologic migration.

What are the physiologic adaptive capacities of the periodontium to occlusal forces?

- Adaptive capacity is referred to as the dynamics of the periodontium to accommodate the forces exerted on the crown

---

- This can vary in different persons and in the same person at different times. This can be explained by four factors which affect the occlusal forces on the periodontium.
- **Magnitude:** When the magnitude of occlusal forces increases the periodontium shows the following:
  - **a.** Thickening of the periodontal ligament.
  - **b.** An increase in the number and width of periodontal ligament fibres.
  - **c.** An increase in the density of the alveolar bone.
- **Direction:** Changes in the direction cause a reorientation of the stresses and strains within the periodontium.
- **Duration:** Constant pressure on the bone is more injurious than intermittent forces.
- **Frequency:** The more frequent the application of an intermittent force, the more injurious to the periodontium.

What is the test done for trauma from occlusion. Explain.

The test done for trauma from occlusion is referred to as Fremitus Test.

- It is a measurement of the vibratory pattern of the teeth when the teeth are placed in contact with each other and in moving positions.
- It is mainly seen in maxillary teeth, but in cases of edge to edge contact or when there is overlap of teeth, mandibular teeth can also be checked.
- In performing this test, the Index finger is placed on the maxillary teeth at the cervical third, and the patient is asked to click the posterior teeth several times.
- There are various grades of fremitus:
  - Class I: Mild vibrations or movements are detected.
  - Class II: Easily palpable vibrations but no visible movements.
  - Class III: Movements are visible with naked eye.

What are the treatment options for TFO?

The treatment for TF O depends on what the cause is. TFO is usually treated with one or more of the below procedures:

- Occlusal adjustments
- Coronoplasty
- Occlusal bite planes
- Orthodontics
- Permanent or temporary splint.

CHAPTER 27

Chronic Periodontitis

Question 1

Define chronic periodontitis, what are in clinical features, how can it be diagnosed? Describe the disease severity, disease distribution, symptoms and disease progression?

Answer

According to Carranza, chronic periodontitis is defined as infections disease resulting in inflammation within the supporting tissues of the teeth, progressive attachment loss and bone loss.

The main aetiological characteristics of the disease are:

- Microbial plaque formation
- Periodontal inflammation
- Loss of attachment and alveolar bone.

Its clinical features are as follows:

- Supragingival and sub-gingival plaque accumulation
- Gingival inflammation
- Pocket formation
- Loss of periodontal attachment
- Loss of alveolar bone
- Suppuration can be seen occasionally
- Gingiva can be slightly to moderately swollen and exhibits alterations in colour ranging from pale red to magenta
- Stippling is lost
- Blunt or rolled out gingival margins
- Flattened or cratered papillae
- Inflammation related exudates of crevicular fluid and suppuration from the pocket may be seen
- Because of long standing, low-grade inflammation, thickness, fibrotic marginal tissue may obscure the underlying inflammatory changes
- Both horizontal or vertical bone loss may be found
- Tooth mobility can be present
- Attachment loss and bone loss seen in severe cases.

Diagnosis

- It can be diagnosed by detecting the chronic inflammatory changes in gingiva like pocket formation, attachment loss.
- Radiographically, bone loss can be detected.
- In some cases, suppuration may be seen.
- In advanced cases, mobility is present.

Disease Distribution

Chronic periodontitis is site-specific, that means a site harbouring chronic microbial plaque would show signs of chronic periodontitis, while other sites would be normal.

Other than this, chronic periodontitis can be localised or generalised.

- Localised periodontitis is when there are less than 30% of sites involved with attachment loss or bone loss.
- Generalised periodontitis is when there are more than 30% of sites involved with attachment loss or bone loss.

Disease Severity

- Disease severity can be described as mild, moderate or severe.
- Mild (slight) periodontitis when attachment loss is not more than 1–2 mm.
- Moderate periodontitis when attachment loss is around 3–4 mm.
- Severe periodontitis when attachment loss is 5 mm or more than 5 mm.

Symptoms

- Patient complains of bleeding gums white brushing or eating.
- Spacing between teeth because of mobility.
- Loosening of teeth

- Usually, there is no pain, but in some cases patient may complain of pain because of exposure of roots due to recession or due to pocket formation.
- Localised dull pain, sometimes radiating deep into the jaws have been reported.
- Areas of food impaction.
- Gingival tenderness or itchiness may be present in some cases.

Disease Progression

- Various models have been described which are related to disease progression.
- Progression is measured by attachment loss during a given period.
- Following models have been prepared.

The Continuous Model

- It suggests that the disease progression is slow and continuous.
- Affected sites show a constantly progressive rate of destruction throughout the duration of the disease.

The Random Model

- According to it, the periodontal disease progresses by short bursts of destruction followed by periods of no destruction.
- This pattern of disease is random with respect to the tooth sites affected and the chronology of the disease process.

Asynchronous, Multiple-burst Model

- It suggests that periodontal destruction occurs around affected teeth during defined periods of life.
- These bursts of activity are interspersed with periods of inactivity or remission.
- Chronology of these bursts of disease is asynchronous for individual tooth or groups of teeth.

Question 2

What are the various risk factors for chronic periodontitis?

Answer

Various risk factors for chronic periodontitis are as follows:
- Prior history of periodontitis
- Local factors
- Systemic factors
- Environmental and behavioural factors
- Genetic factors.

Prior History of Periodontitis

- Patients are at a greater risk if they have a prior history of periodontitis.
- If a patient is not successfully treated he or she will continue pocket formation, attachment and bone loss.
- This reason makes it necessary for continuous monitoring and maintenance of periodontitis patients so that the recurrence of the disease could be prevented.

Local Factors

- Plaque is considered to be the main cause of chronic periodontitis.
- Increase in Gram –ve microorganisms is associated with bone loss and attachment loss.
- Calculus is considered to be the most important plaque retentive factor.
- Other plaque retentive factors are as follows: Sub-gingival and overhanging margins of restorations, carious lesions that extend sub-gingivally, furcation, malalinged or crowded teeth, root grooves or concavities.

Systemic Factors

- When chronic periodontitis occurs in patients who have a systemic disease which may influence the effectiveness of host response, then the rate of periodontal destruction may be high significantly. For example, if a diabetic patient encounters periodontitis, then the rate of disease progression would be much higher as compared to non-diabetic person having periodontitis.
- Synergistic effect of plaque and modulation of host response because of effect of diabetes leads to severe and extensive periodontal destruction, which can be very difficult to manage.

Environmental Behavioural Factors

- Smoking increases the extent and severity of periodontal disease.
- When smoking combines with plaque induced chronic periodontitis, there is an increase is the rate of periodontal destruction.
- Also emotional stress has also been seen to influence the extent and severity of chronic periodontitis.

Genetic Factors

- There is no clear genetic determinant to describe chronic periodontitis, but still a genetic predisposition to more aggressive periodontal breakdown in response to plaque and calculus accumulation might exist.

- A genetic variation or polymorphism in the genes encoding interleukin 1 alpha (IL-1α) and IL-1β is associated with an increased susceptibility to a more aggressive form of chronic periodontitis.
- Therefore, with increased characterisation of genetic polymorphisms that may exist in other target genes, a complex genotype is likely to be identified for many different clinical forms of periodontitis.

CHAPTER 28

Necrotising Ulcerative Periodontitis

Question 1

Describe necrotising ulcerative periodontitis (NUP).

Answer

When acute necrotising ulcerative gingivitis (ANUG) progresses into the underlying periodontal structures leading to the loss of attachment level and bone, it is termed as necrotising ulcerative periodontitis (NUP).

Clinical Presentation

- Ulceration and necrosis of interdental papilla and gingival margin.
- Painful bright red marginal gingiva, that bleeds easily.
- Periodontal attachment and bone loss.
- Deep interdental osseous craters.
- Advanced lesions can lead to severe bone loss, sensitivity, tooth mobility and tooth loss.
- Absence of conventional deep periodontal pockets as the ulcerative and necrotising nature destroys the marginal epithelium and connective tissue.
- Oral malodour, fever, malaise and lymphadenopathy is also seen.

Necrotising Ulcerative Periodontitis In HIV/AIDS Patients

- This disease is much more destructive and causes complications that are rarely seen in a non-HIV/AIDS patient.
- Periodontal attachment and bone loss is extremely rapid and patients can loss 90% of periodontal attachment and 10 mm bone in 3–6 months.
- Other complications include progression of lesion involving large areas of soft tissue necrosis which leads to exposure of bone and sequestration of bone fragments.

- This lesion when extends into vestibular area and palate is termed as necrotising ulcerative stomatitis.

Aetiology

- **Predisposing factors:** Poor oral hygiene, pre-existing periodontal disease, smoking, viral infections, immunocompromised status, psychosocial stress and malnutrition.
- **Microbial flora:** Candida albicans, P. intermedia, P. gingivalis, Fusobacterium nucleatum, Campylobacter spp.
- **Immunocompromised status:** NUP lesions are more prevalent in patients with compromised or suppressed immune system.
- **Psychological stress:** Studies have shown that emotional stress leads to the development of NUP.
- NUP patients having anxiety, higher depression scores under emotional or physical stress are more prone and predisposed to development of NUP.

Treatment

- Thorough medical history and examination to rule out any underlying systemic disease.
- Administration of local anaesthesia in the affected area.
- Removal of necrotic hard and soft tissues with scaling, root planning and curettage procedures.
- Ultrasonic instrumentation with 10% povidone-iodine solution irrigation.
- Anti-microbial therapy to reduce Gram-negative anaerobes
- Anti-fungal agents in cases of fungal infection.
- Home care procedures: Brushing and interdental flossing, chlorhexidine rinses, systemic follow-up when the lesion is resolved.

Question 1

Discuss in detail about the classification, clinical characteristics, epidemiology, risk factors, radiographic findings, diagnosis and treatment options for aggressive periodontitis.

Answer

Classification of Aggressive Periodontitis

Aggressive periodontitis may be classified into localised aggressive periodontitis (LAP) and generalised aggressive periodontitis (GAP) forms.

Localised Form

Localised form is characterised by

- Circumpubertal onset of disease
- Localised first molar or incisor involvement on at least two permanent teeth one of which is a first molar
- Robust serum antibody response to infecting agents.

Generalised Form

- Usually affects persons under 30 years of age (however may be older)
- Generalised proximal attachment loss affecting at least three teeth other than first molars and incisors
- Pronounced episodic nature of periodontal destruction
- Poor serum antibody response to infecting agents
- The distinction between localised and generalized form is mainly based on the distribution of periodontal destruction in the mouth

Clinical Characteristics

- The primary characteristic of aggressive periodontitis that differentiates it from chronic periodontitis is the rapid progression of attachment loss and bone loss.

- Other characteristics that are common to patients with aggressive periodontitis are
  - Otherwise clinically healthy patient
  - Rapid attachment and bone loss
  - Amount of microbial deposits inconsistent with disease severity
  - Familial aggregation of cases.

Some characteristics are common but not universal in aggressive periodontitis patients:

- Diseased sites infected with *Actinobacillus actinomycetemcomitans (A.a.)*
- Abnormalities in phagocyte function
- Hyper-responsive macrophages, producing increased prostaglandin E2 (PGE2) and interleukin-1 beta (IL-1b)
- In some cases self-arresting disease progression.

Epidemiology

Prevalence of Aggressive Periodontitis

- Most of the prevalence and incidence data available are from studies done in the US
- Prevalence and incidence of aggressive periodontitis in India is not known clearly due to lack of epidemiological studies
- In the US and other countries prevalence of LAP is estimated at 1%.

Localized Aggressive Periodontitis

Clinical Characteristics

- LAP has an age of onset around puberty
- Clinically, it is characterised as having localised first molar/incisor presentation with interproximal attachment loss on at least two teeth one of which is a first molar, and involving no more than two teeth other than first molars and incisors

❑ This localised distribution is characteristic but unexplained

❑ Possible explanations for this have been suggested—

○ After initial colonisation of the first permanent teeth to erupt, i.e. first molars and incisors, *A.a.* evades host defences by different mechanisms including production of PMN chemotaxis inhibiting factor, endotoxin, collagenase and leucotoxin and other factors that allow the bacteria to colonise the pocket and initiate destruction of the periodontal tissues. After this initial attachment adequate immune defences are stimulated to produce opsonic antibodies to enhance clearance and phagocytosis of the invading bacteria and neutralise leucotoxic activity. This prevents colonisation of other sites. A strong antibody response to infecting agents is one characteristic of LAP

○ Bacteria antagonistic to *A.a.* may colonise periodontal tissues and inhibit *A.a.* from further colonisation of periodontal sites in the mouth. This would localise *A.a.* infection and tissue destruction.

○ *A.a.* may lose its leucotoxin producing ability for unknown reasons. If this happens the progression of the disease may be retarded or arrested and colonisation of new periodontal sites averted.

○ Defect in cementum formation may be responsible for localisation of the lesions. Root surfaces of teeth extracted from patients with LAP have been found to have hypoplastic or aplastic cementum. This was found not only on root surfaces exposed to periodontal pockets but also on roots still surrounded by the periodontium.

Other Features

Another striking feature of LAP is the lack of clinical inflammation despite the presence of deep pockets. Also in many cases the amount of plaque seems to be inconsistent with amount of destruction.

LAP progresses rapidly. Baer et al. have shown that the rate of bone loss is about 3–4 times faster than in chronic periodontitis.

Other features of LAP include distolabial migration of maxillary incisors with diastema formation.

❑ Increased mobility of first molars

❑ Sensitivity of denuded root surfaces to thermal and tactile stimuli

❑ Deep dull radiating pain during mastication

❑ Periodontal abscesses may form and regional lymph node enlargement may occur.

Microbiologic aspects of LAP:

Microbiologic studies of LAP have provided clear evidence of a strong association between disease and a unique bacterial microbiota predominated by *A.a.*

Other organisms that have been associated with LAP include *P. gingivalis, E. corrodens, C. rectus, F. nucleatum, B. capillus* and *Capnocytophaga spp.* and spirochetes.

However, research shows a primary aetiologic role for *A.a.* in LAP.

Evidence supporting *A.a.'s* role in LAP are

❑ Humoral immune response to this organism is elevated in patients with LAP. *A.a.* has been isolated in 97% of LAP patients compared with 21% of adult periodontitis patients and 17% of healthy patients. The prevalence of *A.a.* is six times greater in LAP than in healthy patients. Serotype B is the most common compared to serotype A.

❑ Incidence of *A.a.* is greater in younger LAP patients than in older patients. Younger patients have more destructive activity. The presence of this organism correlates with disease activity.

❑ A large number of *A.a.* organisms occur in lesions in LAP patients but they are absent or occur in low numbers in healthy sites.

❑ *A.a.* can be identified by electron microscopy, immunofluorescence and culture from LAP lesions within the gingival connective tissues.

❑ *A.a.* is quite virulent and produces a leucotoxin, collagenase, phosphatase and bone resorbing factors and other factors important in invasion of host tissue cells, evasion of host defences, immunosuppression and destruction of periodontal tissues.

❑ Elimination of this organism from the sub-gingival flora results in successful clinical treatment of LAP.

Immunologic Considerations in Lap

Numerous mechanisms of serum mediated killing are available to kill bacteria. These include lysis by the membrane attack complex of complement and antimicrobial substances such as lysozyme

There is a decrease in the chemotactic response to chemotactic agents like C5a, N-formylmethionyl-leucyl-phenylalanine and leucotriene B4.

In LAP the main collagenase found in tissues and gingival crevicular fluid (GCF) is matrix metalloproteinases-1 (MMP-1) as opposed to MMP-8 in chronic periodontitis. LAP patients have elevated antibodies to *A.a.* In LAP the dominant serum antibody isotype is immunoglobulin G2 (IgG$_2$). Some individuals possess a variant of the Fc receptor on neutrophils that do not bind efficiently to IgG_2. To compensate for this inefficient binding more serum antibody is present resulting in a robust serum antibody response. This increase in serum antibody limits the progression of the disease.

Radiographic Findings

Vertical loss of alveolar bone around first molars and incisors beginning around puberty in otherwise healthy teenagers is a classic diagnostic sign of LAP. Radiographic findings may include an arc-shaped loss of alveolar bone extending from distal surface of second premolar to mesial surface of second molar.

Burn out phenomena—the property of LAP to resolve by it. The lesion stops progressing.

Generalised Aggressive Periodontitis—Clinical Characteristics

Generally affects individuals under the age of 30, but older patients may also be affected.

They produce a poor antibody response to the pathogens present.

Characterised by "generalised interproximal attachment loss affecting at least three permanent teeth other than first molars and incisors".

Destruction occurs episodically with periods of advanced destruction followed by stages of quiescence.

As in LAP, GAP patients often have small amounts of plaque associated with the affected teeth.

Quantitatively amount of plaque inconsistent with amount of periodontal destruction.

Qualitatively *P. gingivalis*, *A.a.* and *B. forsythus* are frequently detected in the plaque that is present.

Tissue Responses in GAP

Two gingival tissue responses can be found in cases of GAP. One is a severe acutely inflamed tissue often proliferating, ulcerated and fiery red. Bleeding may occur spontaneously or with slight stimulation. Suppuration may also be present. This tissue response is considered to occur in the destructive stage in that attachment and bone are actively lost.

In other cases the second gingival response occurs where the gingival tissues may appear pink, free of inflammation and occasionally with some degree of stippling. But despite the mild clinical appearances, deep pockets can be demonstrated on probing.

Page and Schroeder have considered this tissue response to coincide with periods of quiescence in that the bone level remained stationary.

Other Features

Some patients with GAP may have systemic manifestations such as weight loss, mental depression and general malaise. Patients with a presumptive diagnosis of GAP should have their medical histories updated and reviewed to rule out systemic involvement.

As with LAP, GAP may be arrested spontaneously or after therapy, while some cases may continue to progress inexorably to tooth loss despite intervention with conventional treatment.

Radiographic Findings

Radiographic picture can range from severe bone loss associated with minimal number of teeth to advanced bone loss affecting majority of teeth in the dentition.

Page et al. have described sites in GAP patients that demonstrated osseous destruction of 25–60% during a 9-week period.

Despite this extreme loss, other sites in the same patient showed no bone loss.

Prevalence and Distribution by Age and Sex

In a study of untreated periodontal disease conducted in Sri Lanka by Loe and colleagues, 8% of the population had rapid progression of the disease characterised by yearly loss of attachment of 0.1–1 mm.

In the US a national survey of adolescents revealed a prevalence of 0.13%. Blacks were at much higher risk than whites for all forms of aggressive periodontitis. Males were more likely to have GAP than females.

Risk Factors for Aggressive Periodontitis

Microbiologic Factors

Although several specific microorganisms frequently are detected in patients with LAP such as *A.a.*, Capnocytophaga, *E. corrodens*, *Prevotella intermedia* and *Campylobacter rectus*. *A.a.* has been implicated as the primary pathogen.

The link between *A.a.* and LAP is based on evidence summarised by Mombelli and Tonetti—

- ❑ *A.a.* is found in about 90% of lesions characteristic of LAP.
- ❑ Sites with evidence of disease progression often show elevated levels of *A.a.*
- ❑ LAP patients have increased serum antibody levels to *A.a.*
- ❑ Clinical studies show a correlation between reduction in sub-gingival load of *A.a.* during treatment and a successful clinical response.
- ❑ *A.a.* produces virulence factors that contribute to the disease process.

Immunologic Factors

Some immune defects have been implicated in aggressive periodontitis. Human leucocyte antigens (HLA) that regulate immune responses have been evaluated as candidate markers for aggressive periodontitis. HLA-A9 and B15 have been consistently associated with aggressive periodontitis. Secondly several studies have shown that patients with aggressive periodontitis display functional defects of PMNs monocytes or both. These defects can impair chemotaxis and phagocytosis.

A hyper-responsiveness of monocytes from LAP patients with respect to production of PGE2 in response to lipopolysaccharide (LPS) has also been seen. This leads to increase connective tissue and bone loss. Poorly functional inherited forms of FcrRII which is the receptor for human IgG_2 antibodies have been found in patients with LAP.

Possible immune mechanisms include increased expression of MHC type II, HLA-DR4 altered helper or suppressor T-cell function, polyclonal activation of B cells by microbial plaque and genetic predisposition.

Genetic Factors

Several studies have shown that all individuals are not equally susceptible to aggressive periodontitis. Authors have shown a familial pattern of alveolar bone loss and have implicated genetic factors in aggressive periodontitis. Specific genes have not yet been identified, but segregation and linkage studies suggest the involvement of a major gene that is transmitted through an autosomal dominant pattern.

Also there is a genetic basis for immunologic defects. But it is unlikely that all patients with aggressive periodontitis have the same genetic defect.

Environmental Factors

Amount and duration of smoking are important variables that can influence extent of destruction. Patients with GAP who smoke have more affected teeth and more loss of clinical attachment than non-smokers with GAP. However, smoking may not have the same impact on attachment levels in patients with LAP.

Diagnosis

- Clinical diagnosis based on probing pocket depth, attachment loss, mobility
- Radiographic—LAP arc-shaped bone loss, around first molars; GAP serial radiographs to assess rate of destruction of bone.
- Microbiologic—sub-gingival plaque samples to culture microorganisms; antibiotic sensitivity testing.
- Immunological—done to test antibodies against *A.a.*

Treatment

Based on whether disease is localised or generalised and the degree of destruction present. If diagnosed early respond to standard periodontal therapy.

The following treatment modalities have been considered:

Extraction

- Teeth with hopeless prognosis have to be extracted.
- Transplantation of developing third molars to the sockets of previously extracted first molars has been attempted.

Standard Periodontal Therapy

It includes scaling, root planing, and flap surgery with or without bone grafts, root amputation, hemi-sections, occlusal adjustments and strict plaque control.

Antibiotic Therapy

- In the late 1970s and 1980s the identification of *A.a.* as a major culprit and the discovery that this organism penetrates tissues has formed the basis for therapy.
- LAP can be treated with scaling root planing (SRP) and tetracycline 250 mg four times for 14 days, every 8 weeks for up to 18 months.
- If surgery indicated systemic tetracycline should be prescribed to be taken 1 hour before surgery.
- Chlorhexidine mouth rinses to aid mechanical plaque control.
- Local delivery systems can be used in the localised form of the disease.
- Advantages of this are the smaller dosage required and the reduced side effects associated with systemic antibiotic therapy.
- Antibiotic sensitivity testing is required for cases which are refractory to treatment.
- Based on cultured organisms the antibiotic regimen can be given.
- When the microflora consists of Gram positive organisms: Augmentin (Amoxicillin 250 mg and K clavulanate 125 mg) is given TID for 14 days along with SRP.
- This can be combined with intrasulcular full mouth lavage with 10% povidone-iodine solution.
- Patient's positive for bacteroides in the absence of *A.a.* and *E. corrodens* can be treated with metronidazole 500 mg 3 times a day for 7 days.
- Clindamycin HCl 150 mg QID for 7 days with SRP can also be used.

- It should be used with caution due to the possibility of occurrence of pseudomembranous colitis.
- Azithromycin can be used for patients positive for *P. gingivalis.*
- Combination antibiotic therapy can be used and has been shown to be more effective since no single antibiotic is bactericidal to all microorganisms.
- Combinations of metronidazole/augmentin
- Metronidazole/ciprofloxacin for treatment of recurrent cases.
- Amoxicillin/doxycycline also used.
- Another approach is the use of host modulation therapy using sub-antimicrobial doses of non-steroidal anti-inflammatory drugs (NSAIDs) in conjunction with conventional therapy.
- Low dose doxycycline controls the activity of MMPs.
- Other agents such as flurbiprofen, indomethacin and naproxen may reduce inflammation.

Other Adjuncts

Other than Scaling and Root Planing, Oral Hygiene Instructions, antibiotic therapy both local and systemic other treatment requirements would include

Occlusal Adjustments

- Migration and drifting of teeth is a late characteristic of aggressive periodontitis.
- Premature contacts should be relieved using selective grinding.
- After successful periodontal therapy when the condition is stable gentle orthodontic retraction of labially drifted incisors can be considered.

Prosthetic Management

- Any partial dentures should be carefully designed to avoid further gingival irritation.
- Abutment teeth should be loaded as near axially as possible.
- Chrome cobalt dentures are usually indicated.
- Acrylic dentures should be used only in the immediate replacement phase.

Maintenance

Patients should be recalled every 3 months for Oral Hygiene reinforcement and scaling.

CHAPTER 30

AIDS and Periodontium

Question 1

What are the oral manifestations of human immuno-deficiency syndrome (HIV) infection?

Answer

Oral lesions in HIV infected patients are very common. Commonly associated oral manifestation seen in HIV infected patients are:

- Oral hairy leucoplakia.
- Oral candidiasis.
- Kaposi's sarcoma.
- Bacillary (epithelioid) angiomatosis.
- Oral hyperpigmentation.
- Atypical ulcers and delayed healing.

Oral Hairy Leucoplakia

- It is commonly seen in patients with HIV infection.
- Site of infection is generally lateral borders of tongue, commonly bilaterally distributed and sometimes may extend to the ventrum. Sometimes it also affects dorsum of tongue, buccal mucosa, floor of mouth, retromolar area and soft palate.
- Characterised clinically by asymptomatic, poorly demarcated keratotic areas ranging from few millimetres to several centimetres. Often, vertical striations are seen which give it a corrugated appearance. Sometimes. surface is shaggy and gives a hairy appearance.
- The lesion does not rub off and resembles other keratotic oral lesions.
- Candidal infections are secondary to this and colonies can be seen on surface of the lesion.
- Microscopically, hyperkeratotic surface with projection that resemble hair.

- Below parakeratotic surface, acanthosis and balloon cells resembling koilocytes are seen.
- These cells contain virus particles of herpes group and Epstein-Barr virus.

Differential Diagnosis

- Dysplasia, lichen planus, carcinoma, tobacco-related leucoplakia, frictional and idiopathic keratotis, psoriasiform lesions and hyperplastic candidiasis.
- Microscopic confirmation of oral hairy leucoplakia serves as an indicator that patient will develop AIDS.
- Severity of lesion is not correlated with chances of developing AIDS, thus small as well as extensive lesion are diagnostically significant.

Oral Candidiasis

- It is a fungal infection which is associated with Candida albicans.
- It is the most common oral lesions and is seen in 90% of AIDS patients.
- It is of four types:
  1. **Pseudomembranous candidiasis:** It is also known as oral thrush. It is a white lesion that can be easily scraped and removed from oral mucosa. Commonly seen on hard and soft palate, and buccal and labial mucosa.
  2. **Erythematous candidiasis:** It is a pseudomembranous type lesion. Appears as red patches on buccal and palatal mucosa. May be associated with depapillation of the tongue.
  3. **Hyperplastic candidiasis:** Least common form. Seen on tongue and buccal mucosa. It is resistant to removal.
  4. **Angular cheilitis:** Commissures are erythematous with crusting and fissuring of surface.

- ❑ Microscopically, smear of lesion is obtained by scraping the lesion and viewed in a microscope. The lesion shows hyphae and yeast forms of organisms.
- ❑ Candidiasis in HIV infected patients respond to antifungal treatment but is refractory and recurs within 4 weeks to 3 months due to the decrease in immunocompetency of the individual.

Kaposi's Sarcoma

- ❑ Kaposi's sarcoma is generally a rare, multifocal, slow-growing malignant vascular neoplasm.
- ❑ However, in AIDS patient, it is an aggressive lesion and is reported in almost 70% of the patients affecting oral mucosa mainly palate and gingiva.
- ❑ In early stages, the oral lesions are painless, reddish purple macules of the oral mucosa.
- ❑ As the lesion progress, they become nodular. It manifests as modules, papules, or non-elevated macules generally brown, blue or purple in colour.
- ❑ Microscopically, formed of four components— (1) endothelial cell proliferation with atypical vascular channels, (2) extravascular haemorrhage with hemo-siderin deposition, (3) spindle-cell proliferation with atypical vessels and (4) mononuclear inflammatory infiltrate formed mainly of plasma cells.

Differential Diagnosis

Pyogenic granuloma, atypical hyperpigmentation, sarcoid-osis, angiosarcoma, haemangioma, bacillary angiomatosis, pigmented nevi and cat scratch disease.

Bacillary (Epithelioid) Angiomatosis

Bacillary angiomatosis (BA) is an infectious vascular proliferative disease similar to Kaposi's sarcoma clinically and histologically.

Aetiology

- ❑ Rickettsia-like organisms, Bartonella henselae, Bartonella quintana, etc.
- ❑ Clinically, BA appears as red, purple or blue oedematous soft tissue lesion which causes destruction of periodontal ligament and bone.
- ❑ Differentiation of BA from Kaposi sarcoma is done by biopsy, which shows an epithelioid proliferation of angiogenic cells with acute inflammatory cell infiltrate. Warthin-Starry silver stain reacts with causative organisms in the biopsy specimen.

Oral Hyperpigmentation

- ❑ There is an increased incidence of oral hyperpigmentation in HIV affected individuals. Pigmented areas appear as spots or striations on buccal mucosa, gingiva, palate or tongue.
- ❑ Pigmentation can be due to prolonged use of drugs, such as zidovudine, ketoconazole or clofazimine.

Atypical Ulcers and Delayed Healing

- ❑ Atypical ulcers in HIV infected individual are commonly associated with neoplasms, lymphoma, Kaposi sarcoma, squamous cell carcinoma, neutropenia.
- ❑ Klebsiella pneumoniae, Enterobacter cloacae and Escherichia coli have been seen causing ulcers in oral mucosa.
- ❑ Herpes simplex virus, varicella zoster virus, Epstein-Barr virus or cytomegalovirus have been retrieved from oral ulcers.

Management

- ❑ Neutropenia can be treated with recombinant human granulocyte colony stimulating factor.
- ❑ Prolonged oral ulcers can be managed using prednisone or thalidomide.
- ❑ Viral infection can be treated with zidovudine, trimethoprim-sulphamethoxazole or ganciclovir.

Question 2

What are the periodontal manifestations of HIV infection?

Answer

Periodontal manifestation of HIV infections are:

- ❑ **Linear gingival erythema:**
  - ○ This is characterised by persistent, linear, easily bleeding erythematous gingivitis.
  - ○ May serve as precursor to rapidly progressing necrotising ulcerative periodontitis (NUP).
  - ○ May be localised or generalised.
  - ○ May be limited to marginal tissue.
  - ○ Extends into attached gingiva in a punctuate or diffuse erythema.
  - ○ Extends into alveolar mucosa.
- ❑ **Necrotising ulcerative gingivitis (NUG):**
  - ○ Some reports have shown increase in incidence of NUG in HIV-infected patients.

- **Necrotising ulcerative stomatitis (NUS):**
  - It is characterised by necrosis of oral soft tissue and underlying bone.
  - It can occur alone or in conjunction with NUP.
  - Severe depression of CD4 immune cells is seen.
- **Necrotizing ulcerative periodontitis (NUP):**
  - Characterised by soft tissue necrosis, rapid periodontal destruction and inter-proximal bone loss.
  - Lesions are seen anywhere in dental arches and are generally localised to a few teeth.
  - Generalised NUP can be seen after marked CD4+ cell depletion.
  - Exposed bone undergoes necrosis and subsequent sequestration.
  - It is a severely painful condition and requires immediate treatment.

CHAPTER 31

Clinical Diagnosis

Question 1

Define wasting diseases. Discuss various wasting diseases.

Answer

According to Carranza "wasting is defined as any gradual loss of tooth substance characterised by deformation of smooth, polished surfaces, without regard to the possible mechanism of this loss".

Various wasting diseases are as follows:

- **Erosion:** It is also known as corrosion.
  - It is a wedge-shaped depression which is sharply defined in the cervical area of the facial region of the tooth.
  - It is caused due to intake of acidic or citrous foods.
- **Abrasion:** it is caused due to mechanical wear other than that of the mastication.
  - It causes saucer-shaped depression with a smooth shiny surface.
  - Most common cause is toothbrushing with an abrasive paste in a horizontal direction.
  - It is also caused by holding objects like pins in between the teeth.
- **Attrition:** It is the occlusal wear caused due to functional contacts with opposite teeth.
  - It is most commonly seen in bruxism patient.
- **Abfraction:** It is caused due to occlusion loads because of tooth flexure and mechanical microfractures and tooth substance loss in the cervical area.

Question 2

What are the grades of tooth mobility? Discuss the mechanism of tooth mobility and what are the factors causing tooth mobility?

Answer

Grades of tooth mobility are:

- **Normal mobility.**
- **Grade I mobility:** Slightly more than normal.
- **Grade II:** Moderately more than normal.
- **Grade III:** Severe mobility faciolingually and mesiodistally along with vertical depressibilty.

Mechanism of Tooth Mobility

Tooth mobility occurs in two stages:

1. In the initial stage the tooth moves within the confines of the periodontal ligament. It is due to viscoelastic distortion of the periodontal ligament (PDL) and redistribution of the PDL fluid, interbundle content, fibres.
2. In the secondary stage, there is elastic deformation of the alveolar bone in response to horizontal force.

Factors of Tooth Mobility

- Loss of tooth support.
- Trauma from occlusion.
- Extension of inflammation.
- Periodontal surgery.
- During pregnancy.
- Pathologic processes of the jaws.

Question 3

Discuss periodontal screening and recording system (PSR).

Answer

- It is a method of periodontal screening developed by American Academy of Periodontology and American Dental Association.
- It is a simple and fast method of periodontal screening.

- ❏ It is done with the help of a probe which has a 0.5 mm ball tip and is colour coded from 3.5–5.5 mm.
- ❏ Patient's mouth is divided into six sextants and each tooth is probed and examined at least six points around each tooth.
- ❏ The deepest finding is recorded in each sextant, along with other findings, according to the following codes:
  - ○ **Code 0:** In the deepest sulcus of the sextant the probes colour band remains completely visible.
    - ➤ Gingiva is healthy and no calculus is found.
  - ○ **Code 1:** The colour band is completely visible.
    - ➤ No calculus but slightly bleeding on gentle probing is seen.
  - ○ **Code 2:** The colour band is completely visible, there is bleeding on probing, supragingival or subgingival calculus and defective margins are found.
  - ○ **Code 3:** Colour band is partially submerged.
    - ➤ This suggests there is need of comprehensive periodontal examination.
  - ○ **Code 4:** Colour band completely disappears.
    - ➤ Comprehensive examination, charting and treatment planning are required.
  - ○ **Code * :** There is furcation involvement, tooth mobility, mucogingival problem or gingival recession.

CHAPTER 32

Radiographic Aids in the Diagnosis of Periodontal Diseases

LONG ESSAYS

Question 1

What are the various radiographic changes in periodontitis?

Answer

Radiographic changes in periodontitis are as follows:

1. Fuzziness and a break in the continuity of the lamina dura: The break in the continuity of the lamina dura either on the mesial or the distal aspect of the crest of the intendental septum are considered to be the earliest radiographic changes in periodontitis.
   - It is caused due to extension of gingival inflammation into the bone which causes reduction in calcified tissue at the margin of the septum and also causes widening of the vessel channel.
   - These changes depend a lot on the radiographic technique like angulation of the tube or placement of the film and on the anatomical variation such as thickness and density of the interdental bone and position of the adjoining teeth.
   - Therefore it can be concluded that the intact crestal lamina dura might be an indicator of periodontal health, whereas its absence lacks diagnostic relevance.
2. A wedge shaped radiolucent area is seen either on the mesial or distal aspect of crest of the septal bone.
   - This is caused due to resorption of the bone of the lateral aspect of the interdental septum, with an associated widening of the periodontal space.
3. Height of the interdental septum is reduced: when the destruction process extends across the crest of the interdental septum, the height of the bone is reduced.
4. Finger like radiolucent projection extend from the crest into the septum.
   - When there is deep extension of the inflammation into the bone, there is appearance of radiolucent projection into the interdental septum.

- There is an increase in bone resorption along the endosteal margins of the medullary spaces because of inflammatory cells and fluid, proliferation of connective tissue cells and increased osteoclasis.
- There are composite images of the partially eroded bony trabeculae which separates the radiopaque projection from the radiolucent spaces.
- Because of extension of inflammation and the resorption of bone, the height of the interdental septum gets reduced.

Radiographic Appearance of Interdental Craters

- Craters generally cannot be sharply demarcated from the rest of the bone, with which they blend gradually.
- They can be seen as irregular areas fo reduced radioopacity on the alveolar bone crests.
- Depth or morphology of the interdental craters cannot be depicted accurately on the radiograph.
- They sometimes appear as vertical defect.

Radiographic Appearance of Furcation Involvement

- Naber's probe makes the correct diagnosis of the furcation involvement.
- Following radiographic diagnostic criteria have been suggested to assist in the radiographic furcation detection :
1. If there is bone loss, specially adjacent to roots, then this slightest change in the furcation should be investigates clinically.
2. Diminished radio-density in the furcation area, in which outlines of bony trabeculae are visible suggests furcation involvement.
3. Furcation might be involved, if there is marked bone loss in relation to a single molar.

Radiographic Appearance of a Periodontal Abscess

- There is discreet area of radiolucency along the lateral aspect of the root.
- But, the radiographic picture is not very typical because of the following reasons:
1. Stage of the lesion: Early stages of acute periodontal abscess is extremely painful but there are no radiographic changes.
2. The extent of bone destruction and the morphologic changes of the bone.
3. The location of abscess: Lesion in soft tissue wall of periodontal pocket shows less radiographic changes as compare to lesions which are present deep into the supporting tissues.
- Therefore a clinical diagnosis is important along with a radiographic diagnosis, especially for a periodontal abscess.

Radiographic Appearance of Localized Aggressive Periodontitis

- Bone loss may be seen in the maxillary and mandibular incisor and or first molar areas, usually bilaterally and result in vertical, arc like destructive pattern.
- Loss of alveolar bone may be generalized, but is seen more in molars and incisors and less in premolar area.

Radiographic Changes of TFO

- Injury phase: In this phase, there is a loss of lamina dura along the apex, furcation marginal areas.
- Widening of PDL space is seen.
- Repair phase: There is widened PDL space which can be localized or generalised.
- Advanced traumatic lesion can lead to angular bone loss, along with marginal inflammation may lead to intrabony pocket formation.

Root resorption can be seen in cases of excessive forces like force by orthodontic appliances.

CHAPTER 33

Advanced Diagnostic Techniques

Question 1

What are the advancements in diagnostic techniques?

Answer

Advancements in diagnostic techniques can be divided into the following:

- Advances in clinical diagnosis.
- Advances in radiographic assessment.
- Advances in microbiological analysis.
- Advances in characterization of host response.

Advances in Clinical Diagnosis

- **Gingival temperature:** Periotemp probe enables the calculation of the temperature differential with a sensitivity of .1 degree centigrade between the probed pockets and subgingival temperatures.
- **Periodontal probing:** Florida probe system—this is an automated probe system consisting of probe handpiece, computer interface , foot switch, computer and digital read out:
  - The probe tip is .4 mm in diameter.
  - The measurements are made electronically and transferred to the computer when the foot-control switch is pressed.
  - This method combines the advantage of constant probing with precise electronic measurements, thus eliminating the potential errors.
  - This method has the disadvantage of lack of tactile sensitivity and underestimation of the probing depths.
- **Gingival bleeding:** Bleeding on probing is an indicator for the presence of an inflammatory lesion in the connective tissue:
  - Severity of bleeding increases within increase in size of inflammatory infiltrate.
  - Lack of bleeding indicates periodontal stability; however, this may not be true in heavy smokers.

Advances in Radiographic Assessment

- Conventional radiographs lack sensitivity and show positive readings only when about 30% of bone mass has been lost.
- Newer techniques of radiography are more sensitive and give a clear picture:
  - **Digital radiography:** This technique of radiography has an advantage over conventional radiographs as the radiographic image can be digitally stored or processed and enhanced thus, providing us real or almost real images.
  - **Subtraction radiography:** Relies on conversion of serial radiographs into digital images:
    - These images then can be superimposed and the resultant composite can be reviewed.
    - Studies have shown:
      - A high degree of correlation between changes in alveolar bone, determined by subtraction radiography and clinical attachment level changes in periodontal patients after therapy.
      - Small osseous lesions can be easily detected as compared to conventional radiographs.
      - It facilitates both qualitative and quantitative visualisation of minor density changes in bone.
    - Computer assisted densitometric image analysis (CADIA).
- In this technique, grey scale images are formed by converting the light transmitted through a radiograph with a help of a video camera.
- This technique has shown higher sensitivity and a high degree of reproducibility and accuracy.

Advances in Microbiological Analysis

Bacterial Culturing

In this technique, the plaque samples are cultivated in anaerobic conditions with the use of selective or non-selective media along with several biochemical and physical tests, allowing the identification of different putative pathogens.

Advantage

- Clinician can obtain relative and absolute count of cultured species.
- Clinician can also assess antibiotic susceptibility.

Disadvantage

- This method can only grow live bacteria; therefore, careful sampling and transport are essential.
- Some pathogens are fastidious (*Treponema pallidum* and *Treponema forsythus*), which are difficult to culture.
- These require sophisticated equipment and experienced personnel and is time consuming and expensive.

Immunodiagnostic Methods

- Immunologic assays employ antibodies that recognise specific bacterial antigens to detect microorganisms.
  - **Direct Immunofluorescent Assays (IFA):** These employ both monoclonal and polyclonal antibodies. These antibodies are then conjugated to a fluorescein marker which binds with bacterial antigen to form a fluorescent immune complex which can be detected under a microscope.
  - **Indirect Immunofluorescent Assays IFA:** This technique employs a secondary fluorescence conjugated antibody that reacts with primary antigen antibody complex.
  - **Cytoflorography or flow cytometry:** This technique helps in rapid identification of oral bacteria.
- In this technique bacterial cells are labelled from the patient's plaque sample with both species specific antibody and fluorescein-conjugated antibody.
- This suspension is then introduced into the flow cytometer which will separate the bacterial cells into single-cell suspension with the help of laminar flow through a narrow tube.
  - **Enzyme-linked Immunosorbent Assa:** In this technique enzymatically derived colour reaction is substituted as the label.
- The intensity of the colour is dependent on the concentration of the antigen and is red photometrically for quantification.

- Evalusite is a chair-side clinically diagnostic aid in which there is a linkage between antigen and membrane bound antibody to form an immunocomplex. This complex can be later revealed by a colorimetric evaluation.
  - **Latex Agglutination:** This is a simple immunologic assay based on binding of protein to latex.

DNA Probes

Probe are basically the nucleic acid molecule obtained from a specific microorganism, artificially synthesized and labelled for detection when placed with plaque sample.

- Hybridization is done for the production of a double stranded nucleic acid by pairing of complementary DNA strands.

This method is highly specific and can accurately detect the presence of target microorganism.

- **Checker board DNA DNA hybridization:** This technology uses whole genomic, digoxigenin-labelled DNA probes and facilitates rapid processing of large number of plaque samples with multiple hybridization up to 40 species of microorganisms in a single test.

Polymerase Chain Reaction

Polymerase Chain Reaction (PCR) is the most powerful tool for the amplification of genes and their RNA transcripts.

- The conventional PCR methods only provided qualitative information and therefore were of limited clinical use.
- Because of this drawback, newer methods have emerged which give quantitative information as well.

Advances in Characterising Host Response

Assessment of host response is the study of immunologic or biochemical mediators and methods that are recognised as part of individuals response to periodontal infections.

Sources of Samples

Potential sample sources are saliva gingival crevicular fluid (GCF), gingival crevicular cells, blood serum, blood cells and urine.

Components of GCF have been studied and can be divided into:

1. Host derived enzymes
2. Tissue break-down products
3. Inflammatory mediator

Host-Derived Enzymes

Various enzymes are released from host cells during initiation and progression of periodontal disease:

- **Aspartate aminotransferase (AST):** This enzyme is released from dead cells from a variety of tissues.

- ○ Marked elevation is seen in AST levels from GCF samples which are collected from the sites with severe gingival inflammation.
- ○ Periogard is a commercially available chair side test kit for measuring AST levels.
- ❑ **Alkaline phosphatase (ALP):** Studies have shown that concentration of this enzyme in GCF is significantly higher in diseased sites as compared to normal one.
- ❑ **Beta glucuronidase:** Studies have shown an elevated level of beta glucuronidase at sites with severe periodontal disease.
- ❑ **Elastase:** GCF collections from the sites with periodontitis have shown higher elastase activity.

Tissue Breakdown Products

Analysis of GCF, obtained from sites with periodontal infection, shows higher levels of hydroxyl proline (collagen breakdown) and glycosaminoglycans (matrix degradation).

- ❑ Presence of osteocalcin and type I collagen peptides are seen when there is loss of alveolar bone.

Inflammatory Mediators

Presence of cytokines like TNF alpha, IL-1 alpha, IL-1 beta, IL-6, and IL-8 in GCF are potential diagnostic markers.

- ❑ Increased PGE2 in GCF indicates active phase of periodontal destruction.

CHAPTER 34

Risk Assessment

LONG ESSAYS

Question 1

What is risk assessment? Discuss in detail its various components.

Answer

Risk is the probability that an individual will develop a specific disease in a given period. There are numerous components which define risk assessment.

Various risk elements are:

- Risk factors.
- Risk determinants.
- Risk indicators.
- Risk markers.

Risk Factors

They are the factors which when present increase the likelihood of development of a disease. They can be environmental, behavioural or biologic.

Exposure to risk factors can occur at a single point in time over multiple, separate points in time, or continuously.

Various risk factors are:

- **Tobacco smoking:** There is a direct relationship between smoking and development of periodontal disease. Smoking has a negative impact on response to therapy. Smokers show greater attachment loss.
- **Diabetes:** It is a well-established risk factor for periodontitis. Prevalence of periodontitis is significantly higher in patients with diabetes.
- **Pathogenic bacteria and microbial tooth deposits:** It has been well proven that accumulation of microbial plaque leads to periodontal diseases and if oral hygiene measures are taken properly then this situation can be reversed.

Risk Determinants (Background Characteristics)

This term is used for those risk factors that cannot be modified.

- **Genetic factors:** Some periodontal diseases show familial aggregation, e.g. localised and generalised aggressive periodontitis.
- **Age:** Prevalence and severity of periodontal disease increase with age.
- **Gender:** Various studies have shown that males have more loss of attachment than females because of higher levels of plaque and calculus.
- **Socio-economic status:** It has been seen that poor oral hygiene is related to lower socio-economic status.
- **Stress:** Incidence of necrotising ulcerative gingivitis increases during the period of stress. Studies have shown that emotional stress interferes with normal immune function and result is increased circulating hormone levels which have an effect on periodontium.

Risk Indicators

They are referred as probable or putative risk factors that have been identified in cross-sectional studies but not confirmed through longitudinal studies.

- **HIV/AIDS:** It has been reported that there is an increased susceptibility in periodontal diseases in patients having HIV/AIDS.
- **Osteoporosis:** It has been suggested that reduced bone mass in osteoporosis may aggravate the progression of periodontal disease.
- **Infrequent dental visits:** Infrequent visits to the dentists can increase the risk for periodontitis.

Risk Markers/Predictor

These do not cause the disease but still they are associated with increased risk for disease.

- **Previous history of periodontal disease:** It has been seen that patients with most severe existing loss of attachment are at the greatest risk for future loss of attachment.
- **Bleeding on probing:** It is the best clinical indicator of gingival inflammation. Absence of bleeding on probing is an excellent indicator of periodontal health.

Question 2

Enumerate the various clinical risk assessment for periodontal disease.

Answer

Demographic Data

- Age
- Duration of exposure to risk elements
- Post-menopausal women
- Evidence of aggressive disease
- Male gender
- Preventive practices
- Frequency of care
- Socio-economic status
- Dental awareness
- Frequency of care.

Medical History

- Diabetes.
- Tobacco smoking.
- HIV/AIDS.
- Osteoporosis.
- Stress.

Dental History

- Family history of early tooth loss.
- Genetic predisposition to aggressive disease.
- Previous history of periodontal disease..
- Frequency of dental care.

Clinical Examination

- Plaque accumulation.
- Microbial sampling for putative periodontal pathogens.
- Calculus.
- Bleeding on probing.
- Extent of loss of attachment.
- Plaque retentive areas in tooth.
- Anatomic factors in tooth.
- Restorative factors in tooth.

CHAPTER 35

Prognosis

Question 1

What is the definition of prognosis? What are various types of prognosis? Explain the factors that help in determining overall prognosis of a patient.

Answer

According to Carranza "prognosis is defined as the prediction of the probable course, duration and outcome of a disease based on the general knowledge of the pathogenesis of the disease and the presence of risk factors for the disease and the likelihood of its response to treatment." Prognosis is divided as follows:

- Overall prognosis (concerned with entire dentition).
- Individual tooth prognosis (determined after overall prognosis and is affected by it).

There are various kinds of prognosis:

- **Excellent prognosis:** In this type of prognosis, there is no bone loss, excellent gingival conditions, good patient cooperation, no systemic/environmental factors.
- **Good prognosis:** Any one or more of the following factors could determine good prognosis:
  - Adequate remaining bone support, possibilities to control aetiological factors and establish a maintainable dentition and adequate patient cooperation with no systemic/environmental factors.
- **Fair prognosis:** Any one or more of the following factors could suggest fair prognosis:
  - Less than adequate remaining bone support, some teeth mobility, grade I furcation involvement, acceptable patient cooperation and existence of limited systemic/environmental factors.
- **Poor prognosis:** One or more of the following suggests poor prognosis.
  - Moderate to advanced bone loss, tooth mobility, grades I and II furcation involvement, difficult to maintain areas, doubtful patient cooperation and presence of systemic/environmental factors.
- **Hopeless prognosis:** The following factors suggest hopeless prognosis:
  - Advanced bone loss, non-maintainable areas, extraction indicated, presence of systemic or environmental factor.
- **Questionable prognosis:** The following factors suggest questionable prognosis:
  - Advanced bone loss, grades I and II furcation involvements, tooth mobility, inaccessible areas and presence of systemic/environmental factors.

Factors for determination of prognosis are as follows:

1. Overall clinical factors.
2. Systemic/environmental factors.
3. Local factors.
4. Prosthetic restorative factor.

1. Overall clinical factors:
  - Patient age.
  - Disease severity.
  - Plaque control.
  - Patient compliance and cooperation.

2. Systemic/environmental factors:
  - Patient habits like smoking.
  - Systemic disease/condition.
  - Genetic factors.
  - Stress.

3. Local factors.
  - Plaque/calculus.
  - Sub-gingival restorations.
  - Anatomic variations/factors.
    - Short tapered roots with short curves.
    - Cervical enamel projections (CEP).
    - Enamel pearls.
    - Bifurcation ridges.

> Root concavities.
> Development groves.
> Furcation involvement.
> Tooth mobility.

4. Prosthetic/restorative factors:
- Abutment selection.
- Caries.
- Non-vital teeth.
- Root resorption.

1. Overall Clinical Factors

Patient Age

- In two patients with comparable connective tissue attachment and alveolar bone, prognosis is better in the older of the two.
- When compared within the older patient, the reparative process in a younger individual is more, the amount of bone loss in a span of few years is also more than the bone formed.
- The younger patient would normally be expected to have a greater reparative capacity, but the occurance of destruction is so much in a relatively short period, would exceed any naturally occurring periodontal repair.

Disease Severity

- Patients with a history of previous periodontal disease may be indicative of their susceptibility for future periodontal breakdown.

Prognosis is affected by following factors:
- Level of attachment.
- Pocket depth/endo-perio-relationship.
- Height of remaining bone.
- Types of defect.

1. **Level of attachment:** It means base of the pocket. Level of clinical attachment reveals the clinical extent of root surface devoid of periodontal ligament.
2. **Pocket depth:** A tooth with deep pockets and little attachment loss has better prognosis compared with one with shallow pockets and more attachment loss.
3. **Height of remaining bone:** Prognosis is poor in case of teeth with severe bone loss where there is no sufficient bone to support the tooth.
4. **Type of defect (horizontal or angular):** In case of horizontal bone loss, the prognosis depends upon the exciting bone because it is unlikely to regenerates significant amount of bone.
- In case of angular or infrabony defects, if the contour of the existing bone and the number of osseous walls

are favourable, chances of regeneration of bone after therapy to approximately the level of alveolar crust exist.
- When there is greater bone less on one tooth surface, the bone height on the less involved surfaces should be considered when determining prognosis.

Plaque Control

Active removal of plaque by the patient on a daily basis is critical to the success and prognosis of periodontal therapy.

Patient Compliance and Cooperation

- The prognosis of patients with gingival and periodontal involvement is critically dependent on the patient's attitude and desire to retain the natural teeth and willingness and ability to maintain good oral hygiene.
- If patients are unwilling to perform adequate plaque control, or follow justification and receive timely periodic, maintenance check-ups, then the dentist can refuse to accept the patient for treatment or extract teeth that have a poor prognosis and perform routine oral prophylaxis on remaining teeth.

2. Systemic and Environmental Factors

Genetics

Detection of genetic factors can influence the prognosis in several ways:
- Early implementation of preventive and treatment measures for these patients.
- During the course of treatment, it can influence treatment recommendations.
- Identification of young individuals at risk can lead to the development of interventional strategies.

Patient Habits: (Smoking)

- It is one of the most important environmental risk factors putting an impact on the development and prognosis of periodontal disease.
- Systemic effects of smoking are inhibition of peripheral blood and oral neutrophil function, reduced antibody production and alteration of peripheral immunoregulatory T-cells.
- Patients who smoke, respond very poorly to the periodontal therapy.
- Cessation of smoking can affect the treatment outcome and also the prognosis.

Systemic Disease and Condition

- Patients systemic background can affect overall prognosis in several ways for e.g. in diabetes mellitus, the prognosis is questionable when surgical treatment is required.

❑ Diseases which affect the motor functions like Parkinson's disease limit these oral hygiene performances adversely affecting prognosis.

Stress

Stress can be physical or emotional and may alter the patient's ability to respond to the periodontal treatment performed.

3. Local Factors

❑ Plaque/calculus.
❑ Sub-gingival restorations.
❑ Anatomic variations/factors.

❑ **Plaque/calculus:** Plaque and calculus are the factors which cause periodontal disease. A good prognosis in most of cases depends on the ability of both patient and the clinician to remove these factors.

❑ **Sub-gingival restorations:** Supragingival margin of the restorations are always better than sub-gingival margins, as sub-gingival margins may contribute to increased plaque retention, which further causes inflammation and bone loss.

Therefore supragingival margins have good prognosis than sub-gingival margins.

❑ **Anatomic factors:**
  ○ Short tapered roots with short crowns:
    ➢ Prognosis is very poor in such cases because of poor periodontal health as there is a very less available root surface.
  ○ CEPs (Cemento enamel projections):
    ➢ They are ectopic enamel projections extending beyond the normal cementoenamel junction (CEJ).
    ➢ Most commonly seen on the mandibular molars and rarely on maxillary premolars.
    ➢ Tooth having CEPs also have a poor prognosis as they can be sources of plaque accumulation.
  ○ Enamel pearls
    ➢ Enamel peals are round, large enamel deposits that are present in the furcation areas.

➢ Commonly seen in maxillary third molars and rarely on the permanent molars.
➢ They also lead to plaque accumulation causing periodontitis.
  ○ Bifurcation ridges
    ➢ These bifurcation ridges interfere with the attachment apparatus and prevent regenerative procedures from achieving their potential.
  ○ Root concavities
    ➢ Root concavities creates areas which are difficult to maintain and cause plaque accumulation leading to inflammation.
  ○ Developmental grooves
    ➢ Palatogingival groove is a developmental groove seen most commonly on maxillary lateral incisors and maxillary central incisors.
    ➢ These grooves start from enamel and extend to some distance of the root, making it a plaque retentive area.
    ➢ Attachment apparatus is absent in the region of developmental grooves, therefore a zone is created for bacterial entry and also periodontal regenerative procedures are difficult to perform.
  ○ Tooth mobility
    ➢ Pockets in a non-mobile tooth responds well as compare to pocket in a mobile tooth.
    ➢ If the mobile teeth are splinted, they may have a beneficial effect on the overall and individual prognosis of the tooth.

4. Prosthetic/Restorative Factors

❑ Abutment selection.
❑ Caries.
❑ Non-vital teeth.
❑ Root resorption.

❑ **Abutment selection:** If the bone levels and attachment levels of the tooth are adequate then the prognosis of that tooth is good.

❑ **Caries, non-vital and root resorption:** Carious, non-vital and teeth with root resorption have poor prognosis. Therefore, these teeth should be treated before any periodontal therapy.

CHAPTER 36

Rationale for Periodontal Treatment

SHORT ESSAYS

Question 1

Explain healing after periodontal therapy.

Answer

Healing processes are almost same for all the forms of periodontal therapy, which consist of removal of diseased tissue and replacement of destroyed tissue.

Various techniques to gain attachment and bone level are as follows:

- ❑ **Regeneration:** It is the natural renewal of a structure, produced by growth and differentiation of new cells and intercellular substances to form new tissues.
  - ○ Regeneration is part of healing and it is a continuous physiologic process.
  - ○ It happens by growth from the same type of tissue.
  - ○ Bacteria and plaque hinders regeneration process whereas their removal would be beneficial for regeneration process.
- ❑ **Repair:** It restores the continuity of the diseased marginal gingiva and re-establishes a normal gingival sulcus at the same level on the roots as the base of the pre-existing periodontal pocket.
  - ○ It can halt the disease process but will not form new bone or periodontal ligament.
- ❑ **New attachment:** It is the formation of new periodontal ligament into cementum and the attachment of gingival epithelium to a tooth surface previously denuded by diseases.
- ❑ **Reattachment:** It means repair in areas not previously exposed to disease, e.g. surgical attachment of tissues.

CHAPTER 37

Periodontal Treatment for Medically Compromised Patients

Question 1

What is the management of a patient with cardiovascular diseases?

Answer

Hypertension

- Epinephrine concentration with local anaesthesia (LA) t1 : 1,000,000 should be given.
- If blood pressure (BP) extending more than180/110, then only emergency care should be given prior consultation with physician.
- Frequent change of position should be done to avoid postural hypertension.

Ischeamic Heart Diseases

- Angina pectoris—stress induced, nitroglycerine should be administered as an emergency.
- Myocardial infarction (MI) n frequent episodes of MI, dental treatment should be deferred for 6 months.

Congestive Heart Failure

- Uncontrolled disease not ideal for treatment.
- In case of orthopnoea (inability to breathe unless in upright position), chair position should be adjusted.
- Short stress free visit should be made.
- Profound anaesthesia should be given.

Cardiac Pacemakers and Cardioverter Defibrillators

- Dental consultation should check the underlying cardiac status.
- Older pacemakers—unipolar/unshielded.
- Newer pacemakers—bipolar, electrical.
- Dental equipment should not interfere with the functioning of cardiac pacemakers. For example, in cases of ultrasonic scalars.

Infective Endocarditis

It is caused by Streptococcus viridans, Capnocytophaga, etc.

American Heart Association Guidelines

Antibiotic prophylaxis should be given for procedures associated with bleeding from soft/hard tissues, periodontal surgery, scaling and professional tooth cleaning.

Indications for Prophylaxis

High-risk Patients:

- Previous history of endocarditis.
- Prosthetic heart valves.
- Congenital heart disease.

Moderate-risk Patients:

- Rheumatic heart disease.
- Mitral valve prolapse .
- Prophylaxis not recommended.
- Mitral valve prolapses without valvular or regurgitation.
- Coronary artery bypass graft (CABG) surgery.
- Cardiac pacemaker and implanted defibrillator.
- Patent ductus arteriosus (PDA)/ventricular septal defect (VSD).
- Standard regimens.

Oral

- Amoxicillin 2 g 1 hour before procedure
- Clindamycin/azithromycin/cephalexin 600 mg/500 mg/ 2 g 1 hour before V
- Ampicillin 2 g IM/IV within 30 minutes before procedure.

Preventive Measures for Infective Endocarditis

- ❑ Careful history should be taken
- ❑ Meticulous oral hygiene maintenance (gentle brushing and oral rinses) should be advocated so as to avoid bleeding and bacteraemia
- ❑ Antibiotic prophylaxis to be alternated with other antibiotic for periodontal therapy
- ❑ Reduce the number of visits and avoid developing resistant bacteria plan multiple procedures
- ❑ 7–14 days interval should be there between two visits
- ❑ Absorbable sutures should be used
- ❑ Recall visits are very important.

Stroke

Post-stroke Management

- ❑ No periodontal therapy should be given for 6 months
- ❑ Short stress-free appointments should be kept with 1:100,000 concentration of epinephrine with anaesthetic.
- ❑ Adjust oral anticoagulant doses with physician if any procedure is to be performed involving bleeding,
- ❑ Regular BP monitoring should be done.

Question 2

What are the steps in managing a patient with diabetes?

Answer

Steps in managing a patient with diabetes:

- ❑ If possible surgical treatment should be done at glycosylated less that 10%.
- ❑ In office blood glucose evaluation should be performed.
- ❑ Long procedures should be avoided.
- ❑ Long procedures demand checking for hypoglycaemia.
- ❑ If symptoms of hypoglycaemia arise, then oral carbohydrate/IV (20–30 mL of 50% dextrose)/IM/IV 1 mg glucagon should be given immediately.

Question 3

What is the management of a patient with renal disease?

Answer

In a patient with renal disease following should be done:
- ❑ Physician consent.
- ❑ Blood pressure (BP).
- ❑ Laboratory values for partial thromboplastin time (PTT), prothrombin time (PT), bleeding time (BT), CT, haematocrit.
- ❑ No treatment if blood urea is less than 60 mg/dL, serum creatinine < 1.5 mg/dL.
- ❑ Remove oral infection focus.

- ❑ Good ora l hygiene, frequent recall, poor prognosis teeth to be extracted.
- ❑ Avoid nephrotoxic drugs/those metabolised by kidney, e.g. tetracycline, aminoglycoside, etc.
- ❑ A dialysis patient should be screened for Hepatitis B and C.
  - ○ Heparin anticoagulation given prior to dialysis, hence wait for periodontal treatment.
  - ○ Renal transplant patients who are on immunosuppressive drugs have reduced resistance to infection, hence teeth with septic focus/periodontally involved should be extracted.

Question 4

What is the management of a patient having bleeding disorder?

Answer

Firstly, history of bleeding should be recorded, past and present drug history and family history, etc. should be done.

Clinical Examination

Jaundice, haemarthrosis, ecchymosis, petechiae, spontaneous gingival bleeding, gingival hyperplasia should be checked.

Laboratory tests like BT, CT, tourniquet test, complete blood count (CBC), PT, PTT should be done.

Bleeding disorder can be coagulation disorder (heredity/acquired), thrombocytopenic purpura (TCP).

Heredity Defect

- ❑ Haemophilia A (factor 8)
  - ○ Factor 8 levels = 30%, are desirable to prevent surgical haemorrhage.
  - ○ (Desmopressin) increases levels 2–3 folds.
- ❑ Haemophilia B (factor 9) desirable levels 30–50%.
  - ○ Factor 9 concentrates or purified prothrombin concentrates are given.
- ❑ Von Willebrands disease (vWf factor).
  - ○ Factor 8 concentrates/cryoprecipitate, desmopressin.
- ❑ Probing, scaling may be undertaken but local anaesthesia administration, surgery demands medical modification.
- ❑ Complete wound closure is extremely important.
- ❑ Pressure application, anti-haemostatic agent administration, anti-fibrinolytic (EACA/tranexamic acid).

Acquired Coagulation Defect

- ❑ Liver disease (chronic alcoholics, chronic hepatitis).
- ❑ Vitamin K deficiency (anticoagulants—warfarin vitamin K antagonist)

❑ Look for:
  ○ Physician consent.
  ○ Laboratory test—PT, BT, CBC, PTT.
  ○ Prefer nonsurgical periodontal therapy.
❑ If surgery warranted—platelet count should be minimum 80,000/mm3, international normalised ration (INR) less than 2.
  ○ INR 2–3 anticoagulant therapy patients.
  ○ INR 2.5–3.5 for prosthetic valves patients.
  ○ Infiltration, scaling and root planing INR less than 3.
  ○ Extraction / minor surgery INR less than 2–2.5.
  ○ Complex surgery/multiple extraction INR less than 1.5–2.
❑ Severity of expected intra/post-postoperative.
❑ Bleeding to be informed to physician while planning to adjust INR.
❑ Aspirin more than 325 mg demands discontinue drug 7–10 days prior with physician consent.
❑ Avoid aspirin in patients with anticoagulant therapy/bleeding disorder.

Thrombocytopenic Purpura

If platelet less than 100,000/mm^3—no treatment should be done.

Leukaemia

❑ Delayed healing, prone to infection, bleeding tendency, chemotherapy effects

❑ Blood profile (BT, CT, PT, platelet count)
❑ Antibiotic cover should be given prior to treatment
❑ hopeless teeth extract 10 days prior to chemotherapy
❑ Routine prophylaxis, oral rinses, topical haemostatics should be given
❑ Oral candidiasis is very common therefore nystatin suspension (100,000 units/mL) should be given
❑ In cases of oral ulceration/mucositis, palliative viscous lidocaine should be given.

Question 5

What is the management of a pregnant female?

Answer

Management of a pregnant female:
❑ Conservative treatment should be given, i.e. basic oral care protocol, scaling and root planing
❑ Second trimester is safe time
❑ Long stressful appointment should be avoided
❑ Supine hypotensive syndrome is very common, which can be corrected by changing the chair position
❑ Place patient on her left side with 5–6 degrees of elevation on right side, frequent position change should be done
❑ American dental association (ADA) specification for drugs—cephalosporins, amoxicillin, clindamycin
❑ ADA guidelines for radiation exposure to be kept minimum, if required proper shielding for mother.

LONG ESSAYS

Question 1

What is treatment plan? What is the goal of treatment plan? What are the phases of periodontal therapy?

Answer

Blue print for case management is referred to as treatment plan.

Goal of treatment plan is to eliminate gingival inflammation and correction of the condition that cause or perpetuate it.

Phases of Periodontal Therapy Are

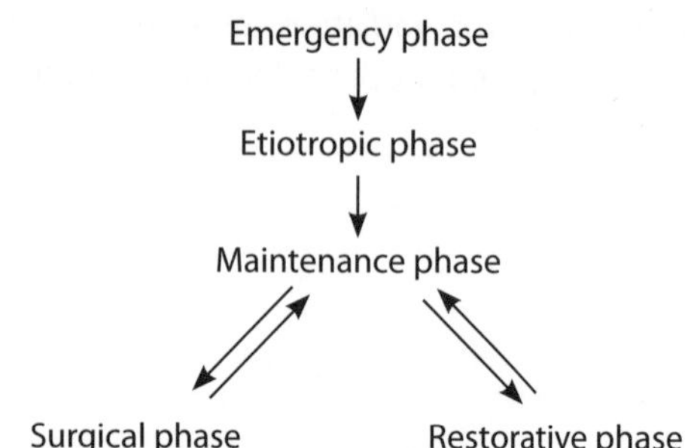

Emergency Phase/Preliminary Phase

- Treatment of Emergencies
- Dental or periapical
- Periodontal
- Other

Hopeless teeth are extracted and provisional replacement is given if needed.

Etiotropic Phase (also known as phase I therapy)

Plaque Control and Patient Education

- Diet control, especially in patients with rampant caries.
- Calculus removal and root planing.
- Correction of restorative and prosthetic irritational factors.
- Excavation of caries and restoration. It can be temporary or final, depending on whether definite prognosis for the tooth has been arrived at and on the location of caries.
- Anti-microbial therapy (local or systemic).
- Occlusal therapy.
- Minor orthodontic movement.
- Provisional splinting and prosthesis.

The patient should be evaluated for the response after aetiotropic phase for:

- Packed depth and gingival inflammation
- Plaque, calculus and caries.

Surgical Phase

This phase is also known as *Phase II therapy*. It includes periodontal therapy, including placement of implant and endodontic therapy.

Restorative Phase

This phase is also known a *Phase III therapy*. It includes final restoration, fixed and removable prosthodontics.

Evaluation should be done in response to restorative procedures by performing periodontal examination.

Maintenance Phase

Maintenance phase (*Phase IV therapy*), it includes periodic rechecking of:

- Plaque and calculus.
- Gingival condition (pockets, inflammation).
- Occlusion, tooth mobility.
- Other pathologic changes.

CHAPTER 39

Phase I Periodontal Therapy

LONG ESSAYS

Question 1

What are the objectives, rationale and steps in Phase I periodontal therapy.

Answer

It is the first step of the periodontal therapy. Phase I periodontal therapy is also known as initial therapy, nonsurgical periodontal therapy, etiotropic phase of therapy and cause relative therapy.

The objectives of this therapy are to eliminate or alter the microbial etiology and the contributing factors for gingival and periodontal diseases.

Rationale

The rationale is complete removal of calculus, correction of defective restorations, treatment of carious lesion and restoration and a comprehensive daily plaque control regime for reduction and elimination of etiologic and contributing factors.

The procedures in phase I therapy are required to solve the patients periodontal problems or may contribute in the preparatory phase of the surgical therapy.

Long term success of the periodontal treatment depends upon the maintenance of the results achieved by Phase I therapy.

Control or elimination of local contributing factors includes the following therapies:

- Complete removal of calculus
- Correction or replacement of poorly fitting restorations and prosthetic devices
- Restoration of carious lesion
- Treatment of food impaction areas
- Treatment of occlusal trauma
- Orthodontic tooth movement
- Extraction of hopeless teeth.

Treatment Sessions

Upon the analysis and diagnosis of the case, the clinician determines the treatment plan for scaling and root planing portion of phase I therapy. However, many patients require several treatment sessions for tooth surface debridement along with amount of calculus visualised, following conditions should also be considered in planning of Phase I periodontal therapy:

- General health and tolerance of patient towards treatment
- Number of teeth present
- Amount of sub-gingival calculus
- Probing pocket depth and attachment loss
- Furcation involvement
- Alignment of teeth
- Margins of restorations
- Developmental anomalies
- Physical barriers to access like limiting opening or gag tendencies.

Sequence of Procedures

- **Step 1:** Limited plaque control instructions
- **Step 2:** Supragingival removal of calculus
- **Step 3:** Recontouring defective restoration and crowns
- **Step 4:** Obturation of carious lesions
- **Step 5:** Comprehensive plaque control instructions
- **Step 6:** Sub-gingival root treatment
- **Step 7:** Tissue re-evaluation.

Results

It has been seen that comprehensive scaling and root planing causes reduction in bleeding on probing and probing depth. Also, caries control and correction of poorly fitting restorations, only augment the positive results of healing gained by plaque control, scaling and root planing.

Healing

About 4 weeks after the completion of phase I therapy, re-evaluation of the case should be done, as this time period permits for epithelial and connective tissue healing and allows the patient to sufficiently practice the oral hygiene instructions.

Gingival inflammation is also reduced substantially within 3–4 weeks after removal of plaque and calculus.

Transient tooth hypersensitivity and recession of gingival margins are seen with the process of healing.

Histologically, there is formation of long junctional epithelium rather than new connective tissue attachment to the root surface. The attachment epithelium reappears within 1–2 weeks.

With decrease in inflammation there is reduction in inflammatory cell population and gingival crevicular fluid (GCF).

CHAPTER 40

Plaque Control

Question 1

Define dental plaque and write in detail about antiplaque and anticalculus agents.

Or

Describe in detail about chemical plaque control.

Answer

Dental plaque is defined clinically as a structured resilient yellow greyish substance that adheres tenaciously to the intraoral hard surfaces including removable and fixed restorations.

It is primarily composed of bacteria in a matrix of salivary glycoproteins and extracellular polysaccharides.

Antiplaque Agents

Idealsrequisites of antiplaque agent are:

- They should be able to reduce plaque and gingivitis to a significant leve
- They should prevent growth of pathogenic bacteria
- Should be biocompatible with the oral tissue
- Should be inexpensive and easy to use
- Should have good retention
- Should not stain teeth or alter taste.

Classification

First Generation

Triclosan

- It is a phenol derivative, non-ionic compound which is used as a topical antimicrobial agent
- It has a broad spectrum of action against both Gram-positive and Gram-negative bacteria
- It acts on the microbial cytoplasmic membrane and uses bacteriolysis

- It delays plaque maturation and inhibits formation of prostaglandins and leukotrienes

Metallic Ions

- Zinc and copper salts are most commonly use
- They act by reducing the glycolytic activity in microorganisms and inhibit bacterial growth.

Quaternary Ammonium Compounds

- These are antiseptics and surface active agents
- They are more effective against Gram positive rather than Gram negative organisms
- They are effective in reducing the development of plaque as it contains mainly Gram-positive microorganisms
- They act by disrupting the cell wall structure of microorganisms, e.g. benzethonium chloride, benzalkonium chloride and cetylpyridinium chloride.

Sanguinarine

- This is an alkaloid which is derived from a plant, *Sanguinaria canadensis*
- These inhibit mainly the Gram-negative organisms
- It has good retentive property when used as a mouth rinse.

Antibiotics

Vancomycin, erythromycin, neomycin and kanamycin are the commonly used antibiotics for plaque control.

Enzymes

- Examples are mucinase, dextranase, lactoperoxidase and thiocyanate synthase enzymes have shown bacterocidal activity when applied topically in the mouth.
- They are able to break down already formed matrix of plaque and calculus.

Second Generation

Bisbiguanides

- Example: 0.2% chlorhexidine gluconate
- It is a cationic bisbiguanide which has a very broad spectrum of action against a wide area of organisms including gram positive, Gram-negative, fungi, yeast, and viruses
- It shows both antiplaque and anti-bacterial action.

Antiplaque Action

Chlorhexidine: It shows antiplaque activity, because of the property of sustained availability that is chlorhexidine is slowly released form all oral surfaces resulting in bacteriostatic activity in oral cavity.

Chlorhexidine inhibits plaque by the following mechanisms:

- **Prevention of pellicle formation:** It blocks acidic groups on salivary glycoprotein thus reducing glycoprotein adsorption on tooth surface
- It binds to the bacteria thus preventing the adsorption of bacterial cell wall on tooth surface
- It displaces calcium from the plaque matrix thus preventing binding of mature plaque
- **Note:** Chlorhexidine prevents the formation of new plaque but has little effect on pre-existing plaque.

Antibacterial Action

- Exhibits a wide spectrum of activity against gram positive, Gram-negative bacteria, fungi, yeast and viruses.
- Chlorhexidine is bacteriostatic in low concentrations and bacterocidal in high concentrations
- After a single mouth rinse with chlorhexidine, saliva exhibits bacterocidal activity for 5shours and bacteriostatic activity for more than 12 hours.
- Regular use of chlorhexidine can reduce the aerobic andcanaerobic bacterial populations in saliva by 80–90%.

Indications

- In moderate to severe inflammation, as an adjunct to mechanical oral hygiene
- Post-periodontal therapy or oral surgical procedures
- Inyphysically, mentally and medically challenged individuals
- Patients undergoing fixed or removable orthodontic treatment
- In patients who have undergone intermaxillary fixation.

Adverse Effects of Chlorhexidine

- Reversible brownish staining of teeth or restorations
- Loss of taste sensation specially bitter and salt sensation
- Some individuals have reported hypersensitivity to chlorhexidine
- The dead bacteria due to use of chlorhexidine may act as the initiator for supragingival, calculus formation
- Can cause oral mucosal erosions when used in high concentrations.

Third Generation

Delmopinol

- It inhibits plaque growth and reduces gingivitis
- It targets dextran producing streptococci by blocking synthesis
- It reduces bacterial adherence by causing weak binding of the plaque to the tooth surface, thus aiding in easy removal by mechanical procedures
- It is used as a pre-brushing mouth rinse
- It can cause transient staining of tongue and teeth
- Taste alteration and mucosal erosions have also been reported.

Anticalculus Agents

Dentifrices containing soluble pyrophosphatase and zinc compounds demonstrate anticalculus effect by absorbing into small hydroxyapatite crystals, thus preventing or inhibiting growth of larger and organised crystals of calculus.

Dentifrices

According to American Dental Association (ADA), a dentifrice is a substance used with a toothbrush for the purpose of cleanin, accessible surfaces of the tooth.

Composition of the Dentifrice

- **Polishing/abrasive agents:** Calcium carbonate, dicalcium phosphate dihydrate, alumina, silica—15 to 45%
- They clean the teeth mechanically, remove pellicle form the tooth surface and abrasive action aids in eliminating plaque
- **Binding/thickening agents (2%):** They contain water soluble agents (alginates, sodium carboxy methyl cellulose) and water insoluble agents (magnesium aluminium silicate, colloidal silica, sodium magnesium silicate)
- These agents bind the solids to form homogenous paste and help in dispersion of dentifrice in mouth.
- **Detergents/surfactants (1–5%):** Sodium lauryl sulphate and sodium dodecyl sulphate. These agents produce foam, which aids in the removal of food debris. These also have antimicrobial property.

- **Humectants (25–40%):** Sorbitol, glycerine, polyethylene glycol. These help in maintaining the consistency of the paste and also prevent loss of moisture from paste.
- **Flavouring agents (1%):** Peppermint oil, spearmint oil, Oil of Wintergreen.
- **Sweeteners and colouring agents (2%):** Saccharin.
- **Water (20–30%):** Acts as vehicle and solvent medium.
- **Preservatives (0.5%):** Benzoic acid.
- **Therapeutic agents (2%):** Tetrasodium, pyrophosphatase, zinc chloride.

Functions of Tooth Pastes

- Removal of food debris, stains and plaque
- Anticaries action
- Mouthrfreshener
- Some tooth pastes are also used for treating sensitivity.

Question 2

Describe the various methods of plaque control or describe oral hygiene aids for plaque control.

Answer

Plaque control is the regular removal of dental plaque and the prevention of its accumulation on the teeth and adjacent gingival surfaces.

Plaque control can be broadly classified into *mechanical*—individual and professional, and *chemical*—individual and professional.

Mechanical Plaque Control

Individual Methods

- Toothbrush (manual or powered)
- Interdental aids- Floss, toothpicks, brushes
- Miscellaneous– Rubber tip stimulator or water irrigator.

Toothbrushes

ADA Specifications

- Head–11¼ inches long
- 24 rows of bristles
- 5/16–3/8 inches wide
- 5–12 tufts per row
- 80–86 bristles per tuft.
- Design–consist of handle, shank and head
  - **Available sizes:** Large medium and small.
- Bristle
  - Nylon (synthetic): Preferred
  - Hog (natural): Susceptible to breakage and fraying.
- Hardness
  - **Soft:** 0.007–0.009 inches (no. 7, 8, 9)
  - **Medium:** 0.010–0.012 inches (no. 10, 11, 12)
  - **Hard:** 0.013–0.014 inches (no. 13, 14)
  - **Extra hard:** 0.015 inches (no. 15).
- Handle design
  - Straight
  - Angulation in the shank
  - Indentation of handle for a better grip.

Interdental Cleaning Aids

These are used for the removal of plaque in interdental areas. The type of embrasure determines the selection of interdental aids:

- **Type 1:** Interdental papilla fills the embrasure. Dental floss is advised.
- **Type 2:** Mild-moderate papillary recession is observed. Miniature interdental brush and wooden tips are advised.
- **Type 3:** Complete loss of papilla and interdental gingiva is tightly bound to bone. Untufted brushes are advised.

Dental Floss

It is most common method for interdental plaque control.

These are of four types:

1. Twisted or non-twisted
2. Bonded or non-bonded
3. Thick or thin
4. Waxed or unwaxed.

Interdental Brushes

Cone shaped or lcylindrical shaped brushes mounted on a handle.

Two types:

1. Single tufted brushe
2. Small conical brushes.

These are used in furcation areas, isolated gingival recession area and on lingual surface of molars and premolars.

Wooden Tips

Two types:

1. With handle, e.g. perio-aid
2. Without handle, e.g. Stim U.

Chemical Plaque Control (*Refer Answer 1*)

Chemicals used of supragingival plaque control (Addy's Classification)

A. Antibiotics:
Penicillin
Vancomycin

Kanamycin
Erythromycin
Spiramycin
Metronidazole

B. Enzymes:
Mucinase
Protease
Lipase
Amylase
Elastase
Lactoperoxidase
Hypothiocynase
Mutanase

C. Quaternary ammonium compounds:
Cetylpyridinium chloride
Benzethonium chloride
Benzalkonium chloride
Domiphen bromide

D. Bisbiguanide:
Chlorhexidine
Alexidine
Octenidine/bispyridine

E. Metallic salts:
Copper
Tin
Zinc

F. Herbal extracts:
Sanguinarine

G. Fluorides
Strontium fluorid

H. Oxygenating agents:
Hydrogen peroxid

I. Phenolic compounds:
Thymol
Menthol
Eucalyptol

J. Othersantiseptics:
Iodine
Povidone Iodine
Sodium hypochlorite
Hexetidine
Triclosan.

Question 3

Describe modified Stillman technique.

Answer

Modified bass technique is a kind of brushing technique which is advocated very frequently.

Technique— the brush should be placed with bristles partly resting on cervical region of teeth and partly on gingiva.

- Bristles are pointed in apical direction with an oblique angle to the tooth long axis.
- Brush is moved in short back and forth motions and simultaneously moving into coronal direction
- Pressure is applied on the gingival margin to produce mild blanching
- The procedure is repeated on all the teeth
- Brush is held in the vertical direction in order to reach the lingual surfaces of maxillary and mandibular anteriors.

Question 4

Describe modified bass technique.

Answer

Bass Method

The head of the brush is placed parallel to occlusal plane covering 34 teeth beginning at the posterior region.

- Bristles are placed at an angulation of 45 degree to the long axis of the tooth along the gingival margin
- Gentle short back and forth movements are used without dislodging the tip of the bristles
- The pressure should be firm enough to blanch the gingiva
- Several strokes should be completed in the same position
- Move the brush to the adjacent teeth and the process is repeated
- After completing the maxillary arch, move mandibular arches
- In the lingual side of anteriors, the brush is held vertically.

Modified Bass

- It combines vibratory and circular motion of bass technique and the sweeping motion of roll technique
- Toothbrush is held to 45degrees to the gingival margin
- Brush is moved in back and forth motion while the bristles are gently vibrated
- In a single motion the brush is moved from side of the teeth to occlusal surface
- This method causes excellent sulcus cleaning and good gingival stimulation.

Question 5

What are disclosing agents?

Answer

These are commercially available solutions, wafers, tablets, lozenges which are capable of staining only bacterial deposits on the surface of teeth, tongue and gingiva.

Examples

- Skinners iodine solution
- Diluted tincture of iodine
- Mercurochrome solution 5%
- Bismarck brown
- Erythrosine
- Fast green
- **Two tone solutions:** FD and C Green number 3; FD and C Red number 3.

   This stains mature plaque in blue colour and immature plaque in red or pink colour.
- Basic Fuchsine.

Question 6

What is PerioChip/chlorhexidine chip?

Answer

It is method of local drug delivery. It is a commercially available local drug delivery system.

   This contains chlorhexidine in a biodegradable device

Advantage

- High concentrations can be achieved in an area with small drug dose
- Systemic side effects of chlorhexidine are reduced

- Antibiotics can also be combined through this chip
- It is area specific.

Question 7

Describe Proxabrush.

Answer

These are small interdental brushes which are indicated in type two embrasures.

   These are used as they provide effective cleaning of concave root depressions exposed due to interproximal gingival recession.

Question 8

Desensitising agents.

Answer

They are used to control tooth/root hypersensitivity.

   These act by reducing the diameter of dentinal tubules thus, limiting the displacement of fluid in them.

Examples

Cavity varnishes, dentin bonding agents, silver nitrate, restorative resins, zinc chloride, potassium ferrocyanide, calcium hydroxide, sodium fluoride, stannous fluoride, etc.

CHAPTER 41

Scaling and Root Planing

Question 1

What is the classification of periodontal instruments? Discuss periodontal probes in detail.

Answer

Classification of periodontal instruments is as follows:

- **Diagnostic instruments:** Includes mouth mirror, probe, explorer and tweezers.
  - **Periodontal probes:** Used to locate, measure and mark pockets.
  - **Explorers:** To locate calculus and caries.
- **Scaling, root planing and curettage instruments:** Used for removal of plaque and calcified deposits from the crown and root of a tooth, removal of altered cementum from the subgingival root surface and debridement of the soft tissue lining the pocket.

  Scaling and curettage instruments can be classified as follows:
  - **Sickle scaler:** They are heavy instrument which are used for the removal of supragingival calculus.
  - **Curettes:** They are fine instruments used for subgingival scaling, root planing and removal of soft tissue lining the pocket.
  - **Hoe-chisel file scaler:** They are the subgingival scalers used for removal of tenacious subgingival calculus and altered cementum. Curettes are used more commonly than these scalers.
  - **Ultrasonic and sonic instruments:** They are used for scaling and cleaning teeth and curetting the soft tissue wall of the periodontal pocket.
- **Periodontal endoscope:** It is used to visualise deeply into the subgingival pockets and furcations, which allow to detect deposits.
- **Cleansing and polishing instrument:** It is used to clean and polish tooth surfaces, e.g. rubber cups, brushes and dental tapes. They can be available in the form of air-powder abrasive system for tooth polishing.

Periodontal Probes

Periodontal probes are used to mark, measure and locate pocket and determine their configuration.

- Probe is a tapered, rod-like instrument which is calibrated in millimetres, with a blunt, rounded tip.
- They are generally thin, shank angled to allow easy insertion into the pocket.
- During measuring the pocket, probe should be held with a gentle firm pressure to the bottom of the pocket.
- The shank should be held parallel to the long axis of the tooth.

Characteristics of an Ideal Probe

According to National Institute of Dental and Craniofacial Research (NIDCR), an ideal probe should have the following criteria:

- Precision of 0.1 mm
- Range of 10 mm
- Constant and standardised probing force
- Non-invasive
- Light weight and easy to use
- Easy to access any location around all teeth
- Proper angulation through a guidance system
- Complete sterilisation of all portions entering the mouth
- Material should not be biohazardous
- No electric shock produced from the material
- Direct electronic reading and digital output.

Classification of Probes

Probes can be classified into five generations:

1. **First generation probes:** Conventional manual (hand-held probes). For Example- Williams probe.

2. **Second generation probes:** Pressure sensitive probes, e.g. true pressure sensitive probes.
   - 30 g of probing pressure is sufficient to determine the probing pocket depth.
   - 50 g of probing pressure is required to detect alveolar bone defects.

   These probes lack tactile sensitivity
3. **Third generation probes:** Computerised probes, e.g. Florida probe, Foster Miller probe and Toronto automated probes.

   Drawbacks of automated probes:
   - Tactile sensitivity is less
   - Patient discomfort is more
   - Expensive.
4. **Fourth generation probes:** They are still under development.
   - These probes, attempt to extend linear probing in a serial manner to take account of the continuous and three dimensional topography of the pocket being examined.
5. **Fifth generation probe:** Without penetrating, they aim at identification of attachment level.
   - They are non-invasive
   - E.g. ultrasound probes.

Various kinds of periodontal probes are as follows:

1. World Health Organisation (WHO) probe, which has a 0.5 mm ball at the tip and millimetres markings at 3.5, 8.5 and 11.5 mm and colour coding from 3.5 mm to 5.5 mm.
2. University of Michigan "O" probe, with William marking at (1, 2, 3, 5, 7, 8, 9 and 10 mm) and marking absent form 4 and 6.
3. **UNC-15 probe:** It is a 15 mm long probe with millimetre marking at each millimetre and colour coding at the fifth, tenth and fifteenth millimetres.
4. **Marquis colour coded probe:** In this probe, the calibrations are in 3 mm section.
5. **Nabers probes:** They are used to detect furcation areas. They are colour coded at 3, 6, 9 and 12 mm marking.
6. **Florida probes:** It is a force sensitive probe.
7. **Foster Miller probe:** This probe detects CEJ automatically. It regarded as a highly accurate reading probe. It has a SD of 0.17 mm and a subject threshold of 0.51 mm.
8. **Toronto automated probe:** It measures clinical attachment levels using occluso incisal surface.
9. **Interprobe:** It has an optical encode transduction element.

Uses of a probe are as follows:

- Most, measure and locate the depth of gingival sulcus and pockets.
- Measures gingival recessions
- Used to measure attached gingiva
- Determines the mucogingival relationship
- Used to check bleeding on probing
- Used for bone sounding or transgingival probing
- Measures the thickness of gingiva
- Can identify tooth irregularities, tissue characteristics, calculus, etc.

Describe sickle scaler in detail.

They are the supragingival scalers which have a blade, handle and connecting shank (**Fig. 41.1**).

- They have a flat surface with two cutting edges which converges of a sharp pointed tip.
- They have two lateral surfaces and one face of the blade.
- Lateral surface and face of the blade join together to form cutting edge (**Fig. 41.2**).
- It is mainly used to remove the supragingival calculus.
- Since its design is large, thus it becomes very difficult to place this instrument subgingivally, without lacerating the gingiva.
- Small, curved sickle scaler blades such as 204SD can be inserted under ledges of calculus a few millimetres below the gingiva.

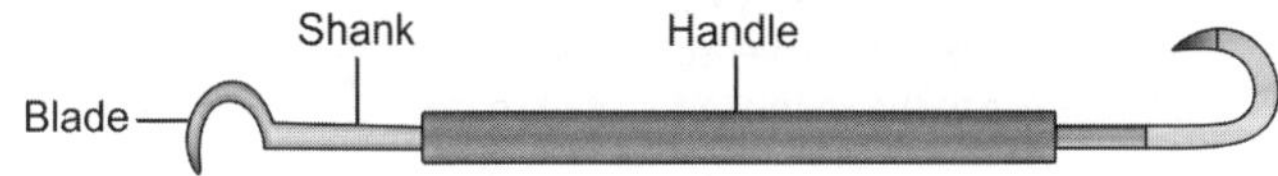

Fig. 41.1: Parts of a sickle scaler.

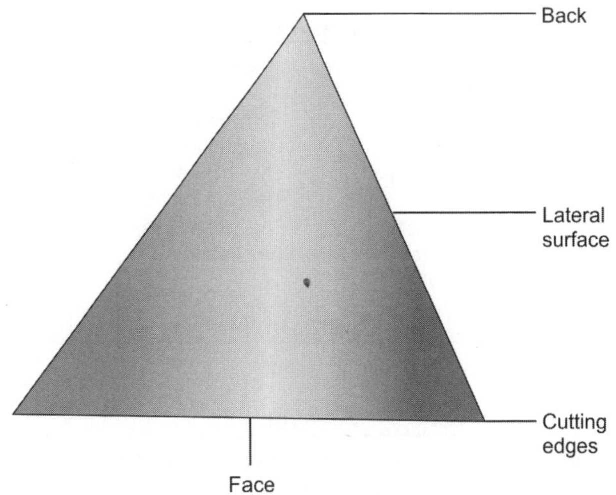

Fig. 41.2: Cross section of a blade of a sickle scaler .

- These scalers are used with a pull stroke.
- Sickle scalers come with different blade size and shanks, but having the same basic pattern.
- For example U15/30, Ball, and Indiana University sickle scalers are large in size, whereas jaquette sickle scalers 1, 2, and 3 have medium blade.
- Curved 204 sickle scalers are available with large, medium or small blade.
- Nevi 2 posterior scaler is thin enough so that it can be inserted several millimetres subgingivally to remove ledges of calculus moderately.
- Sickle scalers can have straight shanks used to scale anterior teeth and premolars.
- Sickle scalers can also have contra angled shank so that it can be adapted to posterior teeth.

Question 3

What are the differences between Gracey curette and universal curette?

Answer

Gracey Curette	Universal Curette
• There are area specific curettes that are used at specific areas.	• They can be used on all areas and surface.
• Only one cutting edge in used, work with outer edge only.	• Both cutting edges can be used, works with either outer or inner edge.
• It is curved in two planes, blade, curves up and to the side.	• Curved in one plane, blade curves up and not to the side.
• They have an offset blade, i.e. the face of the blade is bevelled at 60 degrees to the shank.	• Blade is not offset, i.e. face of the blade is bevelled at 90° to the shank.

Question 4

What are the differences between a scaler and a curette?

Answer

Scaler	Curette
• Scalers are used for supragingival scaling.	• Curettes are used for subgingival scaling.
• They have a pointed tip.	• They have a curved toe.
• They are heavy instruments.	• They are light instruments.
• They cannot be used for curettage procedure.	• They are used for curettage procedure.

Question 5

What is a curette? Explain in detail?

Answer

A curette is a periodontal instrument used for curettage, subgingival scaling and root planing and removal of altered cementum.

- It has sharp cutting edges that converge at a rounded toe.
- In the cross-section of the blade, it appears semicircular with a convex base.
- The lateral border of the convex base forms cutting edges on both sides of the blades.
- It is both single and double ended
- Curette can be of two types:
  1. Universal cutters
  2. Gracey curettes

Universal Curettes

- As the name suggests, these can be used on any area and surfaces of the teeth, i.e. one curette for all areas.
- It does have an offset blade that mean that the face of the blade in at 90° angle to the shank.
- It is curved in one plane, i.e. curved up and not to the side.
- It can be double ended or pair of single ended instruments
- They are difficult to use in furcation areas.
- Examples of universal curettes are Columbia curette No. 13, 14 2R–2L, 4R–4L and Barnhart curette No. 1-2 and 5-6.

Gracey Curettes

- They are referred as area-specific curettes since they are used on specific areas and surfaces.
- They were designed by Dr Clayton H Gracey in the year 1930 at the University of Michigan.
- They are special types of curettes that are designed to permit greater accessibility and adaptability.
- Gracey curettes are as follows:
  - Gracey No. 1-2 and 3-4 for anterior teeth.
  - Gracey 5-6 for anterior and premolar.
  - Gracey 7-8 posterior teeth-facial and lingual surface.
  - Gracey 9-10 posterior teeth facial and lingual surfaces.
  - Gracey No. 11-12 posterior teeth mesial surfaces.
  - Gracey 13-14 posterior teeth distal surfaces.

Recent Additions

- Gracey no. 15-16 (modification of Gracey no. 11-12)
- Gracey no. 17-18 (modifications of Gracey no. 13-14)
  - Gracey curettes can be obtained as a single ended, as a set of 14 instruments.
- They have an offset blade i.e. the face of blade is at 60–70° to the lower shank.
- This angulation allows the blade to be inserted in the precise areas for subgingival scaling and root planing.
- Recent additions of Gracey curette are 15-16 and 17-18
- 15-16 is a modification of standard 11 and 12 and is designated for the mesial surface of the posterior teeth.

❑ It has a Gracey number 11-12 combined with shank of 13-14. New shank of 15-16 allows better adaptation to posterior mesial surfaces from a front position with intra-oral rest.
❑ 17-18 is a modification of 13-14. It has a terminal elongated shank of 3 mm and an accentuated angled shank.
❑ It has better access to all posterior distal surfaces.

Modifications of Gracey Curette

❑ Extended shank curettes
  ○ Hu-Friedy after five curettes are modification of standard Gracey curette design which have an extended shank.
  ○ The terminal shank is about 3 mm longer which allows extension into the deeper periodontal pockets of 5 mm or above.
❑ Miniblade curettes
  ○ Hu-Friedy mini five curettes are modifications of after five curette
  ○ The size of their blades are half the length of the after five or standard Gracey curette
  ○ Mini fives are available in all standard Gracey numbers except for the number 9-10.
❑ Larger and mini larger curettes
  ○ It is a set of three curettes.
  ○ It combines the shank design of the standard Gracey 5-6, 11-12 and 13-14 with a universal blade of 90°.
  ○ These curette can be adapted to both the mesial and distal sides of the tooth without changing the instruments.
❑ American Gracey Curvettes
  ○ Set of 4 Mini bladed curettes
  ○ The length of the blade is 50% of that of the conventional curettes and the blade is slightly curved upward.
  ○ Sub-0 and number 1-2 are for anterior and premolar
  ○ 11-12 for posterior mesial surfaces
  ○ 13-14 for posterior or distal surfaces.

Question 6

What is EVA system?

Answer

It is a prophylaxis instrument used for correcting over hanging and over contoured proximal alloy and resin restoration.
❑ It is the most efficient and least traumatic instrument
❑ Diamond files which are motor driven come in symmetric pairs.

❑ They are made up of aluminium in the shape of a wedge protruding from a shaft.
❑ One side of the wedge is diamond coated whereas the other is side is smooth.
❑ There is a special dental handpiece over which files can be mounted that generates reciprocating strokes of variable frequency.
❑ The oscillating file swiftly planes the contour of the restoration and gives a desired shape when the unit is activated interproximally with the diamond coated side of the file touching the restoration and the smooth side adjacent to the papile.

Question 7

What are HOE scalers?

Answer

They are the subgingival scalers which are used for scaling of ledges or rings of calculus.
❑ The blade is bent at an angle of 99°.
❑ The cutting edge is formed by the junction of the flattened terminal surface with the inner aspect of the blade.
❑ The cutting edge is bevelled at 45°.
❑ Back of the blade is rounded.
❑ Blade is reduced to minimal thickness to permit access to the root without interference from the adjacent tissues.
❑ The blade maintains contact at two points on a convex surface.
❑ HOE scalers can be used in the following manner.
  ○ The blade is inserted to the base of the periodontal pocket so that it can make a two point contact with the tooth, which stabilizes the instrument.
  ○ A firm pull stroke is used to activate the instrument.

Question 8

What are general principles of periodontal instruments? Describe in detail.

Answer

General principles of instruments are as follows:
❑ Accessibility: Proper positioning of patient in the dental chair.
❑ Visibility, illumination and retraction.
❑ Maintaining of clean field.
❑ Sharpening of instrument.
❑ Instrument stabilization: grasp and finger rest.
❑ Instrument activation.
❑ Controlled strokes for scaling and removal of calculus without injury to the tissues.

Accessibility (Positioning of Patients and Operator)

- Accessibility helps in thoroughness of instrumentation.
- The position of the patient and operator should provide maximal accessibility to the area of operation.
- Decreased accessibility impedes thorough instrumentation, prematurely tires the operator and lowers their effectiveness.

Position of Operator

- The back should be straight, head should be erect and shoulders should be relaxed.
- Distance from the patients mouth to the eyes of the clinician should be 14–16 inches
- Forearm and thighs parallel to the floor and hip angle should be 90°
- Weight should be evenly balanced.
- Height of the seat should be positioned low enough so that the heels of feet touch the floor
- When working from 9 to 12 position of the clock, feet should be spread apart so that the legs and the chair base form tripod which creates a stable position.

Patient Position

- Patient should be in a supine position and placed in such a way that the mouth is close to the resting elbow of the clinician
- The back of the chair should be nearby to the floor for maxillary area and the back of chair should be slightly raised for mandible.
- Patients head should be even with the upper edge of the head rest.
- For mandible the position should be chin down and for maxilla, the position should be chin up
- The head rest should be raised or lowered so that the patients neck and head are aligned with the torso.

Visibility, Illumination and Retraction

- Direct vision with direct illumination from the dental light should be present.
- If this is not possible then indirect vision may be obtained by using a mouth mirror to reflect light where it is needed.
- Indirect vision and indirect illumination are often used simultaneously.

Transillumination

- During transilluminating a tooth, the mirror is used to reflect light through the tooth surface.
- The transilluminated tooth almost will appear shiny.
- It is effective only with anterior teeth as they are thin enough to allow the light to pass through them.

- Properly positioned light and the mirror will result in shiny surface of the teeth.

Retraction

- It would provide visibility, accessibility and illumination.
- Following method are effective for retraction.
  - Use of mirror to reflect the cheek while the fingers of the non-operating hand retract the lips and protect the angle of the mouth from irritation by the mirror handle.
  - Use of minor alone to retract the lip and cheek.
  - Use of fingers of the non-operating hand to retract the lips.
  - Use of the mirror to retract the tongue.
  - Combination of above.

Maintaining a Clean Field

A clean field can be maintained by:
- Adequate suction
- By removing all obstacles in the operating area.

Sharpening of Instruments

- All instruments should be inspected to make sure that they are clean, sterile and in good condition.
- The working ends of pointed instruments should be sharp enough to be effective.

Advantages of sharp instruments are as follows:
- Calculus removal is easy
- Patient comfort and improved strokes
- Clinician's fatigue reduces because of reduced number of strokes.

Instrument Stabilization

- Stability of the instruments and the hand are the primarily requisites for controlled instrumentation, stability and control is essential for effective instrumentation and to avoid injury to the patient or clinician.
- The two factors that provide instrument stability are:
  1. Instrumental grasp.
  2. Finger rest.

Instrument Grasp

- A proper grasp is important for precise control of movements made during periodontal instrumentation:
- There are three types of grasps:
  1. Standard pen grasp
  2. Modified pen grasp
  3. Palm and thumb grasp.

- ❑ Standard pen grasp is the grasp in which we hold the instruments in the same manner as we hold a pen.
- ❑ Modified pen grasp is the most effective and stable grasp for all periodontal instruments.
- ❑ This grasp allows precise control of the working end, permits a wide range of movements and facilitates good tactile sensation.
- ❑ Palm and thumb grasp is useful for stabilising instruments during sharpening and for manipulating air and water syringe.

Finger Rest

- ❑ Finger rest helps in stabilising the hand and the instrument by providing a firm fulcrum, as movements are made to activate the instruments.
- ❑ A good finger rest prevents injury and laceration of the gingiva and surrounding tissues.
- ❑ The ring finger is used as finger rest.
- ❑ Minimal control is achieved when the middle finger is kept between the instrument shank and the fourth finger.
- ❑ The built up fulcrum is an integral part of the wrist forearm action that activates the powerful working stroke for calculus removal.
- ❑ Finger rest can be classified as intraoral and extraoral fulcrum.

Types of finger rest are as follows:

- ❑ Intraoral
  - ○ Conventional
  - ○ Cross arch
  - ○ Opposite arch
  - ○ Finger on finger
- ❑ Extra oral
  - ○ Palm up
  - ○ Palm down

Intraoral

- ❑ **Conventional finger rest:** When finger rest is kept on the tooth next to the tooth being involved.
- ❑ **Cross arch:** When finger rest is kept on the arch next the arch involved.
- ❑ **Opposite arch:** Finger rest kept on opposite arch.
- ❑ **Finger on finger.**

Advantages of intraoral finger rest are as follows:

- ❑ It is very stable and secured support for the hand.
- ❑ It provides leverage and power of instrumentation.
- ❑ Excellent tactile sensitivity.
- ❑ Precise stroke control.

- ❑ Allows forceful stroke pressure with least amount of stress to the hand and finger.
- ❑ Injury to the patient is reduced.

Extraoral Finger Rests

- ❑ These are important for effective instrumentation specially for maxillary teeth.
1. Knuckle rest technique or palm up technique.
   - ○ The clinician rests the knuckle against the chin or cheek of the patient.
2. Palm down technique.
   - ○ The clinician rests the palm against the cheek of the patient.

Advantage

Facilitate instrumentation of the proximal root surfaces of maxillary molars

Disadvantage

- ❑ Least effective of all fulcrum techniques
- ❑ Stroke control is more difficult and decreases tactile information.
  - ○ Instrument activation
    - ➤ Adaptation
    - ➤ Angulation
- ❑ Lateral pressure
- ❑ Strokes

Adaptation

- ❑ It is the manner in which the working end of a periodontal instrument is placed against the surface of a tooth
- ❑ Working end of the instrument should conform to the contour of the tooth surface
- ❑ Precise adaptation must be maintained all instruments to avoid trauma to the soft tissues and root surfaces and to ensure maximum effectiveness of instrumentation.
- ❑ Instrument which are bladed-like curette and sharp pointed instruments like explorers are more difficult to adapt.

Angulation

- ❑ It means the angle between the face of a bladed instrument and the tooth surface.
- ❑ To insert beneath the gingival margin, the face to tooth surface angulation should be at an angle between 0° and 40°.
- ❑ For removal of calculus, angulation should be between 45° and 90°.

- The exact blade angulation depends on the amount and nature of calculus, the procedure being performed and condition of tissue during scaling or root planing.
- Angulation should be greater than 90° for curettage.

Lateral Pressure

- It is the pressure created when force is applied against the surface of a tooth with the cutting edge of a bladed instrument.
- Exact amount of pressure depends upon the procedure performed.
- It can be firm, moderate or light.
- If insufficient lateral pressure is applied, rough ledges or lumps may be shaved to thin, smooth sheets of burnished calculus.
- Careful application of controlled and varied amounts of lateral pressure during instrumentation is an important part of effective scaling and root planing techniques.

Strokes

There are mainly three types of strokes, i.e. exploratory stroke, scaling stroke and root planing stroke.
- These strokes can be activated either by a pull or a push motion in a vertical, oblique or horizontal direction.
- Exploratory stroke is a light, feeling stroke.
- It is mainly used with probe and explorers.

- Scaling stroke is a short powerful pull stroke which is mainly used with bladed instrument for removal of subgingival and subgingival calculus.
- Root planing stroke: It is a moderate to light pull stroke which is used for final smoothening and planing of the root surface.

Question 9

What are the principles of sharpening?

Answer

Following are the principles of sharpening:

- Choose a stone suitable for the instrument to be sharpened.
- It the instrument to be sharpened that will be sterilised before it is used on a patient, then use a sterilised sharpening stone.
- A proper angle between the sharpening stone and the surface of the instrument should be established.
- A stable, firm grasp of both instrument and the sharpening stone should be maintained.
- Excessive pressure should be avoided.
- Avoid the formation of a wire-edge, characterised by minute filamentous projections of metal extending as a roughened ledge from the sharpened cutting edge.
- During sharpening lubrication of stone in important.
- If the instruments looks dull, then sharpen the instrument.

CHAPTER 42

Chemotherapeutic Agents

Question 1

What are chemotherapeutic agents? Explain in detail.

Answer

They can be widely classified into systemic and local drug delivery system.

Systemic Drug Delivery

Tetracycline

- Used in treating refractory periodontitis including localised aggressive periodontitis
- Tetracycline's can concentrate in periodontal tissues and inhibit growth of *Actinobacillus actinomycetemcomitans*
- These also have anti-collagenase effect that inhibits tissue destruction. These also help in bone regeneration
- These are derived naturally from certain species of *Streptomyces* or manufactured semi-synthetically
- These have bacteriostatic action and inhibit the growth of rapidly multiplying bacteria
- These are more effective against gram-positive bacteria as compared to gram-negative bacteria
- Studied have shown that long-term regimens of tetracycline are not advisable because of the development of resistant bacterial species. In such cases amoxicillin with metronidazole have been found to be more effective.

Tetracycline

It is usually prescribed four times a day (qid) 250 mg.

Minocycline

- Effective against broad spectrum microorganisms
- It inhibits growth of motile rods and spirochetes and the effect persist up to 3 months after therapy
- Minocycline has less phototoxicity and renal toxicity as compared to tetracycline however may cause vertigo which is reversible.

Dosage

- 200 mg per day for 1 week
- It can also be given for a period of 2 months for complete elimination of spirochetes.

Doxycycline

- Effect is similar to minocycline
- Given only OD therefore has better patient compliance
- 100 mg OD. In patients with gastric irritation the doses can be altered to 50 mg BD.

Metronidazole

- It has a bactericidal action on anaerobic organisms, however it is not the drug of choice against aa infection
- It can be used against aa in combination of other antibiotics
- It is also effective against anaerobic microorganisms such as Porphyromonas gingivalis and Prevotella intermedia
- It is used to treat gingivitis acute necrotising ulcerative gingivitis, chronic periodontitis and aggressive periodontitis.

Doses

- 250 mg three times daily for 7 days
- Metronidazole if consumed with alcohol can cause severe cramps, nausea and vomiting, therefore products containing alcohol should not be consumed till 1 day after the therapy

❑ Patients undergoing anticoagulant therapy should not be given metronidazole as it prolongs prothrombin time.

Penicillin

❑ These act by inhibiting bacterial cell wall formation and thus bactericidal in nature.
❑ Only amoxicillin and Augmentin have been shown to be effective in periodontal therapy
❑ Dose of amoxicillin 500 mg for 8 days.

Azithromycin

❑ Effective against anaerobic and gram negative bacteria
❑ Dose: Initial loading dose of 500 mg followed by 250 mg daily for 5 days.

Local Drug Delivery Systems

These are used to treat those periodontal diseases which require high concentration of antibiotics in a confined area.

Tetracycline containing fibres, e.g. actisite—it is a non-biodegradable ethylene/vinyl acetate copolymer fibre (diameter of 0.5 mm)

❑ It contains tetracycline in the concentration of 12.7 mg per nine inches
❑ When applied in periodontal pocket, it gives concentrations of tetracycline greater than 1300 ug/mL for a period of 10 days.

Sub-gingival doxycycline, e.g. Atridox®—it is supplied as 10% doxycycline in a gel form in a syringe

❑ Studies have shown that Atridox® alone was more effective than other treatment protocols in all time periods

Sub-gingival minocycline, e.g. Ariston—it is supplied in 2% concentration encapsulated in biodegradable microspheres in a gel carrier

❑ These microspheres are placed sub-gingival as an adjunct to scaling and root planing
❑ Studies have shown that there was an increase in clinical attachment levels in patients with pockets of 6 mm or greater than 6 mm.

Sub-gingival metronidazole, e.g.—Elyzol

PerioChip®: Chlorhexidine gluconate—(refer chapter on Plaque Control).

CHAPTER 43

Sonic and Ultrasonic

LONG ESSAYS

Question 1

Explain about powered instruments and their efficacy in Periodontics.

Answer

There are two types of powered instruments:

1. Sonic scalers
2. Ultrasonic scalers:
   - Magnetostrictive
   - Piezoelectric

Sonic Scalers

- They are air-driven. 2000–6500 cps
- The scaler tips are large in diameter and universal in design
- The strokes are elliptical to orbital in shape, therefore can be adapted to all tooth surface.

Ultrasonic Scalers

Piezoelectric Scalers

- When an electric current is applied to a quartz crystal or to a ceramic disc they change in shape due to change in the polarity of the crystal arrangement
- Their tips move in a linear pattern.

Magnetostrictive Scalers

- There are ferromagnetic stacks inside an electromagnetic field changes its shape constantly under an alternating current
- Tip movement is elliptical, therefore all the surfaces are active.

Efficacy of Ultrasonic in Periodontics

Plaque and Calculus

- Both manual and ultrasonic are equally effective

- However in case of deep pockets, ultrasonic micro-inserts are found to be more effective than manual scaling.

Bacterial Reduction and Endotoxin Removal

- Both the sonics and ultrasonics along with manual scaling/root planing (SRP) remove equal amount of endotoxin from the root surface
- Bacterial reduction is also comparable in the same amount
- The ability of ultrasonic to produce cavitation and micro-streaming has shown to reduce the working time to achieve these common objectives.

Reduction in Bleeding On Probing, Probing Depth, and Clinical Attachment

The results as expected are similar to each other.

Furcation Access

- Since the access to furcation is narrower, micro-ultrasonic inserts work more efficiently in these areas.
- Sonics and ultrasonic are equivalent to manual instrumentation in class1 furcations but superior than manual in cases of class 2 or 3 furcations.

Question 2

What is frequency, amplitude, and stroke? Discuss about the water flow in powered scalers.

Answer

Frequency: Number of times a tip moves per second in an elliptical, linear or circular path.

- Higher frequency, lesser working are:
  - **Stroke:** It is the maximum distance travelled by the insert tip during one cycle
  - **Amplitude:** It is one-half of the stroke. Higher power settings produce a longer stroke, with the frequency remaining constant.

Water Flow

- Water flow is primarily required for heat dissipation
- Other beneficial effects of water along with ultrasonics are:
  - **Acoustic micro-streaming:** It is the unidirectional flow of water powered by ultasonics.
  - **Acoustic turbulence:** It is created when the movement of the tip causes the cooling water stream to accelerate and cause an intense swirling effect. This turbulence continues till cavitation occurs.
  - **Cavitation:** When the turbulent water flow reaches the tip of the scaler it gains the energy of the tip and form a bubble. This bubble is however very unstable and implodes on the tooth surface.
- This implosion produces shock waves in the liquid which propagates in the entire area of water flow.
- These three phenomenon together causes breakage of debris, clearance of plaque, and turbulent lavage of the pocket. It also destroys bacterial colonies.

CHAPTER 44

Adjunctive Role of Orthodontic Therapy

Question 1

Describe the benefits of orthodontic therapy in an adult periodontal patient.

Answer

Orthodontic therapy in an adult periodontal patient can be highly beneficial in the following manner:

- The alignment achieved in crowded or malposed dentition permits easy accessibility, thus allowing the patients to clean all surfaces of their teeth.
- Vertical orthodontic tooth repositioning can improve some osseous defect, thus inhibiting the need of osseous surgery.
- Orthodontic therapy can aid in alignment of gingival margins thus avoiding the need of gingival recontouring.
- Fractured tooth can be forced eruption orthodontically allowing enough tooth material for carrying out restorative procedures.
- Open gingival embrasure can be corrected especially in maxillary anterior region by orthodontics root movement, tooth reshaping and restoration.
- Orthodontics therapy can be used to correct the supra-erupted teeth, uprighting of drifted molars in extraction space for the replacement with implants.

Question 2

Describe orthodontic treatment of osseous defects.

Answer

- **Marginal ridge discrepancies:** In such cases, the brackets are placed in a way that the tooth equilibrates according to flat bone ridge. This in some cases may lead to reduction in crown heights, but is acceptable as the periodontal health is improved because of the favourable bone contour. The reduced crown is restored.

- **Advanced horizontal bone loss:** In such cases if the brackets are placed in order to level the crown, it may alter the crown root ratio and cause tooth mobility. Thus, the brackets or bands should be placed according to bone levels. In vital tooth, the equilibration should be performed gradually to allow the pulp to form secondary dentin and insulate tooth during the equilibration process.
- **Root proximity:** Closely-placed roots of the posterior teeth interfere with maintenance of good oral hygiene. Roots can be moved apart orthodontically as this opens up the embrasure spaces, provides additional bone support and enhances the patient's access to interproximal region for hygiene.

The brackets should be placed obliquely to facilitate this process. Generally separation of 2–3 mm provides adequate bone support. These patients may need occlusal adjustment to recontour the crowns.

Fractured Tooth

Extraction or Forced Eruption

The following factors help us in determining the protocol to be followed:

- **Root length:** If the fracture extends to the level of bone, it may erupt 4 mm.

A periapical radiograph is to be taken and 4 mm subtracted from the apex of fractured tooth root. The crown-root ratio should be 1:1 for stability. If it is less than the tooth, should be extracted.

- **Root form:** The root should be broad and non-tapering rather than triangular and tapering, as they provide a narrow cervical region after 4 mm eruption.

The root canal should be one-third of the total width of root, as more than this will cause the crown preparation to be thin.

- **Level of the fracture:** It is difficult to attach a crown to the root of the tooth which has fractures below 2–3 mm apical to the bone.
- **Age:** It is preferable to forced erupt a tooth in a younger individual as compared to an older individual with adjacent having prosthetic crown.
- **Aesthetics:** In patients with high smile line and 2–3 mm of gingival display, restorations are very obvious and thus it may be preferable to extrude the fractured tooth.
- **Endodontic/periodontal prognosis:** In cases of compromised periodontal health or vertical fractures, it is more prudent to extract the fractured tooth.

Question 3

How can gingival discrepancies are treated with orthodontic therapy?

Answer

Gingival Levels

The relationship of the gingival margins of six maxillary anterior teeth plays an important role in aesthetic appearance of the crowns.

Four characteristics contribute to ideal gingival form:

1. Free gingival margin of the two central incisors should be at the same level.
2. Gingival margins of central incisors should be positioned more apically then laterals and at the same level as canines.
3. The contour of labial gingival margins should mimic the cemento-enamel junction CEJ of teeth.
4. There should be a papilla between each tooth and the height of tip of the papilla is usually halfway between incisal edges and labial gingival height of contour over the centre of each anterior tooth.

Gingival marginal discrepancies between the adjacent teeth could be caused by abrasion of incisal edges or delayed migration of gingival levels.

These gingival marginal discrepancies can be corrected either by orthodontic tooth movement or surgical correction of gingival margin discrepancy.

Four criteria to make correct decision:

1. Patients lip line when the patient smiles (if smile line is below the free margin, then requires no correction)
2. **Labial sulcular depth:** If the shorter tooth has a deep sulcus, excisional gingivectomy may be appreciated to move the gingival margins of short tooth apically.
3. **Evaluate the relationship between shortest central incisor and adjacent lateral incisor:** If the short central incisor is longer than laterals then it is possible to extrude the longer tooth and equilibrate the incisal edge.
4. If the incisal edges are attrited and tooth had supra-erupted, then the best method to correct the gingival discrepancy is to intrude the short central incisor and building restoration of incisal edges.

Gingival Form

The presence of papilla between the maxillary central incisors is a key aesthetic factor in any individual.

Occasionally, adults will have open gingival embrasures or black triangles spaces above contact areas that look unaesthetic.

This space is usually due to:

- Tooth shape
- Root angulation
- Periodontal bone loss.

If triangular tooth shape is the cause, then flatten the incisal contact and closing the space.

If the roots angulation is divergent causing excessive space, they should be corrected to descend the papilla down and overcome the dark triangular spaces.

CHAPTER 45

Occlusal Evaluation and Therapy

LONG ESSAYS

Question 1

What are the different occlusal evaluation procedures?

Answer

There are three types of occlusal evaluation procedures as follows:

1. Temporomandibular disorder screening examination.
2. Intraoral evaluation of occlusion.
3. Role of articulated casts.

Temporomandibular Disorder Screening Examination

Maximum inter incisal opening: The patient is instructed to open his or her mouth as wide as possible. A mm scale is kept on the incisal edges of the lower incisor and the interincisal distance between upper and lower incisors are measured.

Opening/closing pathway: The patient is advised to open and close his mouth and the movement is closely watched to record any deviation or deflection from the midline.

Temporomandibular joint sounds: Light finger pressure is applied bilaterally over the temporomandibular joint (TMJ) pre-auricularly or post-auricularly and the patient is asked to open and close the mouth. Joint sounds like clicking or crepitus are to be recorded.

Temporomandibular joint tenderness: Light, bilateral palpation over the lateral aspect of condyle is used to elicit TMJ tenderness in mild moderate or severe categories.

Muscle tenderness: Moderate finger pressure is applied bilaterally to check for tenderness in masseter, pterygoid and temporalis muscle. These are recorded as mild, moderate or severe.

Intraoral Evaluation of Occlusion

- Identification of occlusal contacts in maximum intercuspation.
- Unhindered mandibular guidance should be noted in excursive movements.
- Initial contact in centric relation closure arch.
  - Guidance of patients mandible will allow the first occlusal contact in centric relation with minimal masticatory muscle recruitment.
  - If tooth to tooth contact occurs, before maximum intercuspation is acquired, a deflection of mandible is seen.
- **Tooth mobility:** Mobility is recorded as a part of initial occlusal evaluation and any changes over a period of time are closely monitored.
- **Attrition:** It is defined as wear caused by tooth to tooth contact. A certain amount of physiologic attrition is normal.
  - Any accelerated attrition should be noted in the form of wear facets
  - Significant attrition of the teeth generally implies chronic occlusal habits, clenching of the teeth and bruxism.

Question 2

Describe temporomandibular disorder (TMD) screening.

Answer

The patients with TMDs can be placed in one of the following three categories:

- Jaw function status is in normal limits:
  - The patient in this category have no complains or jaw pain or dysfunction.
  - They have minimal incisal opening of at least 40 mm, with no significant joint or muscle tenderness and minimal joint sounds.

- Patients present with a history of jaw problems after long appointments which involve wide opening of the mouth.
  - These patients report with several sites of mild to moderate muscle tenderness.
  - They may also show TMJ clicking after long appointment which was previously benign.
- These cases show restricted incisal opening, significant pain in the jaw, severe joint or muscle pain and progressive locking of the jaw episodes.
  - These patients indicate comprehensive evaluation or referral before any non-emergency treatment.

Question 3

What are the requirements for oral stability?

Answer

- Maximum intercuspation with:
  - Light or absent anterior contacts.
  - Well-distributed posterior contacts.
  - Coupled contacts between opposing teeth.
  - Cross tooth stabilisation.
  - Forces directed along the long axis of each tooth.
- Smooth excursive movements without interferences.
- No trauma from occlusion.
- Favourable subjective response to occlusal form and function.

Question 4

What are the indications and steps of coronoplasty/occlusal equilibration?

Answer

Coronoplasty is the selective reshaping of occlusal surfaces with the goal of establishing a stable, non-traumatic occlusion.

Indications

- It is indicated in patients with evidence of trauma from occlusion.
- It is performed after elimination of gingival and infra bony pockets.

Procedure

- Removal of retrusive pre-maturities.
- Adjustment of intercuspal position (ICP).
- Test for excessive contact on incisor teeth in ICP.
- Remove posterior protrusive supra-contact.
- Correct pre-maturities on balancing sid.
- Reduce supra-contacts on working sid.
- Eliminate undesirable gross occlusal feature.
- Recheck the occlusal contact relationship in all position.
- Finishing and polishing.

46 Periodontic-Endodontic Continuum

Question 1

Classify pulpo-periodontal problems. Describe aetiology, diagnosis and treatment.

Answer

Pulpo-periodontal problems can be classified as:

- Primary endodontic lesions.
- Primary periodontal lesions.
- Independent periodontal and endodontic lesions.
- Combined periodontal and endodontic lesions.
- Primary endodontic, secondary periodontic.
- Primary periodontic, secondary endodontic.

Primary Endodontic Lesions

- Patients history, periodontal probing, radiographs and pulpal testing are performed.
- Clinically caries would be present and radiographically periapical radiolucency and dental caries would be present.
- Patients experience active episodes of pain.
- Sign and symptoms are almost similar to initial signs and symptoms of abscesses.
- Debridement of the pulp chamber and canal and completion on of appropriate, endodontic therapy, result in healing of the lesion.

Primary Periodontal Lesions

- History probing and radiographs are performed.
- Tooth looks clinically healthy, but may be mobility and pockets are present.
- Radiographically there is presence of bone loss.
- Patient complains of dull pain which can be intermittent or continuous in nature.
- Scaling, root planing followed by flap surgery with or without grafting is the treatment of choice.

Independent Periodontal and Endodontic Lesions

- Patients with pulpal disease may have periodontal inflammation also.
- Pulpal problems are more easily noticeable with noticeable signs and symptoms, where the progression of periodontitis is low, except acute diseases like periodontal abscesses or necrotising ulcerative gingivitis.
- Thus, prompt management of pulpal lesions become important.
- Pulp extirpation and canal filling usually eliminates the patients' acute symptoms.
- Treatment for periodontitis or gingivitis can be delayed until the acute symptoms of pulpal diseases get resolved.
- Another situation might arise, if a patient with chronic periodontitis has loss of pulp vitality.
- Such patients have both the symptoms of periodontitis and apical periodontitis.
- Involvement of apical periodontium by a pulpal lesion may obscure the symptoms of periodontitis.
- Therefore sequence of therapy becomes difficult to make as to treat which problem first.
- Patient may also present with both abscesses, i.e. pulpal and periodontal, but the apical lesion tends to be more painful.
- Thus, endodontic therapy would result in resolution of endodontic lesion but a little or no effect on pocket, and thus periodontal therapy would be required for a successful result.

Combined Periodontal and Endodontic Lesions

- When there is an extension of an endodontic lesion into an existing periodontal lesion, it is referred to as combined periodontal and endodontic lesion.
- Such lesions have features of both the diseases.
- History, clinical radiographic examinations are important to formulate a treatment plan.

- Pain from loss of pulp vitality is the most common feature.
- Probing confirms presence of periodontal pocket.
- In such cases, endodontic therapy is most predictable.
- Periodontal component is a difficult component of the combined lesion.
- Even with periodontal treatment, the periodontal defect typically does not resolve to the same extent as the endodontic lesion.
- After a successful endodontic treatment, the residual periodontal pocket can be more predictably treated.
- Periodontal treatment includes scaling, root planing and surgical treatments.

SHORT ESSAYS

Question 1

What is retrograde pulpitis and retrograde periodontitis?

Answer

If periodontitis progresses to involve the lateral canal or the apex of a tooth then secondary pulpal infection may be initiated, which is referred to as retrograde pulpitis **(Fig. 46.1)**. When a long standing periapical lesion drains through periodontal ligament, secondarily complicated, is referred to as retrograde periodontitis **(Fig. 46.2)**.

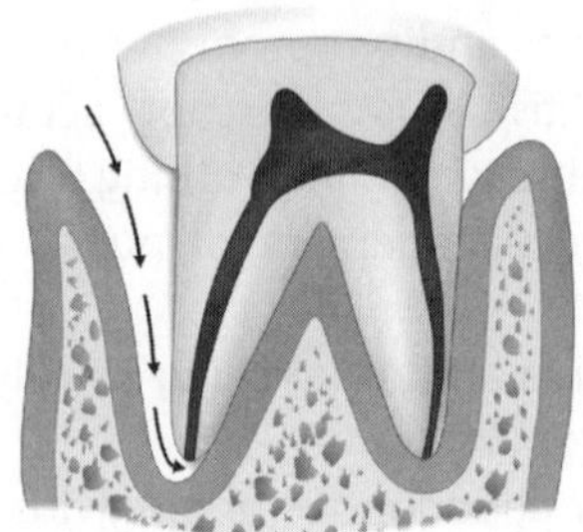

Figs 46.1: Retrograde pulpitis.

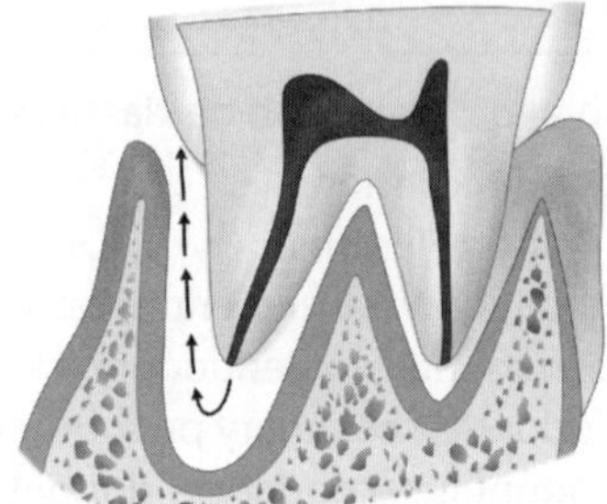

Figs 46.2: Retrograde periodontitis.

CHAPTER 47

Preparation of the Periodontium for Restorative Dentistry

Question 1

Discuss crown lengthening procedures. What are its indications and contraindications. Discuss the importance of biologic width in crown lengthening.

Answer

Crown lengthening are the procedures that are performed to increase the clinical height of a crown for restorative or aesthetic purpose.

Indications are as follows:

- Subgingival caries or fracture.
- Inadequate clinical crown length for retention.
- Unequal or unaesthetic gingival height.

Contraindications are as follows:

- Cases where surgery would cause an unaesthetic outcome.
- Deep caries or fracture would require excessive bone removal on contiguous teeth.

Importance of biologic width:

- While performing crown lengthening, one should take care of preserving the biologic width.

- Biologic width is defined as the physiologic dimension of the junctional epithelium and connective tissue attachment.
- It measures about 2.04 mm (**Fig. 47.1**).
- If the biologic width is violated while performing any kind of restorative procedure then it may cause following problems:

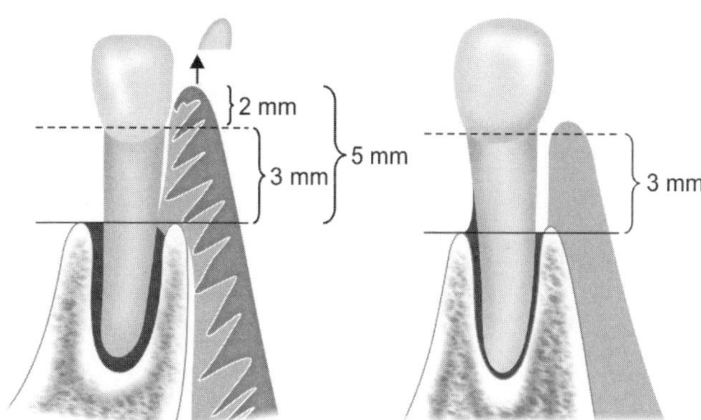

Fig. 47.2: More than 3 mm of soft tissue present above the crest of the alveolar bone, along with adequate attached gingiva, allows crown lengthening by gingivectomy.

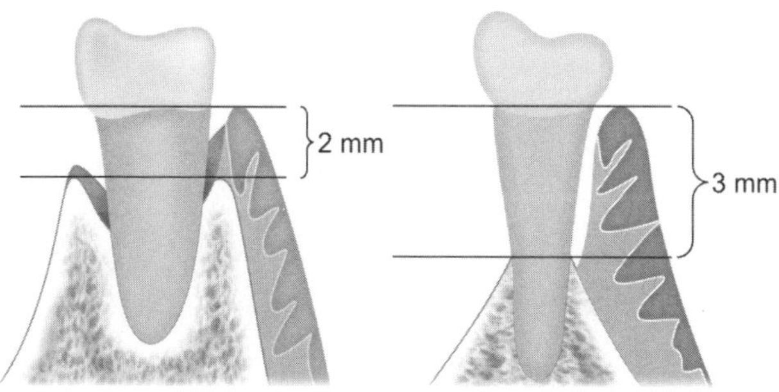

Fig. 47.3: Less than 3 mm of soft tissue present above the crest of the alveolar bone or inadequate gingiva, therefore a flap procedure with osseous recontouring is done for crown lengthening.

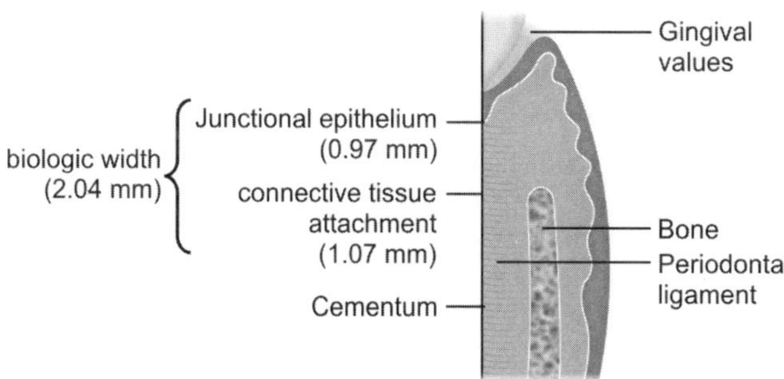

Fig. 47.1: Diagram depicting biologic width.

- Gingival inflammation.
- Pocket formation.
- Alveolar bone loss.

Therefore, biologic width should be preserved while performing any restorative procedure.

Surgical crown lengthening requires removal of gingiva or both gingiva and bone.

- **Situation 1:** If there is adequate attached gingiva and more than 3 mm of tissue coronal to the crest of the bone, then external bevel gingivectomy alone can be performed **(Fig. 47.2)**.
- **Situation 2:** If there is inadequate attached gingiva and less than 3 mm of soft tissue present coronal to the crest of the alveolar bone then it requires a flap procedure and bone recontouring **(Fig. 47.3)**.

CHAPTER 48

Phase II Periodontal Therapy

Question 1

What are the objectives of surgical phase? What is the purpose of surgical pocket therapy and what are the critical zones in pocket surgery?

Answer

Objectives of surgical phase are:

- Improvement of the prognosis of teeth and their replacement.
- Improvement of aesthetic.

Purposes of surgical pocket therapy are:

- To eliminate the pathologic change in the pocket walls.
- To create a stable, easily maintainable state.
- To perpetuate periodontal regeneration.

Critical zones in pocket surgery are as follows:

- **Zone 1:** Soft tissue pocket wall.
- **Zone 2:** Tooth surface.
- **Zone 3:** Underlying bone.
- **Zone 4:** Attached gingiva.

Zone 1: Soft Tissue Packet Wall

One should determine the persistence of inflammatory changes in the pocket wall and the clinical features, and outcome of therapy of the soft tissue pocket wall.

Zone 2: Tooth surface

- One should identify the presence of deposits and alteration on the cementum surface.
- Accessibility of the root surface instrumentation should be determined.

Zone 3: Underlying Bone

- Thorough careful, clinical and radiographic examinations should be done. One should establish the height of the alveolar bone to the pocket wall.

- Important criteria in selection of the treatment technique could be of bony craters, horizontal or angular bone loss and other bone deformation.

Zone 4: Attached Gingiva

Presence or absence of an adequate width of attached gingiva should be considered while selecting a pocket treatment method.

Question 2

What are the indications for periodontal surgery?

Answer

Various indications of periodontal surgery are as follows:

- Pocket and teeth in which a complete removal of root irritant is not considered clinically possible may call for surgery. It is seen mostly in molars and deep molar areas.
- Areas with irregular bony contours, deep craters and other defects usually require surgery.
- In cases of intrabony pocket and distal aspect of last molar, frequently complicated by mucogingival problems.
- Furcation involvement of Grade II and III.
- Persistence of inflammation in areas with moderate to deep pocket may require surgery.

Question 3

What are the methods of pocket therapy and what all are the criteria for method selection?

Answer

Methods of pocket therapy are as follows:

- New attachment technique: They are the ideal result since they eliminate the pocket depth by reuniting the

gingiva to the tooth at a position coronal to the pre-existing pocket.
- ❑ New attachment basally means filling in new bone and regeneration of periodontal ligament and cementum.
- ❑ Removal of the pocket wall.
- ❑ It is the most common method of pocket therapy.
- ❑ It can be removed by following methods:
- ❑ Shrinkage or retraction: This can be achieved non-surgically through scaling, root planing which resolves the inflamed gingiva.
- ❑ The gingiva shrinks, which further reduces the pocket depth.

Surgical removal by means of :
- ❑ Apical displacement of flap.
- ❑ Removal of the tooth side of the pocket.
- ❑ This is achieved by tooth extraction or by partial tooth extraction which is referred to as hemisection or root resection.

Criteria of Method Selection

Selection of a technique for treatment of a particular periodontal problem depends upon following considerations:
- ❑ Characteristics of pocket depth and its relation to bone and its configurations.
- ❑ Response to instrumentation, presence of furcation involvement.
- ❑ Response to phase I therapy.
- ❑ Presence of mucogingival or perioplastic problems.
- ❑ Age and overall health of the patients.
- ❑ Patient cooperation which includes ability to perform effective oral hygiene and for smoker, their willingness to quit their habit at least for some time.
- ❑ Socioeconomic considerations.
- ❑ Overall diagnosis of the case for various types of periodontitis like chronic, aggressive or various types of gingival enlargements.
- ❑ Previous periodontal treatments.

CHAPTER 49

General Principles of Periodontal Surgery

LONG ESSAYS

Question 1

What is haemostasis? Describe management of periodontal bleeding in detail.

Answer

Controlling of bleeding during surgery is referred to as haemostasis.

- Haemostasis is necessary as it permits an accurate visualisation of the extent of disease, pattern of bone destruction and anatomy and condition of the root surfaces.
- It is important for wound debridement and scaling and root planing.
- It also prevents excessive loss of blood into mouth, oropharynx and stomach.
- Periodontal surgery can lead to profuse bleeding which can be managed by following methods:
  - Continuous suctioning of the surgical site.
  - Application of pressure to the surgical wound with a moist gauze.
  - Proper design of the flaps and incisions, can avoid excessive bleeding.
  - If a vessel gets lacerated, suturing around the bleeding end would control the haemorrhage.
  - Applying cold pressure to the site with moist gauze can be helpful.
  - Local anaesthetic with a vasoconstrictor can also be used to control bleeding.
  - Haemostasis can also be achieved by various haemostatic agents, such as absorbable gelatin sponge (gelfoam), oxidised cellulose (Oxycel), oxidised regenerated cellulose (surgical absorbable hemostat) and microfibrillar collagen hemostat (CollaCote, CollaPlug and CollaTape).
  - Drug called thrombin can also be used for achieving haemostasis. It can be applied as topically as a liquid or powder.

Question 2

Describe about periodontal dressings.

Answer

- Periodontal dressings can also be referred as periodontal packs.
- They are generally used to cover the surgical areas after the surgery is completed.

Advantages of Packs

- They assist in healing by protecting the tissue rather than providing healing factors.
- They can minimise post-operative infection and haemorrhage.
- They can facilitate healing by preventing surface trauma during mastication.
- Protect against pain induced by contact of the wound with food or tongue during mastication.

Disadvantages of Pack

- Can be discomforting to patient.
- If applied on anterior teeth, can be unaesthetic for the patient.
- Can cause allergy to the patient.
- Can be a source of plaque accumulation.

Types of Packs

They can be zinc oxide eugenol packs or non-eugenol packs.

- **Zinc oxide eugenol packs:** Example is wonder pack developed by Ward in 1923.

- These packs are based on the reaction of zinc oxide and eugenol.
- Addition of accelerators like zinc acetate can give the dressing a better working time.
- Eugenol can be allergic which can produce a reddened area and burning pain in same patients.
- **Non-eugenol packs:** Example is Coe Pak which is most widely used.
  - These packs work by a reaction between metallic oxide and fatty acids.
  - It is available in form of two tubes.
  - One tube contains zinc oxide, oil (for plasticity), a gum (for cohesiveness), and lorothidol (a fungicide).
  - The second tube consists of liquid coconut fatty acids thickened with colophony resin and chlorothymol (a bacteriostatic agent).
  - This pack does not contain eugenol, therefore, avoiding the side-effects of eugenol.
  - Examples of other non-eugenol packs are cyanoacrylate, methylacrylate gels.

Retention of Packs

They are retained by mechanically inter-locking in inter-dental spaces and connecting the lingual and facial portion of the pack.

Anti-Bacterial Properties and Packs

- Antibiotics, like bacitracin, oxytetracycline, neomycin and nitrofurazone have been tried for improved healing and patient comfort with less odour and taste.
- These drugs have been shown to produce hypersensitivity reaction.

Preparation and Application of Dressings

- A wax paper pad is taken and components from both the tubes are dispensed in equal amount.
- Both are mixed with a spatula to form a thick paste of uniform colour.
- The pack is placed in a cup of water at room temperature.
- In 2–3 minutes, the tackiness of the paste is lost and it remains workable for 15–20 minutes.
- The pack is then rolled into two strips of approximately equal length.
- The end of one strip is fixed around the distal surface of last tooth.
- The remaining strip brought forward along the facial surface to the midline and interproximally.
- The second strip is applied on this lingual surface.
- The strips are then joined interproximally by applying gentle pressure on the pack.
- Overextension of the pack should be avoided.
- Since excess of pack can irritate the mucobuccal fold and floor of the mouth and interferes with the tongue.
- Pack should be trimmed, if it interferes with occlusion.
- The patient should be asked to move the tongue forcibly out and to each side, and the cheek and lips should be displaced in all directions to mould the pack while it is still soft.
- Once the pack is set, it should be trimmed to remove the excess.
- Pack should be kept on for one week after surgery.
- If a portion of the pack is lost from the operated area and the patient is uncomfortable, it is usually best to repack the area.

SHORT ESSAYS

Question 1

What are the complications which can arise in the first post-operative week?

Answer

Following complications may arise in the first post-operative week:

- Persistent bleeding after surgery.
- Sensitivity to percussion.
- Swelling.
- Feeling of weakness.

Question 2

What is the treatment for sensitive roots?

Answer

- It occurs when the root becomes exposed as a result of gingival recession or pocket formation.
- It can also appear after scaling, root planing and surgical procedures.
- It occurs more commonly in the cervical area of the root, where the cementum is extremely thin.
- Scaling and root planing procedures remove this cementum, inducing the hypersensitivity.

❑ A number of agents have been proposed to control root hypersensitivity.

❑ These desensitising agents can be applied by the patient or in office by the dentist.

❑ Agents used by patients can be desensitising dentifrices which contain strontium chloride, potassium nitrate and sodium citrate.

❑ Fluoride rinsing solutions and gels can also be used after the usual plaque-control procedure.

Agents used in office are:

❑ Cavity varnishes.
❑ Anti-inflammatory agents.
❑ Treatment that partially obturate dentinal tubules.
❑ Burnishing of dentin.
❑ Silver nitrate.
❑ Zinc chloride and potassium ferrocyanide.
❑ Formalin.
❑ Calcium compounds:
  ○ Calcium hydroxide.
  ○ Dibasic calcium phosphate.
❑ Fluoride compounds:
  ○ Sodium fluoride.
  ○ Stannous fluoride.
❑ Iontophoresis.
❑ Strontium chloride.
❑ Potassium oxalate.
❑ Restorative resins.
❑ Dentin binding agents.

Question 3

What are the various surgical instruments?

Answer

Various surgical instruments are as follows:

❑ Excisional and incisional instruments, such as gingivectomy knives, interdental knives, and surgical blade.
❑ B P Handle.
❑ Surgical curettes.
❑ Periosteal elevators.
❑ Surgical chisels.
❑ Surgical files.
❑ Scissors.
❑ Haemostat and tissue forceps.
❑ Needle holder.
❑ Castroveijo needle holder and scissors.

CHAPTER 50

Gingival Surgical Techniques

Question 1

What is gingivectomy? What are its indications and contraindications? Explain surgical gingivectomy with its healing and various methods of performing gingivectomy.

Answer

Gingivectomy refers to excison of the gingiva.

Indications of gingivectomy are as follows:

- To eliminate suprabony pockets.
- To eliminate gingival enlargement.
- To eliminate suprabony periodontal abscess.

Contraindications of gingivectomy are as follows:

- When bone surgery is required or when need to examine the bone shape and morphology.
- In cases when the base of the periodontal pocket lies apical to the mucogingival junction.
- In case of anterior region, where esthetic is a consideration.

Gingivectomy Technique

Following steps are performed for gingivectomy procedure:

- **Step 1:** The pockets are probed with a periodontal probe and then they are marked with pocket markers to create bleeding points (**Figs 50.1 and 50.2**).
- **Step 2:** For incisions on the facial and lingual surfaces, periodontal knives, such as Kirkland knives are used. For supplemental interdental incision Orban knives can be used.
  - If necessary, BP knives and scissors can also be used as auxiliary instruments.
  - The incision is made apical to the bleeding points created by the pocket marker (**Fig. 50.3**).
  - These incisions are directed coronally to a point between the bottom of the pocket and the crest of the bone.

- Bone should not be exposed but the incision should be close to the bone.

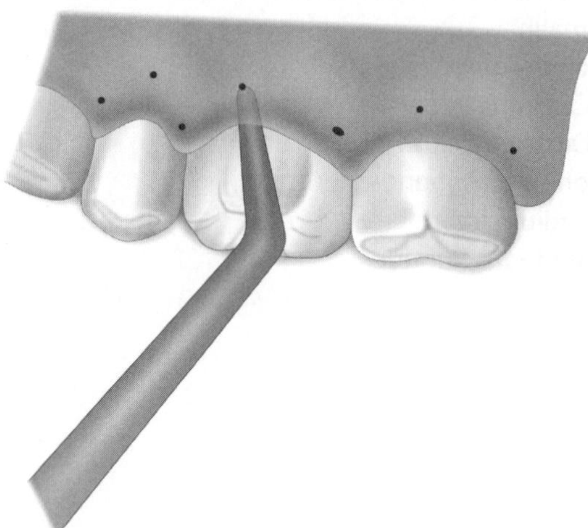

Fig. 50.1: Pocket marker making pin-point bleeding perforations which indicate pocket depth.

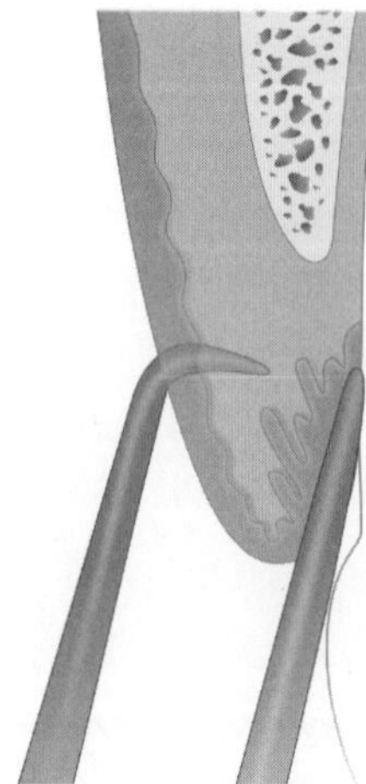

Fig. 50.2: Pocket marker in position.

- ○ Continuous or discontinuous incisions can be made depending upon the choice of the operator (**Figs 50.4A and B**).
- ○ The incisions should be bevelled at an angle of 45° to the tooth surface.
- ○ Normal arcuate pattern of the gingiva should be created.
- ○ If bevelling is not done, it would lead to a broad, fibrous plateau that takes a lot of time to develop into a physiologic contour.
- ❑ **Step 3:** Excised pocket wall should be removed.
  - ○ Area should be cleaned and the root surface should be examined thoroughly.
  - ○ Upon examination, some calculus remnant, root caries or root resorption may be found.
  - ○ Over the excised soft tissue, granulation tissue can be found.
- ❑ **Step 4:** Granulation tissue should be curetted out carefully, and any remaining calculus or necrotic cementum should be removed to achieve a smooth and clean surface.
- ❑ **Step 5:** The area should be covered with a periodontal pack.

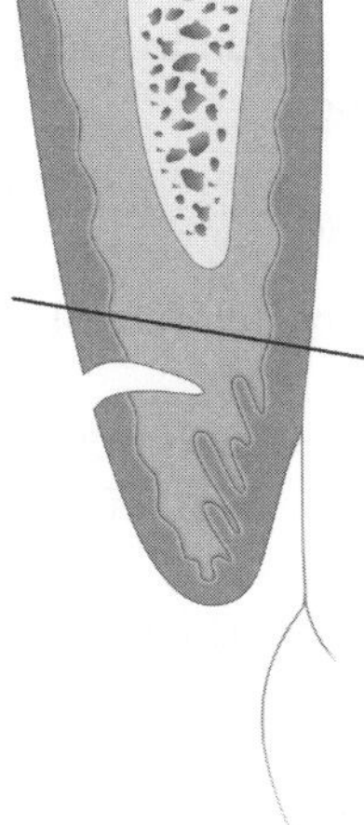

Fig. 50.3: Bevelled incision extending apical to the perforation made by pocket marker.

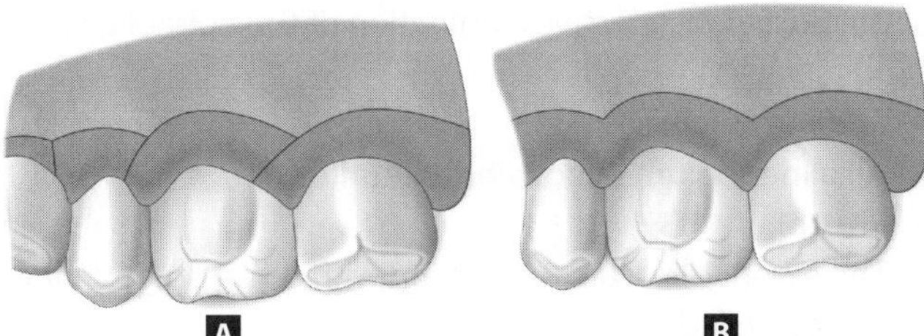

Figs 50.4A and B: (A) Discontinuous incision; (B) Continuous incision.

Healing After Gingivectomy

- ❑ There is formation of protective surface clot as an initial response after gingivectomy.
- ❑ There is some necrosis and underlying tissue is acutely inflamed.
- ❑ Clot is replaced by granulation tissue.
- ❑ In first 24 hours, there is an increase in new connective tissue, particularly angioblasts just below the layer of necrosis and inflammation.
- ❑ By third day, several fibroblasts are seen.
- ❑ Granulation tissue grows coronally, creating a new, free gingival margins and a sulcus.
- ❑ Capillaries from blood vessels of the periodontal ligament migrate into the granulation tissue and within 2 weeks, they connect with gingival vessels.
- ❑ After 12-24 hours, epithelial cells at the margins of the wound start to migrate over the granulation tissue, separating it from the contaminated surface layer of the clot.
- ❑ Within 24-36 hours, the epithelial activity reaches at a peak at the margins.
- ❑ After 5-14 days, epithelisation of the surface is almost complete.
- ❑ Vasodilation and vascularity begin to decrease after the fourth day of healing, but by the 16th day, it appears almost normal.
- ❑ In about 7 weeks, there is a complete repair of the connective tissue.

Methods of Performing Gingiveletomy

Various methods of performing gingivectomy are as follows:

- ❑ By scalpels and periodontal knives, such as Kirkland knives or Orban's knives.
- ❑ By electrosurgery.
- ❑ By lasers: Most commonly used lasers are carbon dioxide (CO_2) or neodymium-doped yttrium aluminium garnet (Nd:YAG) lasers.
- ❑ By chemosurgery: Removal of gingiva using chemicals, such as 5% paraformaldehyde or potassium hydroxide.
  - ○ Disadvantages of using chemosurgery are:
    - ➤ Depth of action cannot be controlled.
    - ➤ Gingival remodelling cannot be accomplished.
    - ➤ Reformation of junction epithelium and epithelialisation occurs slowly.

Question 2

Define Gingival Curettage . What are the aims of curettage? What are the Indications and contraindications of curettage? Explain in detail about the basic procedure and other procedures of curettage.

Answer

According to Carranza curettage is used in Periodontics to mean the scraping of the gingival wall of a periodontal pocket to separate diseased soft tissue.

- ❏ It is one of the oldest periodontal treatment methods. It was performed widely and almost routinely in treating periodontal pockets.

Aims of Curettage

- ❏ To reduce pocket depth by enhancing gingival shrinkage, new connective tissue attachment.
- ❏ Combination of the above.

Indications

- ❏ Curettage can be done as a part of new attachment attempts in cases of moderately deep intrabony pockets.
- ❏ Curettage can be done as a non definitive procedure to reduce inflammation prior to pocket elimination.
- ❏ In patients in whom aggressive surgical techniques (eg. flaps) are contraindicated
- ❏ Curettage is also frequently performed on recall visits as a method of maintenance.
- ❏ In supra bony pockets that are relatively shallow (4-6 mm).

Contraindications

- ❏ Firm, fibrotic pockets.
- ❏ Infrabony pockets.
- ❏ Acute necrotizing ulcerative gingivitis.
- ❏ Mucogingival involvements.

Procedure

Basic technique

- ❏ Gingival curettage always requires some of local anaesthesia.
- ❏ The curette is selected according to the area involved. The cutting edge should be against the tissues.
- ❏ The instrument is inserted so as to engage the inner lining of the pocket wall and carried along the soft tissue, usually in a horizontal stroke.

The curette is then placed under the cut edge of the junctional epithelium to undermine it.

The area is flushed to remove the debris, the tissue is partly adapted to the tooth by gentle finger pressure.

Suturing of separated papillae & application of periodontal pack may be needed.

Other Techniques

- ❏ Excisional new attachment procedure.
- ❏ Ultrasonic curettage.
- ❏ Chemical curettage (caustic drugs).

Excisional New Attachment Procedure (ENAP)

This procedure has been developed & used by the U.S Naval dental corps.

It is a definitive subgingival curettage procedure performed with a knife.

Technique

- ❏ After adequate anaesthesia, an internal bevel incision is made from the margins of the free gingiva apically to a point below the bottom of the pocket. The incision is carried interproximally on both the facial & lingual sides, attempting to retain as much interproximal tissue as possible.

  The intention is to cut the inner portion of the soft tissue wall of the pocket all around the tooth.
- ❏ Remove the excised tissue with a curette & carefully root plane all exposed cementum, preserve all connective tissue fibres that remain attached to the root surface.
- ❏ Approximate the wound edges, place sutures & periodontal dressing.

Ultrasonic Curettage

- ❏ Ultrasound is effective for debriding the epithelial lining of the pocket.
- ❏ It results in a narrow band of necrotic tissue (micro cauterization) which strips of the inner lining of the pocket.
- ❏ The Morse scaler shaped end ultra sonic instrument is used.
- ❏ It has been reported that ultrasonic instruments to be as effective as manual instruments for curettage.

Caustic Drugs

Caustic drugs lead to chemical curettage of the lateral wall of the pocket or selective elimination of the epithelium.

Drugs such as

- ❏ Sodium sulphide.
- ❏ Alkaline sodium hypochlorite (Antiformin).
- ❏ Phenol.
- ❏ The extent of tissue destruction with these drugs cannot be controlled.

SHORT ESSAYS

Question 1

What is gingivoplasty?

Answer

It is reshaping of the gingiva to create physiologic gingival contours, with the main purpose of recontouring of gingiva in the absence of pockets.

- ❑ Gingivoplasty can be performed using a scalpel, periodontal knives, rotary burs, electrodes or lasers.
- ❑ It helps in achieving a tapered gikngival margin, a scalloped marginal outline, thinned attached gingiva, vertical interdental grooves, and helps in shaping the interdental papillae such that they provide sluiceways for the passage of food.

Question 2

What is ENAP procedure ?

Answer

This procedure has been developed & used by the U.S Naval dental corps.

It is a definitive subgingival curettage procedure performed with a knife.

Technique

- ❑ After adequate anaesthesia, an internal bevel incision is made from the margins of the free gingiva apically to a point below the bottom of the pocket. The incision is carried interproximally on both the facial & lingual sides, attempting to retain as much interproximal tissue as possible **(Figs 50.5)**.

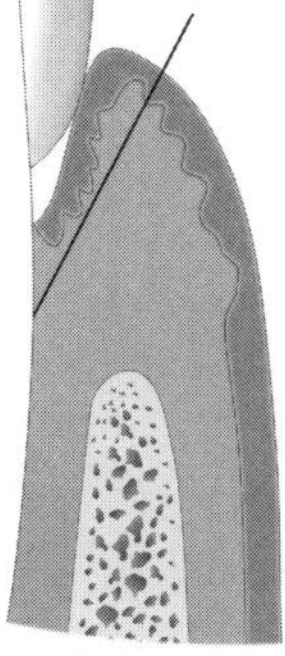

Figs 50.5A and B: (A) Internal bevel incision to a point below the bottom of the pocket; (B) After excision of tissue, scaling and root planing are performed.

The intention is to cut the inner portion of the soft tissue wall of the pocket all around the tooth.

- ❑ Remove the excised tissue with a curette & carefully root plane all exposed cementum, preserve all connective tissue fibres that remain attached to the root surface.
- ❑ Approximate the wound edges, place sutures & periodontal dressing.

Question 3

Discuss the healing after curettage ?

Answer

Healing after curettage is as follows ?

Immediately after the procedure (0hrs):- Gingiva is hemorrhagic, blue- red & blood clot within the pockets are visible.

- ❑ **1-2 days:** Gingiva appears edematous & swollen it still has bluish red color, clots are seen at the margin .PMNs are found at the wound surface beneath the blood clot.

  A well organised blood clot covers the wound surface, which is still devoid of epithelium (after a lag of 12- 24 hrs) epithelial cells from the gingival margin begin to migrate apically between the blood clot and the connective tissue.

- ❑ **4 days:** Edema has diminished , color is normal , clot can be seen sloughing from the gingival crevice. This area will still bleed on probing.
  - ○ Histologically, the acute inflammatory reaction is replaced by granulation tissue at the wound surface.
  - ○ Connective tissue is disorganized but edematous.
  - ○ Epithelization is progressing but incomplete.
  - ○ The epithelium covers the connective tissue separating it from the clot.

- ❑ **6-7 days:** Clinically edema is absent, shrinkage occurs producing recession of the gingival margin.
  - ○ Colour is normal.
  - ○ There is little or no bleeding on probing.
  - ○ Connective tissue is organized, collagen is being produced.

- ❑ **10-14 days:** Gingiva appears normal, pink in colour, firm. No evidence of bleeding on probing.

  Connective tissue maturation continues for 21-28 days. Keratinization of the oral aspect of the gingiva increases.

Problems in Healing

- ❑ Disturbances in healing may indicate some systemic problem. However in most cases they represent

contamination of the curettage wound by plaque/calculus left on the tooth surface.
- Evaluating the success of gingival curettage
- Re-examination & re-evaluation of the gingiva following curettage is an integral part of the procedure.
- This should be done 1-2 weeks after curettage has been completed and healing has occurred.
- Evaluate the gingiva, measure pocket depth &observe bleeding Evaluate plaque control & re-instrument if necessary.

CHAPTER 51

Treatment of Gingival Enlargements

SHORT ESSAYS

Question 1

How can a chronic inflammatory enlargement treated?

Answer

- They are firstly treated by non-surgical means, such as scaling and root planing.
- The inflammatory component is reduced through scaling and root planning only.
- If the gingiva does not undergo shrinkage after scaling and root planing, then it is removed surgically either by gingivectomy or by flap procedure, depending upon the case.

Question 2

How is a drug-induced enlargement treated?

Answer

Treatment of drug induced enlargement should be based upon the medication used and the clinical features of the case.

- Firstly the drug should be discontinued or a substitute for that drug can be given.
- For example, patient taking nifedipine can take a substitute calcium channel blocker, such as diltiazem or verapamil.
- Secondly, the clinician should give importance to plaque control.
- Adequate plaque control would lead to suppression of inflammatory component, which leads to decrease in the, size of the enlargement.
- Thirdly, in some patients, even after careful consideration, the gingival enlargement might persist.
- So in such patients, surgery is required which could either be in a form of gingivectomy or in a form of periodontal flap.
- **(Fig. 51.1)** shows the treatment chart for drug-induced gingival enlargement.

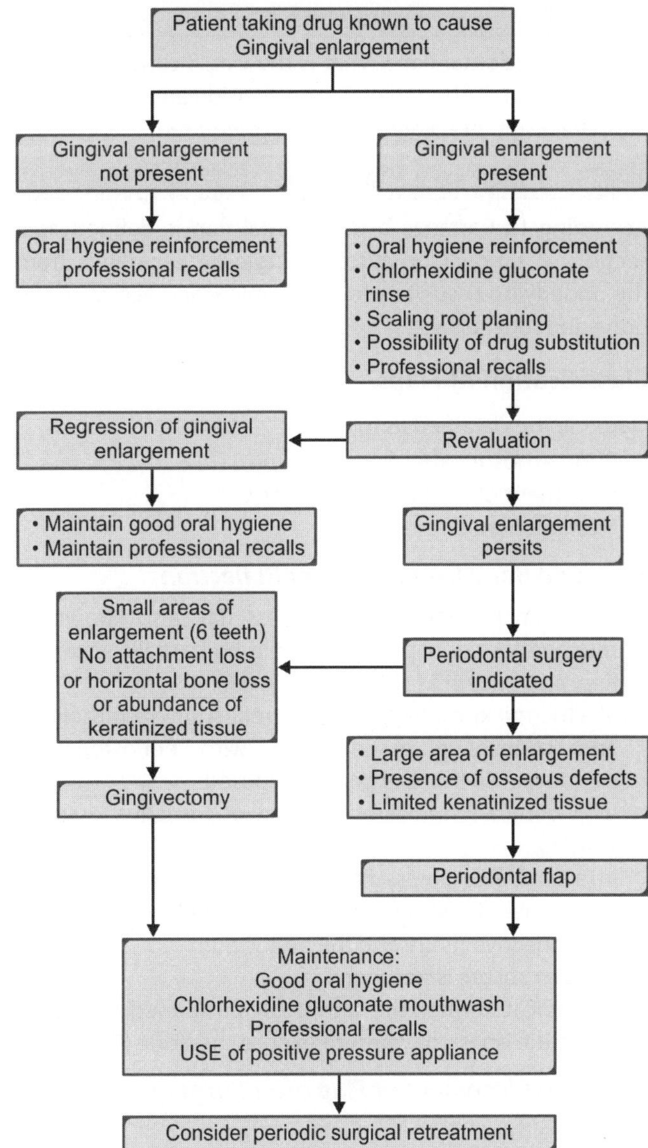

Fig. 51.1: Treatment chart for drug induced gingival enlargement.

The Periodontal Flap

Question 1

Define periodontal flap? What is the classification of flaps? Discuss in detail about flap design, incision and elevation of flap. Draw suitable digrams wherever required?

Answer

According to Carranza a periodontal flap is defined as a section of gingiva or mucosa surgically separated from the underlying tissue to provide visibility and access to the bone and root surface.

Classification of Flaps

Flaps can be classified as follows:

- Bone exposure after flap reflection.
- Placement of the flap after surgery.
- Management of the papilla.

Based on Bone Exposure after Reflection

- They can be either full-thickness flap also known as mucoperiosteal flap or they could be partial-thickeness flap, also known as split thickness flap.
- In a full-thickness flap, complete reflection of epithelium, and connective tissue along with periosteum is performed so that the bone is exposed.
- It is generally indicated in case of resective osseous surgery.
- In a partial thickness flap only epithelium and part of connective tissue is reflected, leaving behind some part of connective tissue and the periosteum.
- Bone exposure is not there.
- It is indicated when the flap is to be positioned apically or when the operator wants to expose the bone **(Fig. 52.1)**.

Based on Placement of Flap after Surgery

It can be either:

- Non-displaced flap.

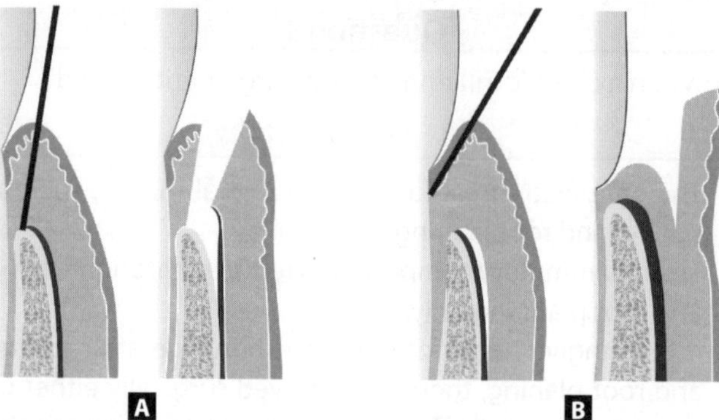

Figs. 52.1A and B: (A) Internal bevel Incision to reflect a full thickness flap. (B) Internal bevel incision to reflect a partial thickness flap.

- Displaced flaps.
- Non-displaced flaps are returned back to then original position and sutured.
- Displaced flaps can be displaced either coronally, apically or laterally depending upon the requirement of the case and sutured in the desired position.
- Full thickness or partial thickness—both the flaps can be displaced.

Based on Management of the Papilla

- It could be either conventional flap or papilla preservation flap.
- In a conventional flap the interdental papilla is split beneath the contact point and allows the reflection of flap in both buccal and lingual directions.
- In a papilla preservation flap, the entire papilla is incorporated in one of the flaps by the means of crevicular interdental incision to sever the connective tissue attachment and a horizontal incision at the base of the papilla, leaving it connected to one of the flaps.

Flap Design

Basic requirement of a flap are:

❑ A good blood supply to the flap is an important consideration.
❑ The flap should provide a good acess for instrumentation.
❑ The flap should provide a good acess to underlying structures, i.e. bone and root surface.
❑ Judge the final position.
❑ The two basic flap designs are conventional flap (in which the papillae are split) and second one is papilla preservation (in which the papillae are preserved).
❑ Before proceeding with any flap procedure, the operator must decide the exact location, type of flap, type of incision, management of the underlying bone and final position of flap and sutures.

Incisions

Incision could be horizontal or vertical.

Horizontal Incisions

There are three types of horizontal incision in a periodontal flap procedure.

❑ **The internal bevel incision**, which is also known as reverse bevel incisions or 1st incision.
   ○ It starts from a distance from the gingival margin and is aimed at the crest of the bone.
❑ **Crevicular incision** which is the known as 2nd incision or sulcular incision.
   ○ It starts from the base of the pocket and is directed towards the crest of the bone.
❑ **Interdental incision** which is also known as 3rd incision, is given to separate the collar of the gingiva that is left

around the tooth (**Fig. 52.2**).

Vertical Incision

Vertical incisions are also known as releasing incisions or oblique incisions.

❑ They are given on one end or both the ends of the horizontal incision depending upon the purpose of the flap.
❑ Advantages of vertical incision are:
   ○ They make the flap tension-free.
   ○ They make the flap movable because it can be displaced in the desired position.
   ○ They aid in better visualization of underlying structures.
❑ Disadvantages of vertical incision are:
   ○ They compromise the blood supply.
   ○ They may lead to delayed healing.
❑ Incision should not be made at the centre of an interdental papilla or over the radicular surface of a tooth, rather they should be made at the line angles of a tooth either to include the papilla in the flap or to avoid it completely. (**Fig. 52.3**).

Elevation of a Flap

❑ A blunt dissection is required when a full-thickness flap is raised, whereas a sharp dissection is required when a partial thickness flap is to be raised.
❑ Elevation of flap is accomplished by a periosteal elevator by moving it mesially, distally and apically until the desired reflection is accomplished.
❑ Sometimes, a combination of partial thickness and full thickness is done.

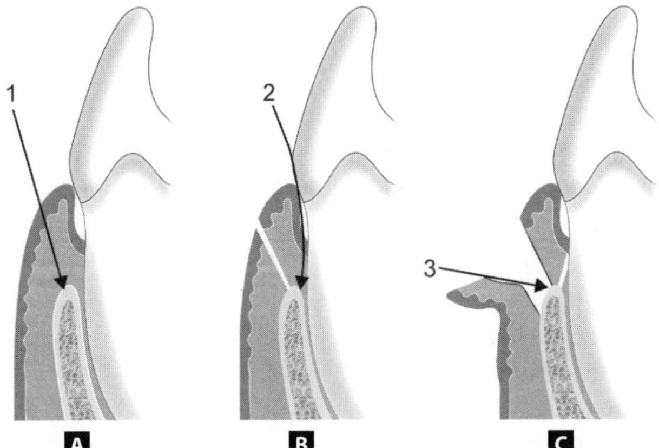

Figs 52.2A to C: Three different types of horizontal incision (A) Internal bevel or first incision; (B) Crevicular or second incision; (C) Interdental or third incision.

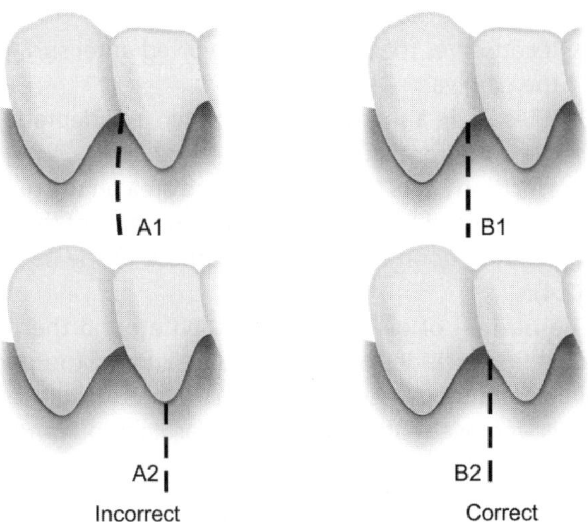

Figs 52.3: (A1 and A2) Incorrect location of a vertical incision; (B1 and B2) Correct location of a vertical incision.

SHORT ESSAYS

Question 1

What are envelope flaps?

Answer

When a flap is raised using only horizontal incision and no vertical incision are given, then the flap is known as envelope flap.

If sufficient access is obtained and apical, lateral or coronal displacement of the flap is not required, then envelope flaps are ideal choice.

Question 2

Describe the internal bevel incision.

Answer

- ❑ It is a type of horizontal incision, which starts at a distance from the gingival margin and is aimed at the crest of the bone.
- ❑ It is also known as the first incision as it is the first incision given in a modified widman flap procedure.
- ❑ It is also referred to as reverse bevel incision because the bevel of the blade, while giving this incision, is in a reverse direction from that of the gingivectomy incision.
- ❑ A #11 or #15 surgical scalpel is used most commonly for this incision.
- ❑ This is the most basic incision for maximum of the flap procedures.
- ❑ It aims at exposing the underlying bone and root.
- ❑ There are three main objectives of internal bevel incision. They are as follows:
  1. It removes the pocket lining.
  2. It conserves the relatively uninvolved outer surface of the gingiva.
  3. It results in a sharp, thin flap margin for adaptation to the bone-tooth junction.
- ❑ The incision starts from a designated area on the gingiva and is directed to an area at or near the crest of the bone depending upon the type and purpose of the flap **(Fig. 52.4)**.
- ❑ The portion of gingiva, which is left around the tooth after first incision, consists of epithelium of the pocket lining and the adjacent granulomatous tissue.
- ❑ It is removed after the crevicular incision and the interdental incision are performed.

Question 3

Classify suture materials and enumerate various types of suturing techniques.

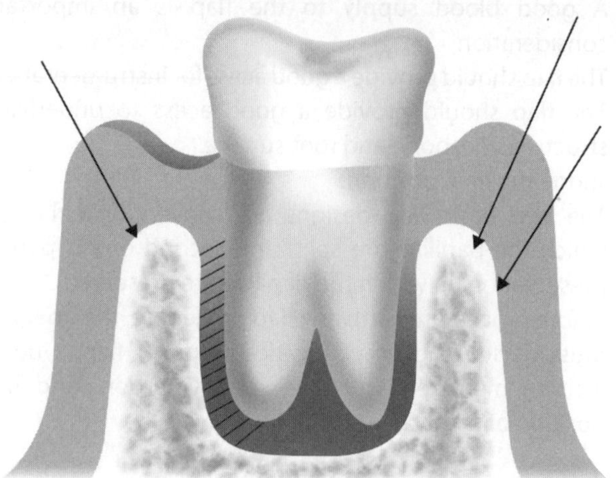

Figs 52.4: Internal bevel incision can be made at different locations and angles depending upon various anatomic and pocket situations.

Answer

Classification of sutures are is as follows:

- ❑ Non-absorbable (Non-resorbable)
  - ○ Silk-braided
  - ○ Nylon-monofilament (Ethilon)
  - ○ ePTFE-monofilament (Gore-Tex)
  - ○ Polyester-braided (Ethibond)
- ❑ Absorbable (resorbable)
  - ○ Surgical: Gut
  - ○ Plain gut: Monofilament (30 days)
  - ○ Chronic gut: monofilament (45–60 days)
- ❑ Synthetic
  - ○ Polyglycolic-braided (16–20 days)
  - ○ Vicryl
  - ○ Polyglecaprone-monofilament (90–120 days)
  - ○ Monocryl (Ethicon)
  - ○ Polyglyconate-monofilament (Maxon™)

Various types of suturing techniques are as follows:

- ❑ Interdental ligation.
- ❑ Sling ligation.
- ❑ Horizontal mattress suture.
- ❑ Vertical mattress suture.
- ❑ Anchor suture.
- ❑ Closed anchor suture.
- ❑ Periosteal suture.
- ❑ Continuous suture.
- ❑ Figure of 8 suture.

Question 4

Discuss the healing after flap surgery.

Answer

- Upto 24 hours, that is immediately after suturing, a blood clot is formed between the flap and the tooth or bone surface.
- This clot consists of a fibrin reticulum with many polymorphonuclear leucocytes, RBCs, injured cells and capillaries at the wound edge.
- 1–3 days after flap surgery, the space between bone and tooth is thinned and over the border of the flap, epithelial cells migrate.
- There is only a minimal inflammatory process, when the flap is closely adapted to the alveolar process.
- A week after the flap surgery, an epithelial attachment to the root is established by the means of a basal lamina and the hemidesmosomes.
- The blood clot gets replaced by granulation tissue which is desired from the gingival connective tissue, bone narrow and the periodontal ligament.
- 2 weeks after the flap surgery, collagen fibres begin to appear.
- There is still a weak union between the flap and tooth because of presence of immature collagen.
- 1 month after the flap surgery, crevice gets fully epithelised and a well-defined epithelial attachment is developed.
- Supracrestal fibres begin to arrange functionally.

CHAPTER 53

Flap Technique for Pocket Therapy

Question 1

What are the aims of a flap procedure for pocket therapy? Enumerate various techniques for access and pocket depth reduction or elimination. Describe modified Widman flap procedure in detail with diagrams.

Answer

Aims of a flap procedure for pocket therapy are as follows:

- To increase accessibility to root deposits.
- To eliminate or reduce pocket depth by resection of the pocket wall.
- To expose the area to perform regenerative methods.

Various techniques for access and pocket depth elimination are as follows:

- Modified Widman flap
- Undisplaced flap (or unrepositioned flap)
- Apically displaced flap.

Modified Widman flap: This procedure is aimed at exposing the root surfaces for efficient instrumentation and removal of pocket lining.

Undisplaced flap: It is an excisional procedure of gingiva.

It improves accessibility for instrumentation along with removal of pocket wall, thereby reducing or eliminating the pocket.

Apically displaced flap: It improves the accessibility for instrumentation and also removes the pocket, by apically positioning of the soft tissue wall of the pocket.

Thus it preserves or increases the width of attached gingiva by converting the previous unattached keratinized pocket wall into attached gingiva.

Modifed Widman Flap

- Originally, in 1965, Morris described this technique and named it as "unrepositioned mucoperiosteal flap".

- Same procedure was described in 1974 by Ramfjord and Nissle and termed it as "Modified Widman flap".

Objectives of this technique are as follows:

- It provides accessibility for instrumentation of the root surfaces and immediate closure of the area.
- It provides an intimate postoperative adaptation of healthy collagenous connective tissue to the tooth surfaces.

Steps for this procedure are as follows (**Fig. 53.1**):

- **Step 1:** An internal bevel incision is made which starts 0.5 to 1 mm away from the gingival margin, hitting the alveolar crest.
- **Step 2:** Gingiva is reflected using a periosteal elevator.
- **Step 3:** Then the second incision is made which is referred to as crevicular incision from the base of the pocket of the bone.
- **Step 4:** Once the flap is reflected, a third incision referred to as interdental incision is made in the

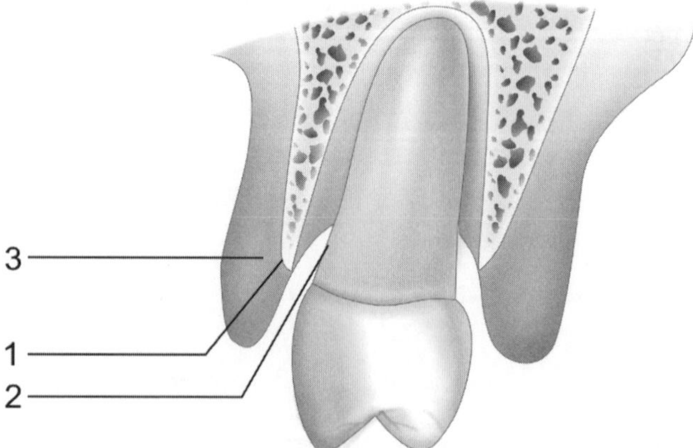

Fig. 53.1: All the three incisions for Modified Widman flap procedure.

interproximal areas coronal to the bone with a BP blade or an orbans knife. Thus the gingival collar is removed.

- **Step 5:** A curette is then used to remove the granulation tissue and tissue tags. Root surfaces are checked and scaling and root planing is performed if required. Residual periodontal ligament fibres which are attached to the tooth surface should not be disturbed.

- **Step 6:** Bone contouring is not done except if it prevents good tissue adaptation of the necks of the teeth.
- **Step 7:** The inside of the flap is trimmed using a Goldman-Fox scissors or a Castroviejo scissors so that tissue tags are removed from the inner surface of the flap and there is a close approximation between the flap and the tooth or the bone.
- **Step 8:** Interrupted direct sutures are placed and covered with a periodontal dressing.

SHORT ESSAYS

Question 1

What are the indications of flap surgery?

Answer

Indications of flap surgery are as follows:

- To increase the accessibility to root deposits.
- To eliminate or reduce the pocket depth by resection of the pocket wall.
- To expose the area to perform regenerative methods.
- To reshape soft and hard tissues to physiologic architecture.

Question 2

Explain apically displaced flap procedure.

Answer

The purpose of apically displaced flap is to:

- Eradicate pocket.
- Widen the zone of attached gingiva.

It can be performed either by a partial thickness or full thickness depending upon the purpose.

The steps in an apically displaced flap are as follows:

- **Step 1:** About 1 mm away from the crest of the gingival margin, the internal bevel incision is made which is directed towards the crest of the bone.

- **Step 2:** Then the second incision, i.e. the crevicular incision is done, after which the flap is reflected. After this the third incision, i.e. the interdental incisions are given and the wedge of tissue that consists of pocket wall is removed.
- **Step 3:** After this, two releasing incisions or vertical incisions are given on both the ends of the flap, which extend beyond the mucogingival junction. If a full thickness flap is to be reflected then a blunt dissection is done, but if a split thickness flap is to be reflected, then a sharp dissection is done.
- **Step 4:** After this is done, all the granulation tissue is removed followed by thorough scaling and root planing and osseous surgery is performed, if required. The flap is then displaced apically. Since the vertical incisions are given beyond the mucogingival junction, it becomes very easy to displace the flap as it becomes freely movable.
- **Step 5:** A sling suture should be given if a full thickness flap is done, but if a partial thickness flap is performed, then a periodontal suturing is done using a direct loop suture or a combination of loop and anchor suture. After suturing, a foil is placed over the flap and then covered with a periodontal dressing.

CHAPTER 54

Resective Osseous Surgery

Question 1

Define osseous surgery. What are its types and what are the rationale of osseous resective surgery? Discuss in detail about the technique for osseous resective surgery.

Answer

According to Carranza, osseous surgery it defined as the procedure by which changes in the alveolar bone can be accomplished to get rid it of deformities induced by the periodontal disease process or other related factors, such as exostosis and tooth supraeruption.

Types of osseous surgery can be:

- Additive osseous surgery.
- Subtractive osseous surgery.

Additive osseous surgeries are the surgeries which aim at restoring the alveolar bone to the original level.

Subtractive osseous surgeries are the surgeries which aim at restoring the form of pre-existing alveolar bone to the level present at the time of surgery or slightly more apical to this level.

Rationales of osseous resective surgery are:

- To reshape the marginal bone to resemble that of the alveolar process undamaged by periodontal disease.
- To convert a periodontal pocket to a shallow gingival sulcus to enhance the patients ability to remove plaque and oral debris from mouth.

Technique

There are four main steps in resective osseous surgery. They are as follows:

- Vertical grooving.
- Radicular blending.
- Flattening interproximal bone.
- Gradualizing marginal bone.

Vertical grooving and radicular blending are osteoplastic techniques whereas last two steps are ostectomy techniques.

Vertical Grooving

It is the first step of resective osseous surgery.

- It is generally performed with rotary instruments, like round carbide burs or diamond burs.
- This step helps to reduce the thickness the alveolar housing and to provide prominence to the radicular aspects of the teeth.
- It also provides continuity from the interproximal surface onto the radicular surface.
- Verticular grooving provides advantage to bones having thick margins, shallow craters or any other area which require maximal osteoplasty and minimal ostectomy.
- This procedure is contraindicated in areas where roots are closely approximated or having thin alveolar housing.

Radicular Blending

- This is the second step of osseous reshaping technique.
- This step is an extension of vertical grooving.
- This steps aims at gradualizing the bone over the entire radicular surface to provide best results from vertical grooving.
- This step provides a smooth, blended surface for good flap adaptation.
- This is also an osteoplastic technique which does not remove the supporting bone.
- Shallow crater formations, thick osseous ledges of bone on the radicular surface and class I and early class II furcation defects are some of the situations which can be treated mainly with these two steps.

Flattening Interproximal Bone

- This is the third step of osseous resective surgery.
- It involves removal of very small amounts of supporting bone.

❑ Therefore it is an ostectomy procedure.

❑ It is performed when the interproximal bone levels vary horizontally.

❑ One-wall defects or hemiseptal defects are most effectively treated with this step.

❑ It can be helpful in good flap closure and improved healing in the three walled defect.

Gradualizing Marginal Bone

❑ This is the last step of this technique.

❑ It is also an ostectomy procedure.

❑ This step requires minimal bone removal, but it is important for a sound, regular base for the gingival tissue to follow.

❑ This step also requires gradualization and blending over the radicular surface.

❑ Instruments used for this technique should be used very carefully as one can tend to over do this step.

❑ Thus instrument used are various hand instruments such as curettes and chisels over rotary instruments for gradualizing the marginal bone.

Various instruments used for resective osseous surgery are as follows:

❑ Both rotary and hand instrument are used for this procedures.

❑ Rotary instruments are mainly used for osteoplastic procedures, whereas hand instruments are used where more precise results are required.

❑ Hand instruments include curettes, rongeurs, interproximal files like schluger and sugarman files, chisels like back action chisels and oschsenbein chisels.

❑ Rotary instruments include carbide and diamond burs.

SHORT ESSAYS

Question 1

What is Widow's peak?

Answer

Widow's peak refers to the peak of bones which are typically seen on the facial or lingual/palatal line angles of the teeth.

Question 2

What is difference between osteoplasty and ostectomy?

Answer

Osteoplasty refers to reshaping of the bone without removing the tooth supporting bone, whereas ostectomy also known as osteoectomy refers to the removal of tooth supporting bone.

Question 3

What is meant by positive, negative and flat architecture?

Answer

❑ Positive architecture means if the radicular bone is apical to interdental bone.

❑ Negative architecture means if the radicular bone is coronal to interdental bone.

❑ Flat architecture means when interdental bone and radicular bone, both at the same level **(Fig. 54.1)**.

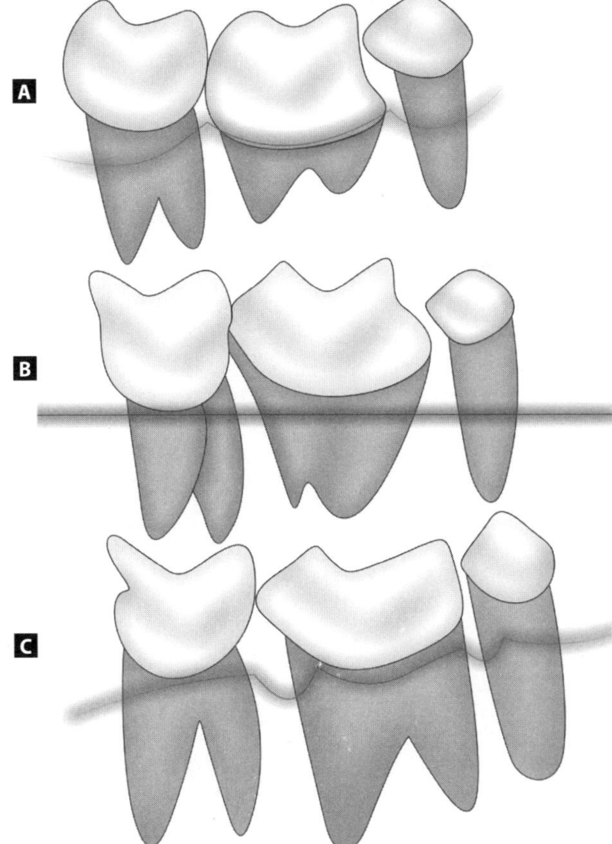

Figs 54.1A to C: (A) Positive architecture; (B) Flat architecture; (C) Negative architecture

Question 4	Answer
What is meant by definitive and compromise osseous reshaping?	Definitive osseous reshaping means that further osseous reshaping would not improvise the overall result, whereas compromise osseous reshaping means that a bone pattern which cannot be improved without significant osseous removal that can be detrimental to the overall result.

CHAPTER 55

Reconstructive Periodontal Surgery

Question 1

What are the possible outcomes of reconstructive periodontal therapy? What are the various methods by which new attachment and periodontal reconstruction can be evaluated? Discuss in detail about reconstructive surgical technique.

Answer

Possible outcomes of reconstructive periodontal therapy are as follows **(Fig. 55.1)**:

- Healing with a long junctional epithelium, which can result soon after filling of bone.
- Ankylosis of bone and tooth.
- Recession.
- Recurrence of pocket.
- Combination of these results.

Various methods for evaluation of new attachment and periodontal reconstruction are as follows:

- Clinical methods.
- Radiographic methods.
- Surgical re-entry.
- Histologic method.

- **Clinical method:** It includes pre and post-treatment pocket probing depths.
    - Probe can be used to determine the pocket depth, attachment level and bone level.
- **Radiographic method:** It includes pre and post-treatment radiograph.
    - Radiographs can depict the entire topography of the involved area before and after treatment.
- **Surgical re-entry:** Surgical re-entry can provide a good view of the state of bone crest of a treated defect after a period a healing.
    - Models from impressions of the bone taken at the initial surgery and later at re-entry can be used to assess the outcome of therapy.

- **Histologic methods:** Pre and post-treatment tissue blocks can be studied and evaluated and it can act as a clear evidence of a new attachment apparatus.

Various techniques for reconstructive surgery are as follows:

- Non-bone graft-associated procedures
    - Removal of junctional epithelium.
    - Prevention or impeding of epithelial migration.
    - Bio-modification of root surface.
    - Biologic Mediators.
    - Enamel matrix proteins.
- Graft-associated procedures.
    - Autogenous bone grafts.
    - Allografts.

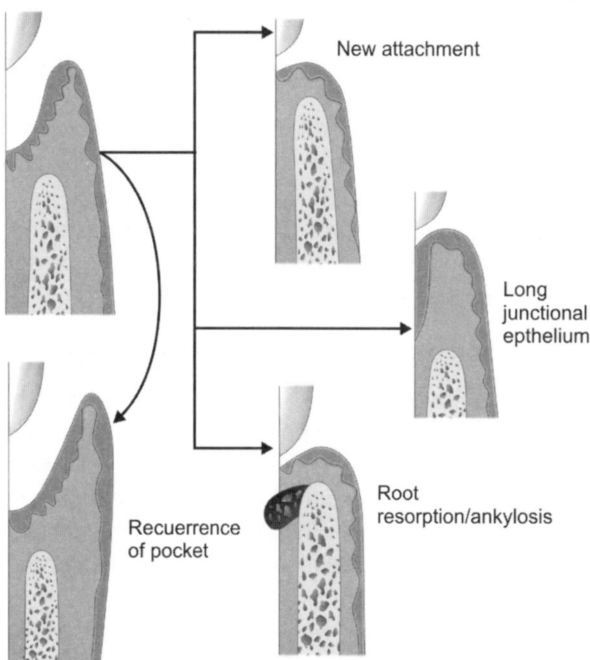

Fig. 55.1: Possible outcomes of reconstructive periodontal therapy.

- ○ Xenografts.
- ○ Non-bone graft materials.
- ❑ Combined techniques.

Non-bone Graft Associated Procedures

Are intended to achieve periodontal reconstruction without the use of bone grafts.

Various techniques used for the above are as follows:

1. Removal of Junctional Epithelium

It is believed that presence of junctional epithelium and pocket epithelium acts as barrier for successful therapy as its presence interferes with direct communication between the connective tissue and cementum, and various methods to achieve this are as follows:

- ❑ **Curettage:** It has not been a reliable procedure as the result of removal of epithelium by means of curettage vary from complete removal to persistence of as much as 50%.
  - ○ Other methods have also been used like ultrasonic methods, rotary abrasives stones and lasers, but because of clinician's lack of vision and lack of tactile sense while using these methods, their effects cannot be controlled.
- ❑ **Chemical agents:** Most commonly used chemical agents for the removal of pocket epithelium are sodium sulphide, phenol, camphor, antiformin, and sodium hypochlorite.
  - ○ Since their depth of penetration cannot be controlled therefore effect of their agents is not limited to the epithelium.
- ❑ **Surgical techniques:** Surgical techniques like excisional new attachment procedure (ENAP) is most oftenly used method.
  - ➢ A gingivectomy procedure can also be performed
  - ➢ Modified Widman flap procedure can also be done to achieve same result.

2. Prevention or Impeding of Epithelial Migration

Since the epithelium from the excised margin may rapidly proliferate to be interposed between the healing connective tissue and the cementum, thus only elimination of junctional and pocket epithelium may not be sufficient.

- ❑ The most common technique which prevents the proliferation of epithelium is referred to as guided tissue regeneration.
- ❑ The method has been derived from the classic studies of Nyman, Lindhe, Karring, and Gottlow which say that only the periodontal ligament cells have the potential for regeneration of the attachment apparatus of the tooth.

- ❑ This technique consists of placing the barrier membranes over the bone and the periodontal ligament, so as to separate them from gingival epithelium.
- ❑ This technique not seperate the gingival epithelium from bone and periodontal ligament but also favours repopulation of the area by the periodontal ligament and bone cells.
- ❑ Two types of barrier membranes are as follows:
  1. Resorbable (e.g. collagen membrane) and non-resorbable membrane (e.g. expanded polytetrafluoroethylene (ePTEF) membrane).
  2. Those membranes can be obtained in different shapes and sizes to suit proximal spaces and facial/lingual surfaces of furcation.

Technique for placing these barriers membranes are as follows:

- ❑ Firstly a mucoperiosteal flap is raised along with vertical incisions.
- ❑ Osseous defects are then debrided thoroughly and granulation tissue is removed.
- ❑ Through scaling and root planning is done
- ❑ The membrane is then trimmed with a sharp scissors to approximate size of the area being treated. The apical border of the material should extend 3–4 mm apical to the margin of the defect and laterally 2–3 mm beyond the defect
- ❑ The occlusal border of the membrane should be placed 2 mm apical to the CEJ.
- ❑ A sling suture is given so that the membrane is tightly bound around the tooth.
- ❑ Flap is then sutured back in its original position or may be slightly coronal to it with the help of independent sutures interdentally and in the vertical incision.
- ❑ Care should be taken that the flap covers the membrane completely
- ❑ Patient should be prescribed antibiotic for 1 week and placement of periodontal dressing is optional
- ❑ 4–6 weeks after the surgery the margins of the membrane becomes exposed
- ❑ The membrane is then removed with a gentle tug 5 weeks after the procedure.

3. Bio-modification of Root Surface

- ❑ Interference with new attachment has been seen because of the presence of degeneration of remnants of sharpy's fibres, accumulation of bacteria and their products, disintegration of cementum and dentin, over the tooth surface wall of periodontal pockets.

- Although these interference to new attachment can be removed through root planing, but root surface of the pocket can be treated to improve it's chances of accepting the new attachment of gingival tissues.

Various substances which are used for this purpose are:

Citric acid: The actions of citric acid are as follows:

1. Citric acid leads to accelerated healing and new cementum formation after detachment of the gingival tissues and demineralisation of the root surface.
2. On root planed roots, citric acid produces a 4mm deep demineralized zone with exposed collagen fibres.
3. On root planed roots, a smear is formed, which can be removed using citric acid, exposing the dentinal tubules. Not only this, citric acid makes the tubules appear wider with funnel-shaped orifices.
4. Citric acid also removes endotoxins and bacteria from the diseased tooth surface
5. Citric acid also prevents the epithelium from migrating over the treated roots.

Citric acid should be used in the following ways:

1. A mucoperiosteal flap should be raised and a thorough scaling and root planing should be done, removing the calculus the underlying cementum.
2. Cotton pledgets soaked in saturated solution of citric acid whose pH is 1.0 for 2–5 minutes should be applied.
3. Pledgets should be removed and root surface should be irrigated profusely with water.
4. Flap should be replaced back and sutured.

- **Fibronectin:** It is a glycoprotein required for fibroblast to attach to root surfaces.
  It is known to promote new attachment.
- **Tetracycline:** It is known to stimulate fibroblast attachment and growth while suppressing epithelial cell attachment and migration.

  It also removes the amorphous layer and exposes the dentinal tubules.

4. Biologic Mediators

- There are various factors which stimulate a series of events and cascades at some point, which can result in the coordination and completion of integrated tissue formation
- Many approaches have been used involving polypeptide growth and differentiation factor, extracellular matrix proteins and attachment factor and proteins involved in the bone metabolism
- These are physiologic molecules released by cells, or derivatives of such molecules, that can regulate events in wound healing.

- These biologic mediators are mainly growth factor which are mostly secreted by macrophages, endothelial cells, fibroblasts and platelets.
- These growth factors are platelet derived growth factor (PDGF), insulin like growth factor (IGF), basic fibroblast growth factor (bFGF), bone morphogenetic protein (BMP) and transforming growth factor (TGF)
- These mediators have shown to stimulate periodontal wound healing or to promote the differentiation of cells to become osteoblasts, favouring bone formation.
- For example, promoting migration and proliferation of fibroblast for periodontal ligament formation.
- Also PDGF has shown to enhance bone formation in periodontal osseous defects.

5. Enamel Matrix Protein

Amelogenin, is the main enamel matrix protein, which is secreted by Hertwig's epithelial root sheath during tooth development and also induces acellular cementum formation.

- These proteins are believed to cause periodontal regeneration
- Emdogain is an enamel matrix protein derivate which is obtained from developing porcine teeth, approved by the US Food and Drug Administration (FDA).
- Emdogain is viscous gel containing enamel derived protein from tooth in a polypropylene liquid, 1 mL of a vehicle solution is mixed with a powder and delivered by syringe to the defect site.
- Amelogenin is the main protein in this mixture, about 90%, with the rest primarily proline rich non-amelogenin, tuft protein, serum proteins, amelin and ameloblastin.

The technique of using Emdogain is as follows:

- A flap for reconstructive purpose is raised.
- All the granulation tissue and tissue tags are removed, exposing the underlying tissues and all the root deposits are removed.
- Bleeding is treated completely within the defect.
- Citric acid (pH of 1.0) is used for conditioning of 24% EDTA (pH of 6.2) for 15 sec. This helps in removal of smear layer and facilitate adherence of the emdogain.
- Wound should be then rinsed with saline.
- Gel should be applied to cover the root surface completely
- Contamination with blood and saliva should be avoided.
- Wound should be closed with sutures.
- Patient should be prescribed with medications, i.e. system antibiotic coverage for 10–20 days (doxycycline, 100 mg daily).

Graft Materials and Procedure

- ❑ The procedure requires placing of graft materials at the site of the defect
- ❑ These graft materials can be evaluated on their osteoinductive or osteoconductive or osteogenic potential.
- ❑ Osteogenesis means to the formation or development of new bone by cells contained in the graft.
- ❑ Osteoinduction means a chemical process by which molecules contained in the graft like BMPs convert their neighbouring cells into osteoblasts, which in turn form bone.
- ❑ Osteoconduction is referred to a physical effect by which the matrix of the graft form a scaffold that favours outside cells to penetrate the graft and form new bone.

Bone graft can be:

1. Autogenous Bone Graft

- ❑ Autogenous grafts are the grafts which are obtained from same individual.
- ❑ Sources of this kind of graft can be bone from healing extraction wound, bone from edentulous ridges, bone trephined from within the jaw without damaging the roots, newly formed bone in wounds especially created for this purpose, and bone removed during osteoplasty and ostectomy.

Various forms of autogenous grafts are as follows:

a. Osseous Coagulum: Mixtures of bone dust and blood is referred to as osseous coagulum.

- ❑ In this technique small particles from cortical bone are used.
- ❑ This particle size provides additional surface area for the interaction of cellular and vascular elements.
- ❑ Sources of the graft material can be lingual ridge on the mandible, exostoses, edentulous ridges, bone distal to a terminal tooth, bone removed by osteoplasty or ostectomy and the lingual surface of the mandible or maxilla. Atleast smm from the roots.

Technique

- ❑ Bone is removed using a carbide bur #6 and #8 using a speed of 500–30,000 rpm
- ❑ It is placed in a sterile dappen dish or amalgam cloth, and used to fill the defect
- ❑ Advantage of the technique is the ease by which bone can be obtained from already exposed surgical site.
- ❑ Disadvantage is its relatively low predictability and the inability to produce adequate material for large defects.

- ❑ Inability to use aspiration during accumulation of the coagulum.
- ❑ Unknown quantity and quality of the bone fragments in the collected material.

b. Bone blend: To overcome the disadvantage of osseous coagulum, the bone bleed technique has been proposed.

Technique: Its technique uses an autoclaved plastic capsule and pestle.

- ❑ Bone is removed from a pre-determined site, triturated in the capsule to a workable, plastic-like mass, and packed into the bony defects.

c. Cancellous bone marrow transplant: Maxillary tuberosity, edentulous areas, and healing sockets are the sites from where cancellous bone can be obtained.

- ❑ Edentulous ridges can be approached will a flap and cancellous bone and marrow can be removed with curettes and back action chisels or trephines.
- ❑ It takes about 8–12 weeks for sockets to heal and apical portion is used as donor material.
- ❑ The particles are reduced to small pieces.

d. Bone swaging: It is a difficult technique.

- ❑ It has a limited use.
- ❑ It requires an edentulous area adjacent to tooth defect, from which the bone is pushed into contact with the root surface without fracturing the bone at its base.
- ❑ Bone can be obtained from extra-oral sites also like iliac autografts, tibia autografts. They have been used in furcations and defects with various numbers of walls.

2. Allograft

- ❑ It is the bone obtained from a different individual of same species.
- ❑ They are commercially available from tissue banks.
- ❑ They are obtained from cortical bone within 12 hours of death of the donor.
- ❑ It is then defatted, cut into pieces, washed in absolute alcohol and then deep-frozen.
- ❑ The material may then be demineralised and subsequently ground and sieved to a plastic size of 250–750 μm and freeze-dried.
- ❑ Finally, it is vacuum-sealed in glass vials.
- ❑ Allografts can be undecalcified or decalcified.
  - ○ Undecalcified freeze-dried bone allograft (FDBA)
    - ➤ It is considered to be a osteo conductive material
    - ➤ It has less osteogenic potential than DFDBA
  - ○ Decalcified freeze-dried bone allografts (DFDBA)
    - ➤ It is considered to be a osteoinductive graft
    - ➤ It has a higher osteogenic potential

- ➤ Components of the bone matrix are exposed, since the bone is demineralised in cold and diluted in hydrochloric acid
- ➤ They are associated with collagen fibrils and have been termed as BMPs
- ➤ DFDBA has shown to have positive results in periodontal defect having significant probing depth
- ➤ DFDBA has also shown a gain in attachment level and osseous regeneration
- ➤ Combination of DFDBA and guided tissue regeneration has also been very successful specially in treating furcation defect.

3. Xenografts

These are the graft obtained from different species.

- ❑ Earlier calf bone, Kiel bone or ox bone were used, but now these materials have been discarded for various reasons
- ❑ Currently, an anorganic bovine derived bone, Bio-Oss has been used in periodontal defects and in implant surgery
- ❑ It is an osteo-conductive, porous bone mineral matrix from cancellous or cortical bone
- ❑ The organic part of the bone is removed but the trabecular part and the porosity are retained.
- ❑ It permits clot stabilization and revascularisation to allow migration of osteoblasts, leading to osteogenesis
- ❑ Bio-Oss is highly compatible with surrounding tissues and elicits no systemic immune responses.

4. Alloplastic Material

- ❑ These are artificial and synthetic materials used for grafting.

They are also referred to as non-bone graft materials:

They include:

- ❑ **Calcium phosphate biomaterials:** There are two types of calcium phosphate ceramics which are being used:
- ❑ Hydroxyapatite (HA) has a calcium to phosphate ratio, similar to that found in bone materials.
- ❑ **Tricalcium phosphate (TLP):** It is with a calcium to phosphate ratio of 1.5.
- ❑ **Bioactive glass:** It consists of sodium and calcium salts, phosphate and silicon dioxide. E.g. perioglass, biogran

  Used in the form of irregular particles measuring 90–170 µm or 300–355 µm.

  Other alloplastic materials are plastic materials, cartilages, sclera and plaster of paris.

Combined Techniques

- ❑ Combination of several technique can also be used
- ❑ Like bone graft and non-bone grafting materials together can be used for regeneration
- ❑ For example enamel matrix derivative like emdogain and xenografts, i.e. Bio-Oss can be combined together and can be used
- ❑ Autogenous bone with guided tissue regeneration results in new attachment and periodontal reconstruction.

CHAPTER 56

Furcation

Question 1

Define furcation involvement. Classify furcation defects. Write in detail about diagnosis and treatment of furcation defects.

Answer

It is defined as the invasion of bifurcation or trifurcation of multi-rooted tooth by periodontitis.

Furcation is an area of complex anatomic morphology which makes it difficult or impossible to clean with regular periodontal instrumentation. Furcation involvement is one of the clinical signs for the diagnosis of advanced periodontitis and potentially less favourable prognosis for the affected tooth.

Classification

Its classification is done in four grades:

1. **Grade 1:** It is an early stage of furcation involvement. Only soft tissue is involved. Early bone loss may be seen because of increase in probing depth but there are no radiological signs.
2. **Grade 2:** In this the lesion is cul de sac having a definite horizontal component. This implies that the bone loss has occurred at one side of the tooth. If multiple defects are present, they do not communicate with each other as the alveolar bone remains attached to the tooth. Radiographically it may or may not be depicted.
3. **Grade 3:** In this the bone is not attached to the dome of the furcation, therefore a multiple defects communicate with each other. In early grade 3, the opening may be filled with soft tissue which is generally not visible. A periodontal probe also cannot be passed through and through completely because of interference with the bifurcational ridges or facial/lingual bony margins.
4. **Grade 4:** In this grade the interdental bone is destroyed and the soft tissue recedes apically, so the furcation can be seen clinically. Therefore, a probe is easily passed through and through in the furcation area.

Diagnosis

Diagnosis can be made with the help of the "Naber's probe". The clinician should be able to identify and classify the extent of furcation involvement and to identify factors which contribute to the furcation defect development.

These factors may include:

- Morphology of the affected tooth.
- Position of the tooth relative to adjacent teeth.
- Anatomy of the alveolar bone.
- Configuration of the bony defect.
- Presence and extent of other dental diseases, like caries and pulpal necrosis.

Treatment

There are three objectives of furcation treatment:

1. To facilitate maintenance.
2. Prevent further attachment loss.
3. Obliterate the furcation defects as a periodontal maintenance problem.

Treatment of Class I Defects

These are early defects which can be treated with conservative periodontal approach. Treatment of choice can be scaling, root planning and maintenance of good oral hygiene. In the presence of thick overhanging margins of restorations, facial grooves or cervical enamel projections, the clinicians must opt for odontoplasty, recontouring or replacement for eradication of such defects.

Treatment of Class II Defects

In the presence of horizontal component, the therapy becomes even more complicated. Odontoplasty and osteoplasty are the treatment of choice for such defects. In cases of isolated deep Class II furcations, flap procedure is used in adjunct with above options.

Treatment of Class II–IV Defects

These are the advanced defects in which there is development of significant horizontal components. Vertical components can also be seen which poses additional problems. Non-surgical therapy is generally not useful in such defects. Endodontics therapy and periodontal surgery may be required to treat the defect.

Surgical therapy can include any of the following:

- **Root resection:** It refers to resection of one of the roots which has the least periodontal and bone support. It is generally indicated in multi-rooted teeth with Grade II–IV furcation involvement. It can be performed on both vital and endodontically treated teeth. Teeth planned for root resection includes the following:
  - Teeth that are critically important to the overall dental treatment plan.
  - Teeth that have sufficient attachment remaining for function.
  - Teeth for which more predictable or cost effective method is not available.
  - Teeth in patients with good oral hygiene and low caries activity.
- Guidelines to determine which root to be resected are as follows:
  - Resect the root or roots which eliminate furcation and allow the production of a maintainable architecture on the remaining side.
  - Remove the root having the maximum amount of bone and attachment loss.
  - Remove the root which will contribute best in the elimination of the periodontal problems.
  - Remove the root having maximum number of anatomic problems.
  - Remove the root which would least complicate the future periodontal maintenance.

- **Hemisection:** It refers to splitting of a multi-rooted tooth into two-rooted tooth and converting them into separate portions. This process can be referred to as bicuspidisation or separation since it converts a molar into two separate teeth. It is generally done in mandibular molars with Class II or III furcation. After sectioning both the roots can be retained and can be given separate crowns or one of the roots can be retained removing the other one on which maximum bone loss has occurred.
- Procedure for root resection or hemisection:
  - After administration of local anaesthesia a full thickness flap is reflected. Adequate access for visualisation and instrumentation to minimize the surgical trauma should be made. After debridement the area of resection or hemisection should be visualised carefully.
  - This procedure might require removal of small amount of facial or palatal bone. A cut is made just apical to the contact point of the tooth, through the tooth, and to the facial and distal orifices of the furcation with the help of a high speed, surgical length fissure or cross cut fissure carbide bur.
  - In case of hemisection a vertically oriented cut is made buccolingually through the pulp chamber and through the furcation.
  - After sectioning the root is elevated from the socket.
  - One should not traumatise the bone remaining on the remaining tooth.
  - Odontoplasty might be required if necessary.
  - Any bony lesion on the adjacent teeth should be resected or regenerated.
  - The flaps are then approximated and sutured.
- **Reconstruction:** It can be achieved with grafting materials. Bone grafts with or without guided tissue regeneration (GTR) membrane can be used to reconstruct the furcation defects.
- **Extraction:** Teeth with through and through furcation defects and advanced attachment loss should be extracted especially for individuals who cannot perform adequate plaque control, who have high level of caries activity, who will not commit to a suitable maintenance program, or who have socio-economic factors that may preclude more complex therapies.

SHORT NOTES

Question 1

What are cervical enamel projections (CEPs).

Answer

These are projections of the enamel seen on the cervical portion of the tooth.

- These are found in 8.6%–28.6% molars.
- These projections interfere with plaque removal, plaque control and therefore, should be removed to facilitate maintenance.

Classification of cervical enamel projection:

- **Grade I:** The enamel projection extends from cemento-enamel junction (CEJ) of the tooth towards the furcation entrance.

- **Grade II:** The enamel projection approaches the entrance to the furcation. It does not enter the furcation, and thus there is no horizontal component.

- **Grade III:** The enamel projection extends horizontally into the furcation.

CHAPTER 57

Periodontal Plastic and Aesthetic Surgery

LONG ESSAYS

Question 1

Enumerate various mucogingival/perioplastic problems and surgery procedures. Define periodontal plastic surgery and what are the objectives of plastic surgery? Enumerate various techniques to increase the width of attached gingiva. Explain in detail about gingival recession along with its treatment. Explain free gingival grafting techniques the root coverage in detail.

Answer

Various mucogingival problems are :

- Shallow vestibule
- Inadequate width of attached gingiva
- Aberrant frenal attachment
- Gingival recession.

Various mucogingival perioplastic surgery procedures are:

- Crown lengthening
- Periodontal prosthetic corrections
- Ridge augmentation
- Root coverage
- Reconstruction papilla
- Aesthetic surgical correction
- Aesthetic surgical correction around implants
- Surgical exposure of unerrupted teeth for orthodontics.

Definition of Periodontal Plastic Surgery

According to Carranza, periodontal plastic surgery is defined as the surgical procedure performed to correct or eliminate anatomic, developmental or traumatic deformities of the gingiva or alveolar mucosa.

Objectives of Periodontal Plastic Surgery

Objectives of periodontal plastic surgery are as follows:
- Problems associated with attached gingiva
- Problems associated with shallow vestibules
- Problems associated with an aberrant frenum.

Problem Associated with Attached Gingiva

- Creation or widening the zone of attached gingiva around the teeth and implants is the ultimate goal of mucogingival surgical procedures.
- The objectives of widening the zone of attached gingiva are as follows:
  - To enhance plaque removal around the gingival margin
  - To improve aesthetics
  - To reduce inflammation around restored teeth.

Problems Associated with Shallow Vestibule

- Adequate vestibular depth is important for placing the toothbrush head and maintaining adequate plaque control.
- In presence of minimal vestibular depth, adequate oral hygiene is not possible.
- Also, adequate vestibular depth is important for proper placement of removable and fixed appliances.

Problems Associated with Aberrant Frenum

An aberrant frenum attachment which on the margin of the gingiva may interfere with plaque removal and tension on this frenum may tend to open the sulcus therefore in such cases surgical removal of frenum becomes important.

Various techniques to increase the width of attached gingiva are as follows:
- Techniques can be classified as follows—
  - Gingival augmentation apical to the area of recession
  - Gingival augmentation coronal to the area of recession (root coverage).

❑ **Gingival augmentation apical to the area of recession**
  ○ In this case no attempt is made to cover the denuded root surface, where there is gingival and bone recession.
  ○ A pedicle or a free graft is placed over the recipient cells apical to the area of recession.

Various techniques of augmentation are:
  ○ Free gingival autografts
  ○ Free connective tissue autografts.

❑ **Gingival augmentation coronal to the area of recession (root coverage)**

Gingival recession: Apical shift of the gingival margin is referred to as gingival recession.

Most accepted classification of gingival recession has been proposed by Miller, it is as follows (**Fig. 57.1**):

1. **Class I:** Marginal tissue recession does not enter to the mucogingival junction
   There is no loss of bone or soft tissue in the intradental area.

2. **Class II:** Marginal Tissue recession extends to or beyond the mucogingival junction
   There is no loss of bone or soft tissue in interdental area.

3. **Class III:** Marginal tissue recession extends to or beyond the mucogingival junction.
   There is interdental bone and soft tissue loss along with malpositioning of the teeth.

4. **Class IV:** Marginal tissue recession extends to or beyond the mucogingival junction.
   There is severe bone loss and soft tissue loss interdentally along with severe malpositioning.

Root coverage options for a gingival recession are as follows:

❑ Free gingival autograft.
❑ Free connective tissue autograft.
❑ Pedicle autograft.
  ○ Laterally (horizontally) positional flap.
  ○ Coronally positioned flap.
❑ Subepithelial connective tissue graft.
❑ Guided tissue regeneration.
❑ Pouch and tunnel technique.

Free Gingival Autograft

Step 1: Prepare the recipient site: The area around the denuded root surface is de-epithelized.

❑ The root surface is scaled and planed thoroughly.
❑ The purpose of this step is to prepare a firm connective tissue bed to receive the graft.

Step 2: Obtain the graft from the donor site.

❑ The classic technique consists of transferring a piece of keratinised gingiva from the donor site to the recipient site.
❑ The dimension of the root in length and breadth along with dimension of the de epithelized recipient site are calculated.
❑ A tin foil template is made by placing the template over the recipient site and cutting it to the size more than the dimensions calculated for the root and de-epithelized area.
❑ Dimension is kept more because the graft would shrink at the time of healing so to compensate this shrinkage, size of the graft should be more than the recipient site.
❑ Then place this transplant over the donor, i.e. the palate between the premolar and molar area, towards the gingival margin and make a shallow incision around this template with a #15 blade.
❑ Insert the blade to the desired thickness.
❑ Elevate one edge and hold with tissue forceps.

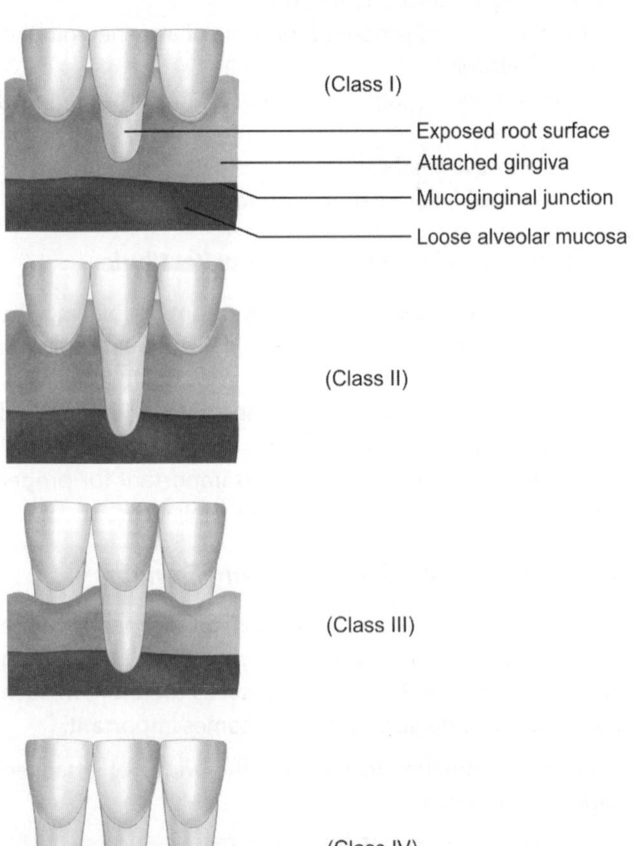

Fig. 57.1: Miller's classification of gingival recession.

❑ Continue to separate the graft with a blade and lift it gently as the separation progresses.

❑ If sutures are placed at the margins of the graft, it helps to control during separation and transfer, and simplifies placement and suturing the recipient site.

❑ For the survival of the graft, it should have proper thickness.

❑ It should be thin enough to permit diffusion of nutritive fluid from the recipient site, which is essential in the immediate post-transplant period.

❑ There may be necrosis of the graft due to exposure of the recipient site, if the graft is too thin.

❑ If, the graft is too thick, its peripheral layer is jeopardized because of the excessive tissue that separates, it from new circulation and nutrients.

❑ Thick grafts also cause deep wounds at the donor site, with the possibility of injuring the major palatal arteries.

❑ Ideal thickness of a graft should be between 1 mm to 1.5 mm.

❑ Once the graft is separated, loose tissue tags should be cleared from the under surface.

❑ Edges should be thinned to avoid bulbous marginal and interdental contours.

❑ Precautions should be taken when harvesting a graft from the palate.

❑ Since the submucosa is in the posterior region, is thick and fatty, so therefore it should be trimmed so that it does not interfere with vascularisation.

❑ Graft can be thinned by holding it between two wooden tongue depressors and slicing it with a sharp # 15 blade longitudinally.

Step 3: Transfer and immobilize the graft.

❑ The gauze should be removed from the recipient site.

❑ Excess clot should be removed.

❑ The graft should be positioned and adapted firmly over the recipient bed so that it covers the root surface and the de-epithelised area completely immobilize.

❑ Graft should be then sutured at the lateral borders and a periosteal suturing can be done if required.

❑ The graft should be completely immobilized.

❑ Excess tension should be avoided, which can lead to distortion of the graft from the underlying surface.

Step 4: Donor site protection.

❑ The donor site should be covered with a periodontal dressing for at least a period of one week.

❑ A modified hawley's retainer is useful to cover the pack on the palate.

Step 5: Recipient site protection.

❑ Once the graft is secured with sutures, the area should be covered by a tempered tin foil, over which the periodontal dressing should be placed.

Healing of the Graft

Survival of the connective tissue, leads to the success of grafts.

❑ The graft in the initial stages, is maintained by a diffusion of fluid from the host bed, adjacent gingiva and alveolar mucosa.

❑ The fluid from the host vessels is transudate and provides nutrition and hydration essential for initial survival of the transplanted tissues.

❑ On first day, the connective tissue becomes oedematous and disorganized.

❑ Connective tissue undergoes degeneration and lysis of some of its elements.

❑ As the healing progresses, the oedema is reduced and degenerated connective tissue is replaced with new granulation tissue.

❑ By the second day, revascularisation of the graft takes place.

❑ Capillaries from this recipient bed proliferates into the graft to form a network of new capillaries and anastomose with pre-existing vessels.

❑ The central portion of the graft revascularises at the last and it is completed by 10th day.

❑ Epithelium undergoes degeneration and sloughing, with complete necrosis occurring is some areas.

❑ It is replaced by new epithelium from the borders of the recipient site.

SHORT ESSAYS

Question 1

Explain laterally displaced flap.

Answer

This technique was given by Grupe and Warren in 1956 for root coverage.

Step 1: Prepare the recipient site.

❑ De-epithelisation is done around the denuded root surface to prepare the recipient site. The root surface should be thoroughly scaled and root planed.

Step2: Prepare the flap.

The donor sites gingiva should have an adequate width of attached gingiva.

❑ Partial thickness or full thickness flap can be raised depending upon the gingival biotypes.
❑ Using a #15 blade vertical incisions are made from the gingival margin to outline ae flap just next to the recipient site.
❑ Periosteum should be incised and the incision should extend into the oral mucosa to the level of the base of the recipient site.
❑ The flap should be wide enough so that it coveres the recipient site completely.
❑ A vertical incision is made along the gingival margin and interdental papilla and separate a flap which consist of epithelium and some part of connective tissue, leaving behind some connective tissue and periosteum.
❑ A releasing incision also known as cut back incision is made to avoid tension at the base of the flap. A short oblique incision is made into the alveolar mucosa at the distal corner of the flap, facing towards the direction of the recipient site.

Step 3: Transfer of flap:

❑ Flap should be slided laterally to the adjacent root, so that it lies flat and firm on the recipient bed.
❑ Flaps should be secured by placing sutures specially sling and interrupted sutures.

Step 4: Protection of flap and the donor site

The involved area should be covered with a tempered tin foil over which a periodontal dressing should be placed. Pack and sutures should to be removed after a period of 1 week.

Question 2

Describe subepithelial connective tissue graft.

Answer

This procedure is indicated for multiple and larger defects with adequate vestibular depth and thick gingival biotype so that a split thickness flap could be raised.

The technique was given by Langer and Langer in 1985.

Techniques

❑ A partial thickness flap should be raised with a horizontal incision at least 2 mm away from the tip of the papilla. Two vertical incisions should also be given 1–2 mm away from the gingival margin of the adjoining teeth.
  ○ These incisions should extend atleast half to one tooth wider mesiodistally than the area of gingival recession.
  ○ Flap should be extended upto the mucobuccal fold.
❑ Root surfaces should be planed through so that if convexity is reduced.
❑ A connective tissue graft is harvested from the palate. It should be taken 5–6 mm away from the gingival margins of molars and premolars.

After taking the graft, the palatal wound is sutured in a primary closure

❑ Connective tissue should be placed over he denuded root surface and sutured using resorbable sutures to the underlying periosteum.
❑ The connective tissue graft is then covered with the outer portion of the partial thickness flap and interdental suturing is done.
  ○ Atleast two-half to two-thirds of the connective tissue graft must be covered by the flap for the exposed portion to survive over the denuded root surface.
❑ The area is covered with a tempered tin foil and over which periodontal dressing is placed.

CHAPTER 58

Recent Advances in Surgical Techniques

SHORT ESSAYS

Question 1

Define lasers in periodontics.

Answer

Laser is an acronym for light amplification by stimulated emission of radiation.

- Laser can concentrate light energy and can exert strong effect targeting tissues at an energy level much higher than the natural light. Once in contact with tissue, laser energy is reflected, scattered, absorbed or transmitted to the neighbouring tissues (**Fig. 58.1**).
- Applications of lasers (**Table 58.1**).

Advantages

- Better haemostasis.
- Bactericidal effect.
- Wound contraction is less.
- Patient and operator comforting.

Disadvantages

- It has strong thermal side effects, leading to melting, cracking and carbonisation.
- Delayed wound healing.
- Plume is generated which has an unpleasant smell.

Precautions

- Use glasses for eye protection (patient operator and assistants).
- Prevent inadvertent radiation.
- Protect the patients' eyes, throat, and oral tissues outside the target area.
- Use wet gauge packs to avoid reflection from shiny metal surfaces.

Potential Risks with Lasers

- Excessive tissue destruction by direct ablation and thermal side effects.
- Destruction of the attachment apparatus at the bottom of the pockets.
- Excessive ablation of root surfaces and gingival tissues within periodontal pocket.
- Thermal injury to the root surface, gingival tissues, pulp and bone tissues.

Question 2

Define microsurgery in periodontics.

Answer

Periodontal microsurgery introduces the potential for less invasive surgical approaches in periodontics.

Magnification systems: It includes:

- Magnifying loupes.
- Microscope.

Magnifying Loupes

- They are the most common mode of magnification.
- They are dual mononuclear telescopes with side by side lenses convergent to focus on the operative field.

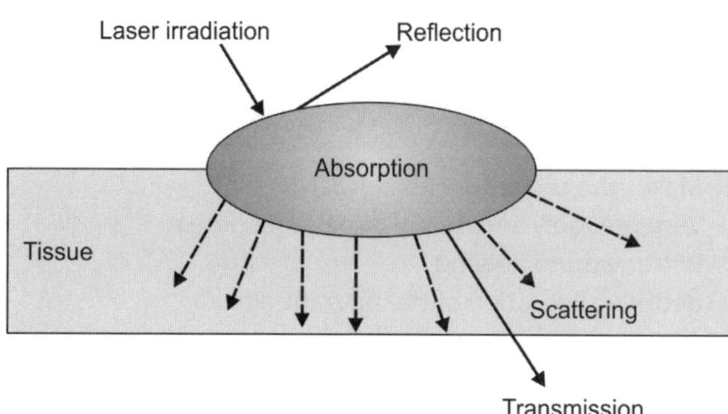

Fig. 58.1: Interaction of human tissue and laser irradiation.

Table 58.1: Application of lasers.

Type (wave length)	Active medium	Dental applications
Excimer laser (193–350)	Argon fluoride (ArF) Xenon chloride (XeCl)	Hard tissue ablation, dental calculus removal
Gas laser	Argon (Ar) (438–515)	Curing of composite materials, tooth whitening, intraoral soft tissue surgery, sulcular debridement (subgingival curettage in periodontitis, and peri-implantitis)
	Helium neon (He Ne) (637)	Analgesia, treatment of dentin hypersensitivity, aphthous ulcer treatment
	Carbon dioxide (CO_2) (10,600)	Intraoral soft tissue and soft tissue surgery, aphthous ulcer, gingival depigmentation , treatment of dentin hypersensitivity, analgesia
Diode lasers (655–980)	Indium gallium arsenide phosphorous (InGaAsP)	Caries and calculus detection
	Gallium aluminium arsenide (GaAlAs) Gallium arsenide (GaAs)	Intraoral general and implant soft tissue surgery, sulcular debridement (subgingival curettage in periodontitis), analgesia, treatment of dentin hypersensitivity, pulpotomy, root canal disinfection, removal of enamel caries, aphthous ulcer treatment, gingival depigmentation
Solid state lasers	Frequency doubled alexandrite	Selective ablation of dental plaque and calculus
	Neodymium: yttrium aluminium garnet (Nd:YAG) (1064)	Intraoral general and implant soft tissue surgery, sulcular debridement (subgingival curettage in periodontitis), analgesia, treatment of dentin hypersensitivity, pulpotomy, root canal disinfection, removal of enamel caries, aphthous ulcer treatment, gingival depigmentation
	Erbium group **Erbium:** yttrium aluminium garnet (Er:YAG) (2940) **Erbium:** yttrium scandium gallium garnet (Er:YSGG) (2790)w Erbium, chromium: yttrium scandium gallium garnet (Er, Cr:YSGG) (2780)	Caries removal and cavity preparation, modification of enamel and dentin surfaces, intraoral general and implant soft tissue surgery, sulcular debridement(subgingival curettage in periodontitis and peri-implantitis), scaling of root surfaces, osseous surgery, treatment of dentin hypersensitivity, analgesia, pulpotomy, root canal treatment and disinfection, aphthous ulcer treatment, removal of gingival melanin and metal–tattoo pigmentation

There are three types of loupes:

1. **Simple loupes:**
   - It has a pair of single meniscus lenses.
   - They are primitive magnifiers with limited capabilities.
   - Weight and size is large because it becomes difficult to handle them.
   - Its magnification is not more than 1.5x.

2. **Compound loupes:**
   - They are multi-element lenses with intervening air spaces to achieve additional refractory surfaces.
   - Its magnification is around 3x.

3. **Prism telescopic loupes:**
   - They are the most advanced system of loupes.
   - They have better magnification, wider depths of fields, longer working distances and larger fields of view.
   - They have a magnification above 4x.

Microscope

As compared to loupes, microscopes provide better magnification and superior optical performance.

- It requires training and practice to gain proficiency.
- Dental microscopes employ Galilean optics with binocular eyepieces joined by offsetting prisms to permit parallel optic axis.
- Surgical microscopes allow the dentist to change the working magnification easily.
- For use in periodontics, the surgical microscope should have both manoeuvrability and stability.

Periodontal Microsurgery

All the kinds of periodontal procedures can be performed with microsurgical techniques. They require surgical loupes, microscope, or both, microsurgical set of instruments which include special microsurgical blades, needle holders, scissors and sutures ranging from 6-0 to 9-0 to approximate the wound edges accurately.

Advantages

- Makes the procedure less invasive
- Very precisely and neatly done procedures
- Better wound healing
- Better visualisation of the operating field.

Disadvantages

- Requires training and practice to gain proficiency
- Expensive equipment.

CHAPTER 59

Dental Implants

Question 1

What is a dental implant? What is osseointegration? Classify dental implants.

Answer

Dental implant is a prosthetic device of alloplastic material(s) implanted into the oral tissues beneath the mucosal and/or periosteal layer, and on/or within the bone to provide retention and support for a fixed or removable prosthesis.

Osseointegration

This concept proposed by Branemark in 1960.

"The apparent direct attachment or connection of osseous tissue to an inert, alloplastic material without intervening connective tissue."

Glossary of Prosthetic Terms

Structurally Oriented Definition

"Direct structural and functional connection between the ordered, living bone and the surface of a load carrying implants."

Branemarks and Associates (1977)

Histologically

Direct anchorage of an implant by the formation of bone directly on the surface of an implant without any intervening layer of fibrous tissue.

Albrektson and Johnson (2001)

Dental implants can be classified as:
- Based on Placement within the Tissues
  - Transosteal implants.
  - Endosteal implants.
  - Sub-periosteal implants.
- **Transosteal implants:** A dental implant that penetrates both cortical plates and passes through the entire thickness of the alveolar bone.
- **Sub-periosteal implant:** An implant that is placed beneath the periosteum of the bone, it receives its primary bone support by resting on it.
  - This implant does not osseointegrate.
- **Endosseous implant:** An implant that is present within the bone, extends into basal bone for support.
  - **Types:** Screw form, cylinder form (hollow, solid), blade form.

Depending on the Materials Used

Metallic Implants

- Titanium.
- Titanium alloy.
- Cobalt chromium molybdenum.

Depending on their Reaction with Bone (Meffert)

- Bioactive HA coated, CaP coated.
- Bio-inert implants metals.

Question 2

What are the various complications of implant surgery? What is peri-implantitis? What is its management?

Answer

- Mobility after the healing period.
- Mucosal inflammation.
- Progressive bone loss.
- Mechanical problem—component fracture, abutment screws loosening.
- Peri-implantitis.

Peri-implantitis

- Peri-implantitits is the inflammation around the peri-implant tissues caused primarily due to plaque accumulation around the implant.
- This process is similar to the one seen on natural tooth.
- Peri-implant infections can be classified as peri-implant mucocitis and peri-implantitis depending on severity.
- Peri-implant mucocitis is the reversible inflammatory process in the mucosa of implant. Whereas, irreversible inflammatory reactions leading to loss of supporting bone results in peri-implantitis.

Signs and Symptoms of Peri-implatitis

- Bleeding, suppuration, pocket formation, bone loss.
- Pain is generally absent but when present it is associated with acute infection.

Management

Non-surgical Therapy

Pharmacological therapy: Sub-gingival irrigation for 2–3 weeks for 2–3 times daily. Proper recommendation of oral hygiene instructions.

- Chlorhexidine is prescribed as it has an antimicrobial effect and substantivity at the affected site.
- Tetracycline fibres and systemic antibiotics can also be prescribed.

Mechanical Debridement

Mechanical debridement can be recommended for a failing implant along with coating the implant surface with a super-saturated solution of citric acid for 30–60 seconds, so as to remove endotoxins from the implant surface. Soft tissue lasers can also be used for eradication of bacteria.

Occlusal Adjustments

Surgical Therapy

If the non-surgical therapy is ineffective, then the surgical techniques are indicated. It includes debriding the implant surface along with resective and regenerative techniques.

Question 3

What are the indications and contraindications of implants?

Answer

Indications

- Patients with edentulous sites or jaw.
- Patients with loss of multiple teeth.

Contraindications

- Smokers, diabetic patients, hypertensive patients.
- Patients undergoing radiation therapy.
- Patients on corticosteroid therapy.
- Patients having psychological problems.
- Patients with poor oral hygiene.
- Cost factor.
- Non-motivated patients.

Question 4

Discuss the surgical procedures for placement of implants. What is two-stage and single-stage implants?

Answer

Procedure

- Clinical evaluation.
- Radiographic evaluation: Intraoral periapical radiography, orthopantomography, cone-beam computed tomography.
- Selection of desired implant size depending on clinical and radiographic evaluation.
- Patient preparation.
- Local anesthetic administration.
- Incision and flap reflection at the desired site.
- Preparation of osteotomy site using pilot drills and subsequent drills.
- Upon the preparation of osteotomy site, the implant is placed either mechanically or motor-driven instruments.
- Cover screw is placed over the implant and flap is sutured.

Two-stage Implant

In a two-stage implant, once the implant is placed patient is called after a period of 1 week for suture removal and then after a period of 2–3 months for a second-stage surgery in which the cover screw is exposed by giving an incision and the cover screw is replaced by a healing abutment or a gingival former and then the prosthetic part is done. Therefore, it is termed as two stage implant placement.

Single-stage Implant

In this type of surgery, the implant is loaded with the crown at the time of implant placement surgery, thus preventing multiple visits.

Question 5

Discuss the maintenance of dental implants.

Answer

- The patient should be recalled at regular intervals in order to provide preventive services.

- A plastic probe should be used for checking the probing depth around the implants.
- Plastic curettes are available for the removal of any deposits around the implant surface.
- A rubber cup should be used to polish the implant surface with a non-abrasive polishing paste.
- Proper oral hygiene instructions should be given to the patients, which include a soft sulcular tooth brush, anti-plaque agents and interdental aids.

CHAPTER 60

Question 1

Discuss in detail supportive periodontal treatment.

Answer

This phase is also known as recall / maintenance / supervised recall.

- ❏ It forms an important and integral part of overall periodontal treatment and can be considered as an extension of periodontal therapy.
- ❏ This part of periodontal therapy begins post the completion of active periodontal therapy and is continued regularly at periodic intervals for the lifetime of dentition or implants.
- ❏ Transfer of the treatment from active treatment stage to supportive periodontal therapy (SPT) requires careful planing on the part of the dental team.

Rationale

- ❏ The main rationale of SPT is to prevent recurrence of periodontal disease.

Aims and Objectives

- ❏ The basic aim of SPT is to supervise, control and prevent development of disease by the patient so that he or she can maintain a healthy and functional dentition for life.

Objectives

- ❏ Maintenance of a healthy and functional oral environment.
- ❏ Preservation and maintenance of alveolar bone support and clinical attachment level.
- ❏ Periodic evaluation of home care.

Parts of Maintenance Phase

- ❏ **Part 1:** Examination:
  - ○ Changes in medical history if any, post active periodontal therapy.
  - ○ Oral pathological examination.
  - ○ Status of the present oral hygiene.
  - ○ Check for any gingival change.
  - ○ Pocket depth changes.
  - ○ Development of mobility if any.
  - ○ Changes in the occlusal harmony.
  - ○ Restorative and prosthetic changes.

- ❏ **Part 2:** Treatment:
  - ○ Oral hygiene instructions are given and maintenance of oral hygiene is reinforced.
  - ○ Oral prophylaxis (scaling and polishing) is performed.
  - ○ Chemical irrigation / site-specific antimicrobial placement is done.

- ❏ **Part 3:** Report, clean-up and schedule next procedure:
  - ○ Write report in the case sheet.
  - ○ Discuss the observations with the patient.
  - ○ Schedule next follow-up visit / periodontal treatment visit / refer to restorative or prosthetic treatment.

- ❏ **Part 1:** Examination and evaluation:
  - ○ In this phase, the operator primarily looks for changes post the last appointment.
  - ○ Current oral hygiene condition of patient is evaluated.
  - ○ Any change in the medical or dental history post the last appointment is updated.
  - ○ Gingival status, periodontal pocket depth and peri-implant probing depth are examined.
  - ○ Oral mucosa should be thoroughly examined for any kind of pathological condition.

- Radiographs are repeated and compared with previous radiographs to check bone height, repair of osseous defects, periapical changes, signs of TFO and carious lesions.
- Patients must be advised to perform their respective oral hygiene regimen immediately before the appointment in order to assess the effectiveness of plaque control.
- Hygiene regimen must be reviewed and corrected till the patient shows the necessary proficiency in plaque control.
- Instruction sessions should be scheduled till adequate plaque control is achieved.

- **Part 2:** Treatment:
  - Scaling, root planing and polishing are performed.
  - The operator must be careful not to instrument normal sites with shallow sulci (1–3 mm depth).
  - Remaining pockets either irrigated with antimicrobial agents or site-specific anti-microbial delivery systems are placed.

- **Part 3:** Determination of recall visit intervals:

  Following factors are taken in account to determine the frequency and time interval between the recall visits:
  - **Severity of disease:** More severe the disease, more frequently the patient is recalled.

- **Effectiveness of home care:** A good home-care regimen by the patient decreases the frequency of recalls.
- **Degree of control of inflammation achieved:** As the patient regains the total health of oral mucosa or tissue, the frequency of appointments is reduced.
- **Management of different types of recall patients:**
  - Patients who are uncooperative in maintaining the home-care instructions require frequent office care with thorough root instrumentation.
  - In patients who had refused surgical phase in active periodontal therapy, require regular scheduling of visits at short-time intervals.
  - Patients who have been hospitalised for several weeks are treated with periodic scaling and root planing in the hospital itself if the health condition of the patients permits.
  - Patients who have been fully and successfully treated yet show distinct breakdown in the localised area in recall visits need to be carefully inspected.
  - Careful medical history is performed and if favourable, involved areas are retreated.
  - Flap surgery, curettage and antibiotic therapy should be administered.
  - Recall visits are scheduled at least once in 2–3 months.

SHORT ESSAYS

Question 1

Important factors causing recurrence of periodontal disease.

Answer

The following factors are responsible for the recurrence of periodontal disease:

- In most cases, the aetiology of recurrence is associated with inadequate maintenance of home care oral hygiene instructions or failure to comply with SPT recall visits.
- Incomplete or inadequate or insufficient treatment procedure that failed to remove the potential factors favouring plaque accumulation.
- Persistence of calculus in areas with difficult access.
- Improper restorations post the active periodontal therapy.
- Failure of patient to comply with periodic check-ups.
- Development or presence of some systemic diseases that may affect host resistance to maintain previously acceptable levels of plaque.

SECTION 2

RECENTLY ASKED QUESTIONS

Recently Asked Questions

GINGIVA

Long Essays

1. Describe the normal clinical features of gingiva. [RGUHS]
2. Describe briefly the importance of attached gingiva. [NTR-OR]
3. Define gingiva. Describe its macroscopic and microscopic appearance and functions. Add a note on the importance of gingival fluid. [NTR-OR]
4. Write about histological and functional features of normal gingiva. Add a note on the role of epithelial attachment in periodontal disease. [NTR-OR]
5. Describe the normal structure of gingiva. Write in detail about the electron microscopic structure of gingival epithelium. [RGUHS]
6. Describe the clinical and histological features of normal healthy gingiva. [MUHS]
7. Define gingiva. Give different clinical features, between normal and diseased gingiva. [MUHS]
8. Define oral mucosa. Describe the clinical and microscopic features of normal gingiva. [NTR-UHS]
9. Define and classify oral mucosa. Describe the anatomical and histological features of gingiva. [NTR-UHS]
10. Correlate clinical and microscopic features of healthy gingiva. [GOA]
11. Define gingiva. Discuss the macroscopic features of gingiva. [GOA]
12. Define gingiva. What are the parts of normal gingiva? Describe the microscopic picture of normal gingiva. [MUHS]
13. Define gingiva. Write in detail the microscopic features of normal gingiva. [GOA]

Short Essays

1. Compare attached gingiva and alveolar mucosa. [RGUHS]
2. Histology of gingival surface epithelium. [RGUHS]
3. Gingival fibres. [NTR-OR; MUHS]
4. Attached gingiva. [NTR-OR]
5. Sulcular epithelium. [NTR-NR]
6. Enzymes in gingival fluid. [NTR-NR]
7. Junctional epithelium. [NTR-OR]
8. Dentogingival junction. [NTR-NR]
9. Gingival pigmentation. [NTR-OR]
10. Histology of gingival surface epithelium. [RGUHS]
11. Compare attached gingiva and alveolar mucosa. [RGUHS]
12. Microscopic features of healthy gingiva. [MUHS]
13. Gingival fluid. [MUHS]
14. Difference between attached gingiva and alveolar mucosa. [MUHS]
15. Describe the various concepts of formation of the gingival sulcus and give its significance. [MUHS]
16. Interdental papilla. [RGUHS]
17. Factors affecting gingival crevicular fluid flow. [NTR-UHS]
18. Inflammatory cell granuloma. [NTR-UHS]
19. Gingival crevicular fluid. [GOA]
20. Clinical features of healthy gingiva. [RGUHS]

Short Notes

1. Col. [RGUHS]
2. Gingiva. [RGUHS]
3. Gingival fibres. [RGUHS]
4. Gingival sulcus. [RGUHS]
5. Attached gingiva. [RGUHS; GOA]
6. Mast cell in gingiva. [RGUHS]
7. Gingival innervations. [RGUHS]
8. Blood supply to gingiva. [RGUHS]
9. Long junctional epithelium. [RGUHS]
10. Role of mast cells of gingiva. [RGUHS]
11. Classification of gingival fibres. [RGUHS]
12. Functions of gingival fibre system. [RGUHS]
13. Gingival fibres and its importance. [RGUHS]

14. Clinical significance of keratinized gingival. [RGUHS]
15. Gingival col. [NTR-NR; RGUHS]
16. Free gingiva. [NTR-NR]
17. Microscopic features of healthy gingiva. [MUHS]
18. Gingival crevicular fluid. [MUHS; RGUHS]
19. Definition and functions of gingival fibres. [MUHS]
20. Gingival collagen fibres. [MUHS]
21. Gingival blood supply and innervation. [MUHS]
22. Consistency of gingiva. [MUHS]
23. Defence mechanism of gingiva. [MUHS]
24. Mention about macroscopic and microscopic structures of normal gingiva. [MUHS]
25. Define periodontology and periodontics. [MUHS]
26. Neutrophils. [RGUHS; NTR-UHS]
27. Define and classify embrasures. [RGUHS]
28. Cells of gingival epithelium. [RGUHS]
29. Lamina dura. [RGUHS; NTR-UHS]
30. Mucogingival junction. [RGUHS; NTR-UHS]
31. Gingival stippling. [RGUHS]
32. Define hypertrophy, hyperplasia and neoplasia. [RGUHS]
33. Biologic width. [RGUHS]
34. Transgingival probing. [RGUHS]
35. Dentogingival unit. [RGUHS; NTR-UHS]
36. Functions of periodontal ligament. [RGUHS]
37. Stillman's clefts: [NTR-UHS]
38. McCall's festoons. [NTR-UHS]
39. Orogranulocytes. [NTR-UHS]
40. Langerhans cells. [NTR-UHS]
41. Prostaglandins. [NTR-UHS]
42. Palatogingival groove. [NTR-UHS]
43. Importance of attached gingiva. [GOA]
44. Saliva. [GOA]
45. Role of saliva as a defence mechanism of gingiva. [GOA]
46. Mast cell. [GOA]
47. Attached gingival. [RGUHS]
48. Fenestration and dehiscence. [RGUHS]

TOOTH SUPPORTING STRUCTURES (PERIODONTAL LIGAMENT, ALVEOLAR BONE, CEMENTUM)

Long Essays

1. Describe the functions and the structure of periodontal membrane. [RGUHS]
2. Discuss in detail about the anatomy, histology and functions of periodontal ligament. [RGUHS]
3. Describe the structure of cementum and add note on clinical significance of cementoenamel junction. [RGUHS]
4. Describe the histology and functions of the principal fibres of periodontal ligament. What are the periodontal ligament changes in trauma from occlusion? [RGUHS]
5. Write in detail the functions of periodontal ligament. [RGUHS]
6. Describe the structure and functions of periodontal ligament. [NTR-OR]
7. Describe briefly the various gingival and periodontal fibre groups. [NTR-OR]
8. Describe in detail the role of alveolar bone in health and periodontal disease. [NTR-OR]
9. Define periodontal ligament. Describe the microscopic and macroscopic features of periodontal ligament. [NTR-NR]
10. Define cementum. Describe the structure, composition and clinical significance of cementum. [NTR-OR]
11. Define periodontal ligament. Describe the microscopic features and add a note on its functions. [NTR-OR]
12. Enumerate the principle groups of periodontal ligament fibres. Add a note on its cellular elements and functions of periodontal ligament. [NTR-NR]
13. Discuss in detail the functions of the periodontal ligament. [MUHS]
14. Describe the normal structure and functions of cementum. Discuss the histologic importance of cementum in periodontal therapy. [MUHS]
15. What is periodontium? Name the different tissues that constitute the periodontium. Describe different tissues of the periodontium. [MUHS]
16. Define periodontal ligament. Describe in detail the functions of periodontal ligament. [MUHS]
17. Enumerate the components of periodontium. Describe the structure of periodontal ligament. [RGUHS]
18. Define cementum. Write in detail the microscopic structure of cementum. [RGUHS]
19. Describe the structure of periodontal ligament. [GOA]
20. Define cementum. Classify and give its microscopic structure. Add a note on clinical significance of cementum. [GOA]

Short Essays

1. Functions of periodontal ligament. [RGUHS; MUHS; NTR-UHS]
2. Alveolar bone. [RGUHS]

3. Define periodontal ligament and describe its function. [RGUHS]
4. Enumerate the various groups of principal fibre bundles with diagrams. [RGUHS]
5. Dehiscence. [NTR-OR]
6. Fenestration. [NTR-OR]
7. Lamina dura. [NTR-OR]
8. Oxytalan fibres. [NTR-OR]
9. Acellular cementum. [NTR-OR]
10. Cellular cementum. [NTR-NR]
11. Intermediate plexus. [NTR-OR]
12. Mediator of alveolar bone. [NTR-OR]
13. Composition of cementum. [NTR-NR]
14. Cementoenamel junction. [NTR-NR]
15. Fenestration and dehiscence. [NTR-OR; MUHS]
16. Dehiscence and fenestration. [NTR-OR]
17. Cementoenamel junction relationships. [NTR-OR]
18. Physical functions of periodontal ligament. [NTR-OR]
19. Describe the mechanisms by which periodontal ligament resists occlusal forces. [MUHS]
20. Cementum and its biologic importance. [MUHS]
21. Hypercementosis. [MUHS]
22. Oblique fibres. [NTR-UHS]
23. Functions of periodontal ligament. [NTR-UHS]
24. Principal fibres of the periodontal ligament. [NTR-UHS]
25. Describe the ultrastructure of junctional epithelium. [GOA]
26. Write about supportive periodontal treatment. [GOA]
27. Junctional epithelium. [GOA]

Short Notes

1. Physical function of periodontal ligament. [GOA]
2. Oxytalan fibres. [RGUHS]
3. Sharpey's fibres. [RGUHS]
4. Functions of cementum. [RGUHS]
5. Cementoenamel junction. [RGUHS; NTR-UHS]
6. Histology of periodontal fibres. [BUHS]
7. Causes of hypercementosis. [RGUHS]
8. Blood supply to periodontal ligament. [RGUHS]
9. Principal fibres of periodontal ligament. [RGUHS]
10. Fenestration and dehiscence. [RGUHS]
11. Define fenestration and dehiscence. [RGUHS]
12. CEJ. [RGUHS]
13. Define periodontium. What does it comprise of? [MUHS]
14. Hypercementosis. [MUHS; NTR-UHS]
15. Cemental tear. [RGUHS]
16. Clinical significance of gingival crevicular fluid. [RGUHS]
17. Enamel pearls. [RGUHS]
18. Functions of periodontal ligament. [GOA]
19. Junctional epithelium. [GOA]
20. Periosteum. [NTR-UHS]
21. Bundle bone. [NTR-UHS]
22. Functions of periodontal ligament. [GOA]
23. Periodontal fibres. [GOA]
24. Cementum. [GOA]
25. Types of cementum. [GOA]
26. Types CEJ. [RGUHS]
27. Schroeder's classification of cementum. [RGUHS]

AGE-RELATED CHANGES IN PERIODONTIUM

Long Essays

1. Describe the effects of ageing upon the periodontal tissues. [RGUHS]
2. Describe the microscopic and macroscopic appearance of human keratinized oral mucous membrane. [RGUHS]
3. Describe the changes in the periodontal tissues due to ageing. [MUHS]
4. Age changes in the periodontium. [NTR-NR]

Short Notes

1. Age changes in gingiva. [RGUHS]
2. Nature of periodontal disease. [RGUHS]
3. Age changes in the periodontium. [NTR-NR]
4. Enumerate the factors for prognosis of individual tooth in periodontal diseases. [MUHS]
5. Bruxism. [RGUHS]

CLASSIFICATION OF DISEASES OF THE PERIODONTIUM

Long Essays

1. Discuss the role of anatomical factors in aetiology of periodontal disease. [RGUHS]
2. Classify inflammatory diseases of periodontium and describe in detail anyone of them. [RGUHS]
3. Classify periodontitis. Describe the clinical and radiographic features of chronic periodontitis. [RGUHS]

Short Notes

1. Classify periodontal diseases. [MUHS]

EPIDEMIOLOGY OF GINGIVAL AND PERIODONTAL DISEASES

Long Essays

1. Define dental epidemiology and write in detail about the indices used in assessing gingival inflammation. [NTR-OR]

2. "Periodontal health for all by 2000 AD". What do you understand by this statement? How are you going to implement it by systematic manner? [NTR-OR]

3. Describe the possible causes as to why the incidence and prevalence of periodontal diseases are very high in India. [GOA]

Short Essays

1. Indices used to measure periodontal destruction. [RGUHS]

2. CPITN probe. [NTR-OR; RGUHS]

3. Russell's periodontal index. [NTR-OR; RGUHS]

4. Silness and Loe index. [NTR-OR]

5. Bleeding Point index. [NTR-OR]
6. Oral hygiene simplified. [NTR-OR]
7. Russell's periodontal index. [NTR-OR]
8. Periodontal disease index. [NTR-NR]
9. Ideal requirements of an index. [NTR-NR]
10. Oral halitosis. [RGUHS]
11. Gingival index. [RGUHS]
12. Community periodontal index. [RGUHS]
13. Name any two plaque indices. Describe in detail any one of them. [RGUHS]

Short Notes

1. OHIS. [RGUHS]
2. Silness and Leo index. [RGUHS]
3. Investigations for gingival bleeding. [RGUHS]
4. Miller's tooth mobility index. [RGUHS]
5. Define risk factor and risk determinant. [RGUHS]
6. CPITN Index. [NTR-UHS]

PERIODONTAL MICROBIOLOGY

Long Essays

1. Discuss supragingival and subgingival plaques. [RGUHS]

2. Discuss the role of plaque in aetiology of periodontal disease. [RGUHS]

3. Describe in detail steps in the formation of dental plaque. Add a note on specific plaque hypothesis. [RGUHS]

4. Define dental plaque. Describe its types, composition, bacteriology and role in aetiology of periodontal disease. [RGUHS]

5. Define dental plaque. Write in detail about the formation of plaque. Add a note on specific plaque hypothesis. [RGUHS]

6. Write bacterial composition of different types of plaque. Describe mechanisms of bacteria-mediated periodontal tissue destruction. [RGUHS]

7. Describe the role of microorganisms in the aetiology of periodontal diseases. [NTR-OR; MUHS]

8. Define and classify dental plaque. Write in detail about its composition and ill effects. [NTR-NR]

9. Define and classify microbial plaque. Discuss the role of microbial plaque in the aetiology cff gingival and periodontal diseases. [NTR-NR]

10. Define and give broad classification and composition of dental plaque. Describe the characteristics of the gel-like matrix of 'biofilm'. [MUHS]

11. What is dental plaque? Give its composition. Describe its role in the initiation and progression of gingival and periodontal diseases. [MUHS]

12. What are the signs and symptoms of periodontal diseases? Describe the general aspects of microbiology and immunology of periodontal diseases. [MUHS]

13. Define plaque. Describe the classification, composition, structure and formation of dental plaque in detail. [MUHS]

14. Define plaque. Describe the composition and formation of dental plaque. [RGUHS]

15. Describe in detail the plaque retention factors in the aetiology of periodontal disease. [RGUHS]

16. Discuss the role of microorganisms in periodontal disease. [GOA]

17. Define and classify plaque. Describe the formation of plaque and its role in the aetiology of periodontal disease. [NTR- UHS]

18. Define dental 'biofilm'. Highlight the properties of the same and add a note on various plaque hypotheses. [RGUHS]

Short Essays

1. Structure and composition of plaque.　　[RGUHS]
2. Compare supragingival and subgingival plaque.　　[RGUHS]
3. Composition of dental plaque in adult periodontitis.　　[RGUHS]
4. Materia alba.　　[NTR-OR]
5. Acquired pellicle.　　[NTR-NR]
6. Subgingival plaque.　　[NTR-OR; GOA]
7. Specific plaque hypothesis.　　[NTR-NR]
8. Differences between supra- and subgingival plaque.　　[NTR- OR]
9. Formation of plaque.　　[RGUHS; GOA]
10. Oral microorganisms in health and disease.　　[MUHS]
11. Dental plaque.　　[RGUHS]
12. Socransky's modification of Koch's postulates.　　[RGUHS]
13. Diagnostic methods used for bacterial identification.　　[RGUHS]
14. Specific and non-specific plaque hypothesis.　　[NTR-UHS; RGUHS]
15. Microbial specificity of periodontal disease.　　[NTR-UHS]
16. Socransky's criteria for identification of periodontal pathogens.　　[NTR-UHS]
17. Define plaque. Classify plaque and add a note on its mechanism of formation.　　[GOA]
18. Chemical plaque control.　　[RGUHS]

Short Notes

1. Dental pellicle.　　[RGUHS]
2. Acquired pellicle.　　[RGUHS]
3. Aetiological significance of microbial plaque.　　[RGUHS]
4. Specific plaque hypothesis.　　[NTR-NR; MUHS; GOA]
5. Define and classify dental plaque.　　[MUHS]
6. Stages of plaque formation.　　[MUHS]
7. Socransky's postulates.　　[RGUHS]
8. Giemsa's stain.　　[RGUHS]
9. Co-aggregation.　　[NTR-UHS]
10. Spirochaetes.　　[NTR-UHS]
11. Radius of action.　　[NTR-UHS]
12. Prevotella intermedia.　　[NTR-UHS]
13. Subgingival plaque.　　[GOA]
14. Normal oral bacterial flora.　　[RGUHS]

DENTAL CALCULUS, IATROGENIC AND OTHER LOCAL PREDISPOSING AETIOLOGICAL FACTORS

Long Essays

1. Define calculus mention its composition. Discuss various theories of calculus formation.　　[RGUHS]
2. Define calculus composition formation and its aetiological significance in periodontal disease.[RGUHS]
3. What is calculus, what are the theories of calculus formation? Write about composition, types of calculus, and also anticalculus agents.　　[RGUHS]
4. Define calculus. Give its classification, prevalence, composition, formation and aetiologic significance in detail.　　[MUHS]
5. Discuss the various local aetiologic factors that are responsible for initiation and progress of periodontal disease.　　[MUHS]
6. Define and classify gingival recession. Discuss in detail the procedure for free gingival autografts in the treatment of gingival recession.　　[RGUHS]
7. Describe the role of iatrogenic factors in aetiology of periodontal disease.　　[RGUHS]

Short Essays

1. Plaque retention factors.　　[RGUHS; NTR-UHS]
2. Theories of calculus formation.　　[RGUHS]
3. Calculus.　　[NTR-OR]
4. Food impaction.　　[NTR-OR]
5. Subgingival calculus.　　[NTR-NR]
6. Attachment of calculus.　　[NTR-OR]
7. Theories of calculus formation.　　[NTR-OR; RGUHS]
8. Difference between supra- and subgingival calculus.　　[NTR-OR; MUHS; RGUHS]
9. Dental calculus.　　[MUHS]
10. Mode of attachment of dental calculus.　　[MUHS]
11. Dental stains.　　[MUHS]
12. Mechanism of calculus formation.　　[MUHS]
13. Mouth breathing habit and the periodontium.　　[MUHS]
14. Sequelae of food impaction.　　[MUHS]
15. Mechanism of food impaction and its role in periodontal diseases.　　[MUHS]
16. Composition of dental plaque.　　[RGUHS]
17. Define dental calculus. Discuss theories of mineralization of dental calculus.　　[RGUHS]
18. Bruxism.　　[RGUHS]
19. Role of iatrogenic factors in periodontal disease.　　[GOA]
20. Suprabony and infrabony pockets.　　[GOA]
21. What is calculus? What is the role of calculus in periodontitis? List the features of subgingival calculus.　　[GOA]
22. Write about composition and formation of calculus.　　[GOA]

Short Notes

1. Aetiological significance of calculus. [RGUHS]
2. Food impaction. [NTR-NR; MUHS; RGUHS]
3. Enumerate various theories of mineralization of calculus. [MUHS]
4. State the composition of dental calculus. [MUHS]
5. Dental calculus. [MUHS]
6. Theories of mineralization of calculus. [MUHS]
7. Composition of calculus. [MUHS]
8. Theories of calculus formation. [MUHS]
9. Sequelae of food impaction. [MUHS]
10. Iatrogenic factors. [MUHS]
11. Hypersensitivity. [MUHS]
12. Epitactic concept in calculus formation. [RGUHS]
13. Any 5 methods to treat dental hypersensitivity and overhanging restorations. [RGUHS]
14. Ill effects of overhanging restorations. [RGUHS]
15. Supragingival calculus. [GOA]
16. Composition and attachment of calculus. [GOA]
17. Theories regarding mineralization of calculus. [GOA]
18. Iatrogenic factors in the aetiology of periodontal disease. [GOA]

SMOKING AND PERIODONTIUM

Short Essay

1. Smoking and periodontal disease.

HOST RESPONSE—BONE CONCEPTS

Short Essays

1. Cytokines. [RGUHS]
2. Mast cells. [RGUHS]
3. Role of macrophages in periodontal disease. [RGUHS]
4. Complement system. [RGUHS]
5. IgG. [NTR-OR]
6. Mast cell. [NTR-OR]
7. Lymphocyte. [NTR-OR]
8. Immunoglobulins. [NTR-NR]
9. Arthus reaction. [NTR-OR]

Short Notes

1. Type 1 hypersensitivity. [RGUHS]
2. Cytokines. [RGUHS]
3. Lymphocytes. [RGUHS]
4. Lymphokines. [RGUHS]
5. Define cytokines. [RGUHS]
6. Cytokines. [NTR-NR]
7. Neutrophils. [NTR-NR]
8. Name the functional defects of leukocytes. [NTR-NR]
9. Antibacterial factors in saliva. [RGUHS]

HOST-MICROBIAL INTERACTIONS IN PERIODONTAL DISEASES

Short Notes

1. Prostadlandins [NTR UHS]

TRAUMA FROM OCCLUSION

Long Essays

1. What is trauma from occlusion? Give the signs, symptoms and treatment of primary traumatic occlusion. [MUHS]
2. What is trauma from occlusion? Give the signs, symptoms and histopathological features of trauma from occlusion. [MUHS]

3. Discuss the aetiopathogenesis of pathologic migration and mobility of teeth. [MUHS]
4. What is traumatic occlusion? What is trauma from occlusion? Classify and give its signs and symptoms. [MUHS]
5. Define trauma from occlusion and discuss its aetiology, clinical features and management. [NTR-OR]
6. Define trauma from occlusion. Discuss the pathology, clinical and radiographic features of trauma from occlusion. [NTR-NR]
7. Describe the role of trauma from occlusion in case of periodontal diseases. Describe the physiological and pathological tooth mobility seen in the teeth involved in trauma from occlusion. [NTR-OR]
8. Discuss the pathology, clinical futures, and diagnosis of trauma from occlusion. [RGUHS]
9. Define trauma from occlusion and traumatic occlusion. Discuss role of trauma from occlusion. [BUHS]
10. Define trauma from occlusion. Describe in detail clinical manifestations of trauma from occlusion. [BUHS]
11. Define and classify trauma from occlusion. Write the various stages of trauma from occlusion. Add a note on the influence of trauma from occlusion on the spread of inflammation. [RGUHS]

Short Essays

1. Primary traumatic occlusion. [MUHS]
2. Pathological migration of teeth. [MUHS]
3. Difference between primary traumatic occlusion and secondary traumatic occlusion. [MUHS]
4. Secondary trauma from occlusion. [MUHS]
5. Forces of occlusion. [NTR-NR]
6. Pathology migration. [NTR-NR]
7. Pathological tooth migration. [NTR-OR]
8. Define and classify trauma from occlusion. [NTR-NR]
9. Classification and diagnosis of trauma from occlusion. [NTR-NR]
10. Concepts of trauma from occlusion. [BUHS]
11. Tissue response to increased occlusal forces. [RGUHS]
12. Differentiate between primary and secondary occlusion trauma. [BUHS]
13. Bruxism. [NTR-OR]
14. Night guard. [NTR-OR]

15. Masticatory cycle. [NTR-NR]
16. Clinical features of bruxism. [RGUHS]
17. Injury phase in trauma from occlusion. [RGUHS]
18. Management of dentinal hypersensitivity. [RGUHS]
19. Soft tissue changes to increased occlusal forces. [NTR-UHS]
20. Tooth mobility. [NTR-UHS]
21. Trauma from occlusion. [NTR-UHS]

Short Notes

1. Define trauma from occlusion. What are the various stages of tissue response in trauma from occlusion? [MUHS]
2. What is adaptive remodelling of the periodontium in response to external force? List various changes produced in the periodontium due to remodelling. [MUHS]
3. Pathological migration of teeth. [MUHS]
4. Clinical and radiological changes in trauma from occlusion. [MUHS]
5. Traumatic occlusion. [MUHS]
6. What is adaptive remodelling of the periodontium in response to external force? List various changes produced in the periodontium due to remodelling. [MUHS]
7. Causes of and changes produced by primary trauma from occlusion. [MUHS]
8. Pathologic migration. [MUHS]
9. Primary and secondary trauma. [RGUHS]
10. Trauma from occlusion. [RGUHS]
11. Define acute and chronic trauma from occlusion. [RGUHS]
12. Facets. [NTR-NR]
13. Parafunctional condition and periodontium. [RGUHS]
14. Define trauma from occlusion. [RGUHS]
15. Secondary occlusal trauma. [GOA]
16. Fenestration and dehiscences. [GOA]
17. Therapeutic occlusion. [NTR-UHS]
18. Supra contacts. [NTR-UHS]
19. Acute trauma from occlusion. [GOA]
20. Primary trauma from occlusion. [GOA]
21. Bruxism. [GOA]
22. Passive eruption. [GOA]
23. Fremitus test. [RGUHS]

INFLUENCE OF SYSTEMIC DISEASES ON THE PERIODONTIUM AND PERIODONTAL MEDICINE

Long Essays

1. Discuss the causes of gingival bleeding. How will you proceed to investigate such case? [MUHS]
2. State the systemic conditions modifying the clinical appearance of periodontal tissue. Describe in detail the clinical features of any three such conditions. [MUHS]

3. Write in detail about the systemic diseases causing periodontal manifestations. [RGUHS]
4. Antibiotic prophylaxis for the medically compromised patient. [NTR-NR]
5. Describe pregnancy gingivitis and its management. [GOA]
6. Relationship between diabetes and periodonotal disease and management of a diabetic patient with periodontal disease.

[GOA]

Short Essays

1. Describe in short oral manifestations in scurvy. [MUHS]
2. Possible role of ascorbic acid deficiency in aetiology of periodontal disease. [MUHS]
3. Periodontal manifestations of leukaemia. [MUHS]
4. Describe the relationship between diabetes and periodontitis. [MUHS]
5. Vitamin C. [NTR-NR]
6. Chediak-Higashi syndrome. [NTR-OR]
7. Diabetes and periodontal health. [NTR-NR]
8. Oral lesions in diabetes mellitus. [NTR-OR]
9. Diabetes mellitus and periodontal disease.

[NTR-OR; RGUHS]
10. Periodontal manifestations of diabetes mellitus.

[NTR-NR]
11. Diabetes as a risk factor in periodontal diseases.

[NTR-UHS]
12. Diabetes and periodontal diseases. [NTR-UHS]
13. Periodontal care of patients with cardiac pacemakers.

[RGUHS]
14. AIDS and periodontium. [RGUHS]
15. Effects of smoking on periodontium. [RGUHS]
16. Periodontitis and metabolic control of diabetes mellitus.

[RGUHS]
17. Periodontal management of a dental transplant patient.

[RGUHS]

18. AIDS and periodontal disease. [RGUHS]
19. Periodontal management of diabetic patient. [NTR-UHS]
20. Periodontal manifestations of HIV infection. [NTR-UHS]
21. Kaposi's sarcoma. [NTR-UHS]
22. Risk factors associated with periodontal disease.

[NTR-UHS]
23. Antibiotic prophylaxis for infective endocarditis.

[NTR- UHS]
24. Discuss management of a diabetic patient. [GOA]
25. Influence of diabetes on the periodontium. [GOA]
26. Discuss periodontal findings in AIDS. [GOA]
27. Describe the periodontal features in HIV-positive individuals. [GOA]

Short Notes

1. Scorbutic gingivitis. [RGUHS]
2. Gingiva in leukaemia. [RGUHS]
3. Gingival pigmentation. [RGUHS]
4. Vitamin C in gingival disease. [RGUHS]
5. Periodontal disease in infective endocarditis. [RGUHS]
6. Impact of diabetes and periodontium. [RGUHS]
7. Bruxism. [MUHS]
8. Stress and periodontal diseases. [MUHS]
9. Treatment for bruxism. [MUHS]
10. Oral manifestation of diabetes mellitus. [MUHS]
11. Role of systemic conditions on periodontal health.

[MUHS]
12. Periodontal medicine. [BUHS]
13. Periodontal care of patients on anticoagulant therapy.

[RGUHS]
14. Any five neutrophil disorders causing periodontitis.

[RGUHS]
15. Scurvy. [RGUHS]
16. Pregnancy gingivitis. [GOA]
17. Papillon-Leferve syndrome. [GOA]
18. Gingival changes in pregnancy. [GOA]
19. Impact of diabetes mellitus on periodontium. [RGUHS]

DENTAL IMPLANTS

Short Essays

1. Indications for implant therapy. [RGUHS]
2. Failure of implants. [RGUHS]
3. Osseoinducation, osseoconduction and osseointegration.

[NTR-UHS]
4. Osseointegration. [NTR-UHS]

Short Notes

1. Peri-implantitis. [MUHS; NTR-UHS; GOA; RGUHS]
2. Maintenance of dental implants. [RGUHS]
3. Peri-implant diseases. [RGUHS]
4. Osseointegration. [GOA]
5. Implant bone interface. [GOA]
6. Aetiology of peri-implant disease. [GOA]

DEFENCE MECHANISMS OF THE GINGIVA

Long Essay

1. Describe in detail about the defence mechanism of gingiva. [RGUHS, NTR-OR, NTR-UHS]

Short Essays

1. Role of saliva in oral health. [RGUHS]
2. Methods of collection of GCF. [RGUHS]
3. Gingival fluid. [NTR-OR]
4. Enzymes in gingiva. [NTR-OR]
5. Gingival crevicular fluid. [NTR-OR]
6. Disease activity and inactivity. [NTR-NR]
7. Composition of gingival cervical fluid. [NTR-NR]
8. Methods of collection of gingival crevicular fluid (GCF). [NTR-NR]
9. Role of saliva in oral defence mechanism. [RGUHS]
10. Interleukin-I. [NTUHS]
11. Immunoglobulins. [GOA]

12. Saliva in oral defence. [RGUHS]

Short Notes

1. Gingival fluid. [RGUHS]
2. Functions of GCF. [RGUHS]
3. Intrasulcular drug delivery. [RGUHS]
4. Antibacterial factors of saliva. [RGUHS]
5. Clinical significance of gingival fluid.
6. Clinical significance of crevicular fluid. [RGUHS]
7. Enumerate the protective component of saliva in periodontal disease process. [MUHS]
8. Complement. [RGUHS]
9. Host modulation therapy (HMT). [NTR-UHS]
10. Active immunity. [NTR-UHS]
11. Cytokines. [GOA]
12. Anaphylaxis. [GOA]
13. Proinflammatory cytokines. [RGUHS]

GINGIVAL INFLAMMATION AND CLINICAL FEATURES OF GINGIVITIS

Long Essays

1. Define gingival recession. Enumerate its causes. [RGUHS]
2. Describe clinical and microscopic features of chronic gingivitis. [RGUHS]
3. Define gingival bleeding. Write about causes and management of gingival bleeding. [RGUHS]
4. What is gingival recession? How will you treat a case of localized gingival recession on mandibular left central incisor. [MUHS]
5. Discuss the causes of gingival bleeding. How will you proceed to investigate such a case. [MUHS]
6. Discuss gingival bleeding. [NTR-OR]
7. Define gingival bleeding. Write about causes and management of gingival bleeding. Define and classify gingival recession. [NTR-OR]
8. Discuss in detail the aetiology and management of gingival recession. [NTR-NR]
9. Discuss the causes of gingival bleeding. How will you proceed to investigate such cases. [MUHS]

Short Essays

1. Gingival recession. [MUHS]
2. Treatment of advanced stage of gingivitis. [MUHS]
3. Treatment of localized gingival recession. [MUHS]
4. Enumerate the stages of gingivitis. [NTR-OR]

5. Pathways of gingival inflammation. [NTR-OR]
6. Established lesion of chronic gingivitis. [NTR-OR]
7. Gingival recession. [NTR-OR]
8. Gingival pigmentations. [NTROR]
9. Management of operative bleeding. [NTR-OR]
10. Management of localized gingival bleeding. [NTR-OR]
11. Mucogingival problems. [RGUHS]
12. Enumerate stages of gingivitis. Discuss established lesion. [RGUHS]
13. Gingival bleeding. [NTR-UHS]
14. Describe the clinical features and management of acute pericoronitis. [GOA]

Short Notes

1. Stillman's cleft. [RGUHS; NTR-NR]
2. McCall's festoons. [RGUHS]
3. Gingival recession. [RGUHS]
4. Causes of gingival bleeding. [RGUHS]
5. Causes of gingival recession. [RGUHS]
6. Aetiology of gingival recession. [NTR-NR]
7. Classify the gingival recession. [NTR-NR]
8. Enumerate the stages of gingivitis. [NTR-NR]
9. Plasma cell gingivitis. [NTR-UHS]
10. Gingival abscess. [GOA]
11. Stages of gingivitis. [RGUHS]
12. Transgingival probing. [RGUHS]

GINGIVAL ENLARGEMENTS

Long Essays

1. Classify gingival enlargements. Write in detail drug-induced gingival enlargement. [RGUHS; MUHS]
2. Define gingival abscess. Write in detail about aetiology and treatment of the same. [RGUHS]
3. Classify gingival enlargements. Describe clinical features and histopathology of leukaemic enlargement. [RGUHS]
4. Describe effects of pregnancy on periodontium. Mention the precautions to be taken during pregnancy in periodontal therapy. [RGUHS]
5. Classify gingival enlargement. Discuss in detail signs, symptoms and treatment of dilantin sodium gingival enlargement. [MUHS]
6. Define and classify gingival enlargements. Describe aetiology, clinical features and management of any one type of gingival enlargement. [MUHS]
7. Classify gingival enlargement. What is conditioned enlargement in pregnancy? [MUHS]
8. Classify gingival enlargement and write in detail about phe- nytoin enlargement. [NTR-OR]
9. Classify gingival enlargement and describe the drug-induced gingival enlargements. [NTR-NR]
10. Classify gingival enlargement. Discuss the histopathology and clinical features of drug-induced gingival enlargement (DIGO). [NTR-NR]
11. Define gingival enlargement. Write briefly the differential diagnosis of inflammatory and noninflammatory gingival enlargement. [NTR-OR]
12. Classify gingival enlargements. Write about clinical features and histopathology of dilantin-induced gingival enlargement. [GOA]
13. Classify gingival enlargements. Describe the pathogenesis, histopathology, clinical features and treatment of conditioned gingival enlargement. [NTR-UHS]
14. Classify gingival enlargements. Give indications, contraindications and method of gingivectomy. [GOA]
15. Classify gingival enlargement. Describe drug-induced gingival enlargement in detail. [GOA]
16. Classify gingival enlargement. How will you differentiate between leukaemic and scorbutic gingival enlargement. [GOA]
17. Classify gingival enlargement. Discuss phenytoin-induced gingival enlargement in detail. [GOA]

Short Essays

1. Classify gingival enlargements. Add a note on idiopathic enlargement. [RGUHS]
2. Compare leukaemic gingival enlargement and dilantin sodium hyperplastic gingival enlargement. [RGUHS]
3. Pregnancy gingival enlargement. [MUHS]
4. Give differential diagnosis of epulis. [MUHS]
5. Angiogranuloma. [NTR-NR]
6. Pregnancy gingivitis. [NTR-NR]
7. Benign tumours of gingiva. [NTR-OR]
8. Leukaemic gingival enlargement. [NTR-OR]
9. Conditioned gingival enlargement. [NTR-OR]
10. Drug induced gingival enlargements. [NTR-OR]
11. Classification of gingival enlargements. [RGUHS]
12. Pyogenic granuloma. [NTR-UHS]
13. Drug induced gingival hyperplasia. [NTR-UHS]
14. Peripheral giant cell granuloma. [NTR-UHS]
15. Idiopathic gingival enlargement. [NTR-UHS]
16. Lymphocytes. [NTR-UHS]
17. Non-inflammatory gingival enlargement. [RGUHS]

Short Notes

1. Gingival abscess. [RGUHS]
2. Angiogranuloma. [RGUHS]
3. Gingival enlargement. [RGUHS]
4. Drug induced gingival enlargement. [RGUHS]
5. Pathogenesis of phenytoin sodium gingival enlargement. [RGUHS]
6. What is the difference between gingival abscess and periodontal abscess? [MUHS]
7. Pregnancy tumour. [MUHS; RGUHS; NTR-UHS]
8. Management of periodontal diseases in pregnant patient. [MUHS]
9. What is drug-induced gingival hyperplasia? [MUHS]
10. Gingival enlargement. [BUHS]
11. Familial gingival enlargement. [RGUHS]
12. Pathogenesis of phenytoin sodium gingival enlargement. [BUHS]
13. Developmental gingival enlargements. [RGUHS]
14. Classification of gingival enlargement. [RGUHS]
15. Clinical features of drug-induced gingival hyperplasia. [NTR-UHS]
16. Conditioned enlargement. [GOA]
17. Rapidly progressive enlargement. [GOA]
18. Phenytoin-induced gingival enlargement. [GOA]

ACUTE GINGIVAL INFECTIONS

Long Essays

1. Describe in detail clinical features of ANUG.　　[RGUHS]
2. Describe clinical features and treatment of ANUG.　　[RGUHS]
3. What are acute infections of gingiva? Describe in detail anyone of them.　　[RGUHS]
4. What is a Vincent's infection? Write its aetiology, clinical features and its management.　　[RGUHS]
5. Describe aetiology, clinical features, differential diagnosis and treatment of ANUG in detail.　　[RGUHS]
6. Discuss about clinical features, histopathology and differential diagnosis of acute herpetic gingivostomatitis.　　[RGUHS]
7. Classify gingival lesions and discuss in detail about acute necrotizing ulcerative gingivitis and its management.　　[RGUHS]
8. Give the signs, symptoms, differential diagnosis and treatment of acute herpetic gingivostomatitis.　　[MUHS]
9. Give the signs, symptoms, differential diagnosis and treatment of acute necrotizing ulcerative gingivitis.　　[MUHS]
10. Enumerate acute gingival lesions. Discuss in detail aetiology, clinical features, histopathology and differential diagnosis of acute herpetic gingivostomatitis.　　[MUHS]
11. Discuss the clinical features, histopathology and management of gingivosis.　　[NTR-OR]
12. Describe the aetiology, clinical features and treatment of acute necrotizing ulcerative gingivitis.　　[NTR-OR]
13. Describe the aetiology, clinical features and differential diagnosis of acute herpetic gingivostomatitis.　[NTR-OR]
14. Enumerate the acute infections of gingiva. Describe the aetiology, clinical features and histopathology of acute necrotizing ulcerative gingivitis.　　[NTR-NR]
15. Enumerate the acute lesions of gingiva and write in detail the clinical features, histopathology and management of acute necrotizing ulcerative gingivitis.　　[NTR-OR]
16. Enumerate acute gingival infection. Discuss the aetiopathogenesis, clinical features and treatment of ANUG.　　[GOA]

Short Essays

1. Management of acute pericoronitis.　　[RGUHS]
2. Compare necrotizing ulcerative gingivitis and acute herpetic gingivostomatitis.　　[RGUHS]
3. Enumerate the acute infections of the gingiva.　[MUHS]
4. Pericoronitis.　　[NTR-OR; GOA]
5. Aphthous ulcer.　　[NTR-OR]
6. Gingival abscess.　　[NTR-OR]
7. Hepatic gingivostomatitis.　　[NTR-OR]
8. Acute herpetic gingivostomatitis.　　[NTR-NR]
9. Treatment of ANUG.　　[NTR-OR]
10. Aetiology of ANUG.　　[RGUHS]
11. Necrotizing ulcerative gingivitis.　　[NTR-UHS]

Short Notes

1. Gingivosis.　　[RGUHS]
2. Tzanck test.　　[RGUHS]
3. Aphthous ulcer.　　[RGUHS]
4. Borrelia vincentii.　　[RGUHS]
5. Herpetic gingivostomatitis.　　[RGUHS]
6. Management of pericoronitis.　　[RGUHS]
7. EM findings of necrotizing ulcerative gingiva.　[RGUHS]
8. Clinical features of acute herpetic gingiva stomatitis.　　[RGUHS]
9. Management of acute herpetic gingivostomatitis.　　[MUHS]
10. Laboratory investigations of acute herpetic gingivostomatitis.　　[MUHS]
11. Treatment of acute pericoronitis.　　[MUHS]
12. Porphyromonas gingivalis.　　[NTR-NR]
13. Differential diagnosis of acute herpetic gingivostomatitis.　　[RGUHS]
14. Bacterial flora in ANUG.　　[RGUHS]
15. Gingival abscess.　　[NTR-NR]
16. ANUG.　　[GOA]
17. Acute herpetic gingivostomatitis.　　[RGUHS]

DESQUAMATIVE GINGIVITIS

Long Essays

1. What is desquamative gingivitis? Give the clinical features, histopathological and treatment of severe form of desquamative gingivitis.　　[MUHS]

2. Describe about aetiology, clinical features, pathogenesis and management of chronic desquamative gingivitis.　　[RGUHS]

3. Classify desquamative gingivitis lesions and describe in detail the candidiasis lesions.　　[NTR-NR]

4. Describe the aetiopathogenesis, histopathology, clinical features and treatment of chronic desquamative gingivitis. [NTR-UHS]

4. Define and classify chronic desquamative gingivitis lesions. [NTR-NR]
5. Management of chronic desquamative gingivitis. [RGUHS]

Short Essays

1. Treatment of chronic desquamative gingivitis. [MUHS]
2. Desquamative gingivitis. [NTR-OR]
3. Herpetic gingivostomatitis. [NTR-OR]

Short Notes

1. Acute pericoronitis. [MUHS]
2. Chronic desquamative gingivitis. [MUHS]
3. Pericoronitis. [MUHS]

GINGIVAL AND PERIODONTAL DISEASES IN CHILDREN AND YOUNG ADOLESCENTS

Long Essay

1. Discuss in detail about the gingival diseases in children. [RGUHS]

Short Essays

1. Aetiopathogenesis and clinical features of ANUG. [RGUHS]
2. Iatrogenic factors in periodontal disease. [RGUHS]
3. Endotoxins and periodontal disease. [RGUHS]

4. Aetiology of gingival recession. [RGUHS]

Short Notes

1. Hypophosphatasia. [BUHS]
2. Papillon-Lefevre syndrome. [RGUHS]
3. Aetiology of gingival recession. [RGUHS]
4. Linear gingival erythema. [RGUHS]
5. Gingival recession. [NTR-UHS]
6. Periodontal cyst. [NTR-UHS]

PERIODONTAL POCKET

Long Essays

1. Discuss the pathogenesis of periodontal pocket. [RGUHS]
2. Define and classify periodontal pocket. Describe the pathogenesis. [RGUHS]
3. Describe the pathogenesis of periodontal pocket. Add a note on reattachment concept. [RGUHS]
4. Classify periodontal pockets. Describe how would you treat a suprabony periodontal pocket. [RGUHS]
5. Define pocket. Describe the classification, pathogenesis and histopathology in detail with a note on root surface changes. [RGUHS]
6. Define periodontal pockets. Classify periodontal pockets and methods of eliminating pockets. Write in detail about gingival curettage. [RGUHS]
7. Define pocket. Give its classification and describe various methods of pocket elimination. [MUHS]
8. Describe the signs, symptoms and treatment of acute periodontal abscess. How would you differentiate between acute periodontal abscess and acute periapical abscess. [MUHS]
9. Classify periodontal pockets. Discuss pathogenesis and treatment of pseudopockets. [MUHS]

10. Define and classify periodontal pockets. Add a note on its histopathology and management. [NTR-OR]
11. Define periodontal pocket. Describe its classification, histopathology, pathogenesis and sequale. [NTR-OR]
12. Define periodontal pocket. Classify periodontal pocket and discuss the pathogenesis and contents of periodontal pocket. [NTR-OR]
13. Define periodontal pocket. Describe the nonsurgical treatment regimen, which may help in pocket elimination. [NTR-OR]
14. Classify periodontal pockets. Describe the clinical and microscopic features of the pocket. [NTR-NR]
15. Define and classify periodontal pocket. Describe the pathogenesis of periodontal pocket and enumerate the differences between suprabony and infrabony pockets. [NTR-UHS]
16. Define and classify periodontal pockets. Describe the histopathology and treatment of periodontal pockets. [GOA]
17. Define and classify periodontal pocket. Write the various treatment modalities for pocket elimination procedures. Define and classify periodontal pocket. [NTR-UHS]

18. Define and classify pockets. Discuss the aetiopathogenesis of a periodontal pocket. [GOA]

19. Classify periodontal pockets. Describe in detail the pathogenesis and histopathology of pocket formation. [GOA]

20. Enumerate periodontal pocket management procedures. Discuss the role of 'phase I therapy' in the treatment of periodontal disease. [RGUHS]

21. Define and classify periodontal pocket. Describe in detail about modified Widman's flap. [RGUHS]

Short Essays

1. Suprabony and infrabony pocket. [RGUHS; GOA]

2. Give the aetiology and line of treatment of a chronic periodontal abscess. [MUHS]

3. What is the difference between a gingival abscess and periodontal abscess? [MUHS]

4. Infrabony pockets. [MUHS]

5. Micro flora in periodontal pocket. [MUHS]

6. Acute periodontal abscess. [MUHS]

7. Microtopography of periodontal pocket wall. [MUHS]

8. Periodontal pocket. [MUHS]

9. Suprabony pockets. [NTR-OR]

10. Infrabony pocket. [NTR-OR]

11. Classification of periodontal pockets. [NTR-NR]

12. Root surface changes in periodontal pocket. [NTR-NR; GOA]

13. Histopathology of lateral wall of pocket. [RGUHS]

14. Angular defects. [RGUHS]

15. Aetiopathogenesis of pockets. [RGUHS]

16. Pathogenesis of periodontal pocket. [NTR-UHS]

17. What are the signs and symptoms of pocket formation? [GOA]

18. Define and discuss the aetiopathogenesis of periodontal pocket. [RGUHS]

Short Notes

1. Periodontal cyst. [RGUHS]

2. Periodontal pocket. [RGUHS]

3. Supra- and intrabony pocket. [RGUHS]

4. What is the difference between gingival and periodontal abscess? [MUHS]

5. Classify periodontal pockets. [MUHS]

6. Correlation of clinical and histopathological features of periodontal pocket. [MUHS]

7. Root surface changes in presence of periodontal pocket. [MUHS]

8. Differentiate between suprabony and infrabony pockets. [MUHS; RGUHS]

9. Changes in root surface wall of periodontal pockets. [MUHS]

10. Advances in periodontal probing. [MUHS]

11. Complex pocket. [NTR-UHS]

12. Cemental changes in periodontal pocket. [GOA]

13. Infrabony pocket. [GOA]

14. Root surface changes in periodontal pocket. [GOA]

BONE LOSS IN PERIODONTAL DISEASES

Long Essays

1. Schematically explain bacterial and host-mediated mechanism of bone resorption in periodontitis.[RGUHS]

2. Explain the osseous crates. What are the procedures employed in eliminating osseous craters? [RGUHS]

3. What are different types of osseous defects. Write in detail about the procedure of osseous craters. [RGUHS]

4. Describe the mechanism of bone resorption. Mention the pattern of bone defects in trauma from occlusion. [RGUHS]

5. Classify bony defects in periodontal disease. How would you establish the prognosis of such defects? [MUHS]

6. What is meant by bone defect? Describe the various bones defects observed in periodontal diseases and discuss the various factors that determine the morphology of alveolar bone in periodontal diseases. [MUHS]

7. Enumerate the periodontal osseous defects. Describe the regenerative osseous surgery. [RGUHS]

8. Describe the features of alveolar bone in health. Discuss the various types of osseous defects seen in periodontal diseases. [RGUHS]

Short Essays

1. Osseous defects. [RGUHS]

2. Bone loss in periodontal diseases. [MUHS]

3. Osseous defects in periodontal diseases. [MUHS]

4. Lipping. [NTR-OR]

5. Osseous defects. [NTR-OR]

6. Intrabony defects. [NTR-OR]

7. Osseous deformity. [NTR-OR]

8. Angular bone defects. [NTR-OR]

9. Positive architecture of alveolar bone. [NTR-OR]

10. Mediators of alveolar bone destruction. [NTR-OR]
11. Tooth mobility. [RGUHS; NTR-UHS]
12. Pathological migration. [NTR-UHS]
13. Bone destruction patterns in periodontal disease. [GOA]
14. Discuss osseous defects. [GOA]
15. Patterns of bone destruction in periodontal disease. [RGUHS]

Short Notes

1. Bone factor. [RGUHS]
2. Osseous defects. [RGUHS; GOA]
3. Radius of action. [RGUHS]
4. Bone functional unit. [RGUHS]
5. Buttressing bone formation. [MUHS]
6. Describe in short the various osseous defects seen in periodontal disease. [MUHS]

7. Bone destruction patterns in periodontal disease. [MUHS]
8. Tooth mobility. [MUHS; GOA]
9. Reverse architecture. [NTR-NR; RGUHS]
10. Inconsistent bony margins. [NTR-NR]
11. Enumerate bone destructive patterns in periodontal diseases. [NTR-NR]
12. Pathologic migration. [RGUHS]
13. Hemiseptum. [NTR-UHS]
14. Pathologic tooth migration. [GOA]
15. Mobility. [GOA]
16. Recession. [GOA]
17. Osseous craters. [GOA]
18. Bone sounding. [GOA]
19. Buttressing bone formation and its type. [RGUHS]

PERIODONTITIS: CHRONIC, REFRACTORY AND NECROTIZING ULCERATIVE

Long Essays

1. Discuss the pathology, clinical features, diagnosis of trauma from occlusion. [RGUHS]
2. Define trauma from occlusion and traumatic occlusion. Discuss role of trauma from occlusion. [RGUHS]
3. Define trauma from occlusion. Describe in detail clinical manifestations of trauma from occlusion. [RGUHS]
4. Classify periodontitis. Compare between rapidly progressive and adult periodontitis. [RGUHS]
5. What is 'juvenile periodontitis'? Describe sign, symptoms and treatment of the same. [MUHS]
6. Treatment of acute necrotizing ulcerative gingivitis (ANUG). [MUHS]
7. Classify periodontitis. Describe the clinical features of chronic periodontitis. [RGUHS]

Short Essays

1. Trauma from occlusion. [RGUHS]
2. Pathological tooth migration. [RGUHS]
3. Primary trauma from occlusion. [RGUHS]
4. Concepts of trauma from occlusion. [RGUHS]
5. Tissue response to increased occlusal forces. [RGUHS]
6. Differentiate between primary and secondary occlusal trauma. [RGUHS]

7. Slowly progressive periodontitis. [RGUHS]
8. Refractory periodontitis. [NTR-OR]
9. Necrotizing ulcerative periodontitis. [NTR-OR]
10. Clinical features of chronic periodontitis. [RGUHS]
11. Refractory periodontitis. [GOA]

Short Notes

1. Trauma from occlusion. [RGUHS]
2. Define acute and chronic trauma from occlusion. [RGUHS]
3. Hypophosphatasia. [RGUHS]
4. Papillon-Lefevre syndrome. [RGUHS]
5. Refractory periodontitis. [MUHS; NTR-UHS]
6. Necrotizing ulcerative periodontitis. [MUHS; NTR-NR; RGUHS]
7. Juvenile periodontitis. [MUHS]
8. Treatment of ANUG. [MUHS]
9. Bacteriology of localized aggressive periodontitis. [RGUHS]
10. Periodontal disease activity. [RGUHS]
11. Radiographic findings in LJP. [GOA]
12. Rapidly progressive periodontitis. [GOA]
13. Treatment of localized juvenile periodontitis. [GOA]
14. Clinical and radiologic features of LJP. [GOA]
15. Prepubertal periodontitis. [GOA]

AGGRESSIVE PERIODONTITIS

Long Essays

1. Describe clinical feature, diagnosis and management of localized juvenile periodontitis. [RGUHS]
2. Define and classify plaque. Describe the plaque host interaction in juvenile periodontitis. [RGUHS]
3. Classify juvenile periodontitis. Describe in detail clinical and radiographic features of juvenile periodontitis [RGUHS]
4. Describe aetiology, clinical features, radiographic finding and management of localized juvenile periodontitis. [RGUHS]
5. What do you mean by prognosis? Discuss the doctors you could take into consideration for determining prognosis of juvenile periodontitis. [RGUHS]
6. Define juvenile periodontitis. Write in detail about aetiology, clinical features, radiographic findings and management of such condition. [RGUHS]
7. Describe the signs, symptoms, aetiology and treatment of localized juvenile periodontitis. [NTR-OR]
8. Describe the signs, symptoms, differential diagnosis and treatment of localized juvenile periodontitis. [NTR-OR]
9. Describe in detail about the juvenile periodontitis. Enumerate the differences between the juvenile periodontitis and adult periodontitis. [NTR-OR]
10. Describe the aetiology, clinical radiographic features and treatment of localized aggressive periodontitis. [RGUHS]

Short Essays

1. Aetiology and clinical features of LJR [RGUHS]
2. Localized juvenile periodontitis and its management. [RGUHS]
3. Pre-pubertal periodontitis. [NTR-OR]
4. Localized juvenile periodontitis. [NTR-OR]
5. Localized aggressive periodontitis. [NTR-NR]
6. Microorganisms in juvenile periodontitis. [NTR-OR]
7. Clinical and radiographic features of localized juvenile periodontitis. [NTR-NR]
8. Aetiology, clinical features of localized aggressive periodontitis. [RGUHS]
9. Aggressive periodontitis. [NTR-UHS]
10. Aetiology and radiographic features of localized aggressive periodontitis. [RGUHS]

Short Notes

1. Pre-pubertal periodontitis. [RGUHS]
2. Define juvenile periodontitis. [RGUHS]
3. Plaque in localized juvenile periodontitis. [RGUHS]
4. Role of periodontal disease on systemic health. [RGUHS]
5. Distinguish between localized and generalized periodontitis. [RGUHS]
6. Porphyromonas gingivalis. [NTR-NR]
7. Actinobacillus actinomycetemcomitans. [NTR-NR]

PERIODONTAL ABSCESS

Long Essays

1. Discuss the diagnosis, management of acute periodontal abscess. [RGUHS]
2. Describe the aetiology of periodontal abscess. How would you treat the same? [RGUHS]
3. Give the aetiology, signs, symptoms and treatment of periodontal abscess. [RGUHS]

Short Essays

1. Compare acute periodontal abscess and acute periapical abscess. [RGUHS]
2. Treatment of periodontal abscess. [MUHS]
3. Give the aetiology and line of treatment of a chronic periodontal abscess. [MUHS]
4. Periodontal abscess. [NTR-OR]
5. Management of chronic periodontal abscess. [RGUHS]
6. Difference between gingival, periodontal and periapical abscess. [RGUHS]
7. Periodontal abscess versus periapical abscess. [RGUHS]
8. Periodontal and periapical abscess. [GOA]

Short Notes

1. Treatment of periodontal abscess. [MUHS]
2. Give the aetiology, differences and treatment of gingival and periodontal abscess. [MUHS]
3. Periodontal abscess versus periapical abscess. [MUHS]
4. Periodontal abscess. [NTR-NR]
5. Difference between periodontal and periapical abscess. [NTR-NR]

HALITOSIS

Short Essays

1. Halitosis.   [NTR-NR; RGUHS]
2. Causes and management of halitosis.   [RGUHS]
3. Treatment of oral malodour.   [NTR-UHS]
4. Food impaction.   [NTR-UHS; GOA]
5. Sequelae of food impaction.

[GOA]

Short Notes

1. Food impaction.   [RGUHS; GOA; NTR-UHS]
2. Define food impaction, food lodgement and gingival ablation.   [RGUHS]
3. Mouth-breathing habit.   [GOA]
4. Halimeter.   [NTR-UHS]
5. Food impaction and its sequelae.   [GOA]

CLINICAL DIAGNOSIS AND ADVANCED DIAGNOSTIC METHODS

Long Essays

1. What are diagnosis and differential diagnosis? Write the importance of different aids in diagnosis of gingival and periodontal disease.   [MUHS]
2. Discuss the causes of gingival bleeding. How will you proceed to investigate such a case?   [MUHS]
3. Discuss the importance of history taking in periodontal diagnosis and treatment planning.   [MUHS]
4. Discuss the causes of gingival bleeding. How will you proceed to investigate such case?   [MUHS]
5. Describe the diagnostic aids used in periodontal diseases.   [NTR-NR]
6. Define diagnosis. Describe the various microbiological investigations used in periodontal diagnosis. Add a note on the limitations of the radiographs in periodontal diagnosis.   [NTR-NR]
7. Discuss about the diagnosis and diagnostic aids in periodontics.   [RGUHS]

Short Essays

1. Tooth mobility.   [RGUHS; NTR-OR; MUHS]
2. Diagnostic aids in periodontics.   [MUHS]
3. Root hypersensitivity as a periodontal problem. [MUHS]
4. Tooth mobility test.   [NTR-OR]
5. Halitosis.   [MUHS]
6. Discuss the causes of gingival bleeding.   [MUHS]
7. What are the uses of radiography in the periodontal therapy?   [MUHS]
8. Wasting diseases of teeth.   [NTR-OR]
9. Physiologic tooth mobility.   [NTR-OR]
10. Miller's tooth mobility.   [RGUHS]
11. Roentgenograms in periodontal diagnosis.   [NTR-OR]

12. Importance of radiographs in periodontics.   [NTR-OR]
13. Microbiological tests used in periodontal diagnosis.   [RGUHS]

Short Notes

1. Halitosis.   [RGUHS]
2. Tooth mobility.   [RGUHS; NTR-NR]
3. Wasting disease.   [RGUHS]
4. Causes of tooth mobility.   [RGUHS]
5. Radiographic features of periodontitis.   [RGUHS]
6. DNA probes.   [RGUHS]
7. BANA.   [MUHS]
8. What are the various causes of increased tooth mobility?   [MUHS]
9. Acute episodes of gingival bleeding.   [MUHS]
10. Define and give the aetiology of halitosis. [MUHS]
11. What is halitosis?   [MUHS]
12. What are the uses of radiography in the periodontal therapy?   [MUHS]
13. Uses and limitations of radiograph in periodontics.   [MUHS]
14. Tension test.   [NTR-NR]
15. Transgingival probing.   [NTR-NR]
16. Causes and measurements of tooth mobility.   [NTR-NR]
17. Periotemp.   [NTR-NR]
18. DNA probe.   [NTR-NR]
19. Fremitus test.   [NTRUHS]
20. Perio Aid.   [NTR-UHS]
21. Limitations of radiographs of radiographs in diagnosis of periodontal disease.   [GOA]
22. Use of antimicrobials in periodontal therapy. [GOA]
23. Limitations of radiographs in periodontal diagnosis.   [GOA]

DETERMINATION OF PROGNOSIS

Long Essays

1. Define prognosis. Discuss in detail factors taken in to consideration in overall prognosis. [RGUHS]
2. Define prognosis. Describe factors that help in determining prognosis of a periodontal patient. [RGUHS]
3. Define prognosis. What factors will you consider while evaluating prognosis of periodontally involved teeth? [RGUHS]
4. Define prognosis. What are the points to be considered in a periodontally affected tooth from the point of prognosis? [RGUHS]
5. Define prognosis. What factors will you take into consideration while determining the prognosis of a case? [MUHS]
6. Define prognosis. How will you determine the prognosis of a patient suffering from chronic periodontitis? [MUHS]
7. Define prognosis. Describe in detail the various factors you consider to assess the prognosis. [NTR-OR]
8. Define prognosis. Write in detail the procedures adopted to assess the prognosis for periodontal treatment. [NTR-OR]
9. Define prognosis and discuss the various aspects which influences the prognosis of periodontal therapy. [NTR-OR]
10. Define prognosis. What factors would you consider for determining the prognosis of a tooth with periodontal disease? [NTR-OR]
11. Define prognosis. Write in detail the procedure adopted to assess the prognosis for periodontal treatment. [NTR-OR]
12. What do you understand by the term 'prognosis'? Enumerate the various factors which determine the prognosis of various factors which determine the prognosis of periodontal involved teeth. [NTR-OR]
13. Define periodontal prognosis. What are its types? Outline the factors influencing individual prognosis. [RGUHS]
14. Define prognosis. Discuss in detail factors affecting prognosis. [NTR-UHS]
15. Define prognosis. Discuss the various factors you consider to assess the prognosis of periodontally involved teeth. [NTR-UHS]
16. Define prognosis. Describe the factors affecting overall prognosis of a case of periodontitis. [GOA]
17. Define prognosis. Discuss the various factors which determine the prognosis of a patient with periodontal disease. [GOA]

Short Essays

1. Tobacco use and its effect on periodontium. [MUHS]
2. Overall prognosis. [NTR-OR]
3. Periodontal therapy for pregnant patients. [NTR-NR]
4. Assessment of individual tooth prognosis in periodontitis. [RGUHS]
5. Factors for overall prognosis. [RGUHS]
6. Factors affecting overall prognosis. [GOA]
7. Define prognosis. Describe the various factors which affect individual tooth prognosis. [GOA]

Short Notes

1. Prognosis of teeth with furcation involvement. [RGUHS]
2. Epithelial attachment. [RGUHS]
3. Define new attachment and repair. [RGUHS]
4. Phases of periodontal therapy. [MUHS]
5. Mention the importance of cementum in periodontal therapy. [MUHS]
6. Give definition and factors influencing 'individual prognosis' of periodontal disease. [MUHS]
7. Describe in short the important factors to prevent recurrence of periodontal disease. [MUHS]
8. Role of tooth morphology in assessing prognosis of individual tooth. [MUHS]
9. Enumerate the factors for overall prognosis of periodontal diseases. [RGUHS]
10. Individual prognosis. [NTR-UHS].

PERIODONTAL TREATMENT PLAN

Long Essays

1. Describe the importance of maintenance phase in periodontal therapy. [RGUHS]
2. What is treatment plan? Describe the various phases of treatment plan. Discuss in detail about the 'maintenance phase'. [MUHS]

Short Essays

1. Treatment planning in periodontitis. [RGUHS Apr 2001]

2. Phase 1 therapy?   [NTR-NR Apr 2005]
3. Maintenance phase.   [NTR-NR Oct 2002, Apr 2004]
4. Importance of maintenance phase.   [NTR-OR Apr 1996]

PERIODONTAL INSTRUMENTATION

Long Essays

1. Classify periodontal probes. Add a note on its uses.
                                                  [RGUHS]
2. Classify periodontal instruments and describe anyone of them in detail.   [NTR-OR]
3. Describe the general principles you follow during oral prophylaxis.   [NTR-OR]
4. Describe the general principles of periodontal instrumentation.   [BUHS]

Short Essays

1. Periodontal probe.   [RGUHS]
2. Area specific curette.   [RGUHS]
3. Principle of sharpening periodontal instruments.
                                                  [MUHS]
4. Finger rest.   [NTR-NR]
5. Naber's probe.   [NTR-OR]
6. Kirkland knife.   [NTR-OR]
7. Periodontal probes.   [NTR-OR]
8. Polishing instruments.   [NTR-OR]
9. Area-specific curettes.   [NTR-NR]
10. Sharpening of periodontal instruments.   [NTR-OR]
11. Differences between scalers and curettes.   [NTR-OR]
12. CPITN index.   [RGUHS]

Short Notes

1. Gracey curette.   [RGUHS; NTR-NR; GOA]

2. Universal curette.   [RGUHS]
3. Periodontal probe.   [RGUHS; GOA; NTR-UHS]
4. Gingivectomy knives.   [RGUHS]
5. Periodontal surgical instruments.   [RGUHS]
6. CPITN.   [GOA]
7. Difference between Gracey and universal curettes.
                                                  [RGUHS]
8. What are the principles of sharpening periodontal instruments?   [MUHS]
9. Limitations and contraindications of ultrasonic scalers.
                                                  [MUHS]
10. Classification of periodontal instruments.   [MUHS]
11. Periotron.   [MUHS]
12. Instrument stabilization.   [MUHS]
13. Sharpening of periodontal instruments.   [MUHS]
14. Instrument grasp.   [RGUHS]
15. Hoe scalers.   [RGUHS]
16. Area-specific curettes.   [RGUHS]
17. DNA probe.   [RGUHS]
18. Features of Florida probe.   [RGUHS]
19. Curettes.   [RGUHS]
20. William's periodontal probe.   [NTR-UHS]
21. Langer's curettes.   [NTR-UHS]
22. Periodontal knives.   [NTR-UHS]
23. Naber's probe.   [NTR-UHS]
24. William's probe.   [NTR-UHS]
25. Periotrievers.   [NTR-UHS]
26. Florida probe.   [GOA]

PRINCIPLES OF PERIODONTAL INSTRUMENTATION

Long Essays

1. Describe the general principles of periodontal instrumentation.   [RGUHS]

Short Essays

1. Instrument stabilization.   [RGUHS]
2. Probing techniques in periodontics.   [RGUHS]
3. Finger rest.   [NTR-UHS]

4. General principles of periodontal instrumentation. [GOA]

Short Notes

1. Finger rest.   [RGUHS]
2. Instrument stabilization.   [RGUHS]
3. Finger rest and grasps.   [RGUHS]
4. Principles of instrumentation.   [NTR-UHS]
5. Finger rest in periodontal instrumentation.
                                                  [RGUHS]

SONIC AND ULTRASONIC INSTRUMENTATION

Long Essay

1. What is ultrasonic scaling? Write about indications, contraindications, unit proper and also recent advances. [RGUHS]

Short Essays

1. Hazards of ultrasonic scalers. [RGUHS]

2. Ultrasonic scalers. [GOA]

Short Notes

1. Ultra sonics. [RGUHS; NTR-OR; GOA]
2. Principles of ultrasonic scalers. [RGUHS]
3. Ultrasonic scaling. [NTR-OR]
4. Ultrasonic scaler. [NTR-NR; RGUHS ; GOA]
5. Ultrasonics in periodontics. [NTR-NR]

GENERAL PRINCIPLES AND CONCEPTS OF GROWTH

Long Essay

1. What is phase 1 therapy? Discuss the importance. [NTR-OR]

Short Essays

1. Phase 1 therapy. [NTR-NR]

2. Root planing. [RGUHS]

Short Notes

1. Importance of phase 1 therapy. [RGUHS]
2. Scaling and root planing. [NTR-UHS]
3. Burn-out phenomenon. [NTR-UHS]

PLAQUE CONTROL

Long Essays

1. Write in detail about antiplaque and anticalculus agents. [RGUHS]
2. Define oral hygiene, oral prophylaxis and oral physiotherapy. Describe the various aids available for the plaque control. [MUHS]
3. What is preventive periodontics? Describe the different oral hygiene aids to prevent and control the plaque formation. [MUHS]
4. What is oral physiotherapy? Describe the indications, contraindications, advantages and disadvantages of modified Stillman's method. [MUHS]
5. Describe the various methods of plaque control. [NTR-OR; GOA]
6. What is plaque control? Describe the various aids used for interdental cleaning. [NTR-OR]
7. What do you understand by plaque control? Discuss the various interdental clearing aids. [NTR-OR]
8. Describe various plaque control methods. [NTR-UHS]
9. Dental plaque control in detail. [GOA]

Short Essays

1. Define dental plaque and describe chemical plaque control. [RGUHS]
2. Chemical inhibition of plaque. [MUHS]
3. Merits and limitations of datun and toothbrush. [MUHS]
4. Dental floss. [MUHS; NTR-UHS]
5. Modified Stillman's brushing technique. [MUHS]
6. Factors in selection of a toothbrush. [MUHS]
7. Bass brushing technique. [MUHS]
8. Interdental cleansing aids. [MUHS]
9. Disclosing agents. [MUHS; RGUHS]
10. Abuses of toothbrush. [MUHS]
11. Vehicles of local drug delivery in periodontics. [MUHS]
12. Historical background and current developments in the designs of toothbrushes. [MUHS]
13. Dentifrice. [NTR-OR]
14. Toothbrush. [NTR-NR]
15. Dental floss. [NTR-OR]
16. Ideal toothbrush. [NTR-OR]
17. Interdental clearers. [NTR-NR]

18. Interdental devices. [NTR-OR]
19. Interdental cleaning aids. [NTR-OR]
20. Interdental hygiene aids. [NTR-OR]
21. Disclosing solution. [NTR-NR]
22. Desensitizing agents. [NTR-OR]
23. Chemical plaque control. [NTR-OR]
24. Chlorhexidine. [NTR-OR]
25. Chlorhexidine digluconate. [NTR-NR]
26. Bass technique of tooth brushing. [NTR-NR]
27. Uses and abuses of toothbrush. [NTR-OR]
28. Chemical antiplaque agents. [NTR-OR]
29. Dental floss and technique of flossing. [NTR-NR]
30. ADA specific confiscations of a toothbrush. [NTR-NR]
31. Oral prophylaxis and physiotherapy. [NTR-OR]
32. Adverse effects of chlorhexidine mouthwash. [RGUHS]
33. Various plaque control methods. [RGUHS]
34. Chemical plaque control. [RGUHS; NTR- UHS; GOA]
35. Chlorhexidine as a mouth rinse. [RGUHS]
36. Interdental aids. [RGUHS; GOA]
37. Toothbrush design. [NTR-UHS]
38. Powered toothbrushes. [NTR Feb-UHS]
39. Modified bass technique. [NTR-UHS]
40. Bass method of brushing. [NTR-UHS]
41. Discuss mechanical plaque control. [GOA]

Short Notes

1. Dental floss. [RGUHS; GOA]

2. Plaque control. [RGUHS]
3. Disclosing agent. [RGUHS; GOA]
4. Interdental brushes. [RGUHS]
5. Chlorhexidine gluconate. [RGUHS; GOA]
6. Interdental cleaning aids. [RGUHS]
7. Concepts of brushing teeth. [RGUHS, GOA]
8. Adverse effects of chlorhexidine. [RGUHS]
9. Dentifrices. [MUHS]
10. Interdental cleansers in type II embrasures. [MUHS]
11. Toothbrush. [MUHS; RGUHS; GOA]
12. Controlled release local delivery system. [MUHS]
13. Indications and side effects of chlorhexidine. [MUHS]
14. Enumerate the interdental aids. [MUHS]
15. Oral physiotherapy. [RGUHS]
16. Chemical plaque control. [RGUHS]
17. Subgingival irrigation. [RGUHS]
18. Charters technique of tooth brushing. [RGUHS]
19. Chlorhexidine chip. [RGUHS]
20. Bass technique of brushing. [RGUHS]
21. Dentifrices. [RGUHS; NTR-UHS]
22. Interdental cleaning devices. [NTR-UHS]
23. Chlorhexidine. [NTR-UHS; GOA]
24. Proxabrush. [NTR-UHS]
25. Anticalculus agents. [NTR-UHS]
26. Interdental plaque control devices. [GOA]
27. Interdental aids. [GOA]
28. Stillman's method of tooth brushing. [RGUHS]

CHEMOTHERAPEUTIC AGENTS

Long Essay

1. Enumerate the components of nonsurgical periodontal therapy. Discuss in brief local drug delivery system. [RGUHS]

Short Essays

1. Metronidazole in periodontal therapy. [MUHS]
2. Antibiotics. [NTR-OR]
3. Periodontal pack. [NTR-OR]
4. Periodontal dressing. [NTR-OR]
5. Desensitizing agents. [NTR-OR]
6. Tetracyclines in periodontics. [NTR-NR]
7. Local drug delivery system. [NTR-NR]

8. Antibiotic prophylaxis for the medically compromised patients. [NTR-NR]
9. Metronidazole. [RGUHS]
10. Advantages of local drug delivery system. [RGUHS]

Short Notes

1. Prophylactic antibiotics. [RGUHS]
2. Tetracycline in periodontitis. [RGUHS]
3. Role of tetracyclines in periodontal diseases. [RGUHS]
4. Controlled release local delivery system. [MUHS]
5. Enumerate various controlled release local drug delivery system. [MUHS]
6. Periodontal dressing. [NTR-NR]
7. Desensitizing agents. [NTR-NR]

PERIODONTAL SPLINTS

Long Essays

1. Define periodontal splint. Give classification of periodontal splints. Discuss their role as adjuncts in periodontal therapy. [RGUHS; GOA]
2. Define periodontal splint. Give the indications and contraindication for splinting of teeth. [RGUHS]
3. Define periodontal splinting. Mention ideal requisites of a periodontal splint and write in detail about one periodontal splinting procedure. [RGUHS]

Short Essays

1. Classify periodontal splint. [RGUHS]
2. Periodontal splints. [RGUHS; NTR-UHS; GOA]
3. Periodontal dressing. [NTR-UHS]

Short Notes

1. Function of periodontal splint. [RGUHS]
2. Clinical importance of biologic width. [RGUHS]
3. Treatment of bruxism. [RGUHS]
4. Periodontal packs. [RGUHS; GOA]
5. Permanent splinting. [GOA]
6. Periodontal dressing. [GOA]
7. Splinting. [GOA]

GENERAL PRINCIPLES OF PERIODONTAL SURGERY

Long Essays

1. Describe the general principle of periodontal surgery. [RGUHS]
2. Discuss in detail the role and importance of preoperative management in periodontal surgery. [MUHS]
3. Discuss the rationale and the procedures employed in the 'etiotropic phase' and 'initial phase' of treatment planning in periodontal therapy. [MUHS]
4. Write in detail general principles of periodontal surgery. [MUHS]
5. Discuss in detail the role and importance of adequate preoperative management in periodontal surgery. [MUHS]
6. How will you prepare the patient for periodontal surgery? Discuss in detail the common general consideration to carry out various periodontal surgical procedures. [MUHS]
7. Describe the concept of physiological tissue formation as an essential aspect of periodontal surgery. [NTR-OR]

Short Essays

1. Periodontal dressing. [RGUHS; MUHS; NTR-OR]
2. Objectives of surgical phase in periodontal treatment. [MUHS]
3. Periodontal pack. [NTR-OR]
4. Suture material used in periodontal surgery. [NTR-OR]
5. Difference between frenectomy and frenotomy. [RGUHS]
6. Frenectomy. [RGUHS]
7. Factors that affect wound healing. [NTR-UHS]

Short Notes

1. What are the various indications for hospital periodontal surgery? [MUHS]
2. Indications of periodontal surgery and methods of pocket elimination. [MUHS]
3. Types of periodontal dressings. [RGUHS]
4. Factors influencing the successful outcome of surgery. [NTR-UHS]
5. Horizontal mattress suture. [NTR-UHS]

GINGIVAL SURGICAL PROCEDURES

Long Essays

1. How do you manage a case of soft, oedematous 4 mm deep pocket. [RGUHS]
2. Define curettage and write about indications, contraindications and procedure. [RGUHS]
3. Mention pocket eradication techniques available. Briefly describe the procedure for gingival curettage. [RGUHS]
4. Give the indications and step-by-step procedure in gingi- vectomy. [RGUHS]
5. What are the indications for gingivectomy? Describe the healing affect on gingivectomy. [RGUHS]

6. Define gingivectomy. Give its indications, contraindications and surgical technique with a note on healing. [RGUHS]
7. Define gingivectomy. Write indications, contraindications, step-by-step procedure. Add a note on healing after gingivectomy. [RGUHS]
8. What are the indications and contraindications for gingivectomy? Describe step-by-step procedures for performing gingivectomy. [RGUHS]
9. Describe in detail the procedure of subgingival curettage. [MUHS]
10. Describe various aspects of gingivectomy surgery. [MUHS]
11. Mention different surgical procedures for widening the zone of attached gingiva. Describe any one technique in detail. [MUHS]
12. Define mucogingival surgery. Give the indications for mucogingival surgery. Describe any one technique to cover a localized area of gingival recession. [MUHS]
13. Define mucogingival surgery. Give the classification and indications of it. Describe the free gingival autograft technique for gingival augmentation apical to recession in detail. [MUHS]
14. Define and classify gingival recession. Discuss in detail the procedure for free gingival autografts in the treatment of gingival recession. [RGUHS]
15. Define gingivectomy. What are the indications and contraindications for gingivectomy? Describe the gingivectomy procedure. [NTR-UHS]
16. Define periodontal plastic surgery. Discuss the techniques to increase the width of attached gingiva. [NTR-UHS]
17. Define mucogingival surgery. Describe the classic technique of free gingival autograft. [GOA]
18. Give indications and contraindications for gingivectomy. Describe in detail conventional gingivectomy technique. Add a note on its healing. [GOA]
19. Enumerate mucogingival surgeries. Write in detail about free gingival autograft procedure. [GOA]

Short Essays

1. Define curettage and add a note on ENAR [RGUHS]
2. Healing after gingivectomy. [RGUHS]
3. Rationale of subgingival curettage. [MUHS]
4. Merits and demerits of electrosurgery. [MUHS]
5. Describe the healing process after gingivectomy. [MUHS]
6. Gingivoplasty. [MUHS; RGUHS; NTR- UHS]
7. Indications and contraindications of gingivectomy. [MUHS; NTR-UHS; RGUHS]
8. High frenal attachment sequelae and" treatment. [MUHS]
9. Definition and indication of mucogingival surgery. [MUHS]
10. HMT. [NTR-UHS]
11. Free gingival graft. [GOA]

Short Notes

1. ENAP. [RGUHS]
2. Gingivoplasty. [RGUHS; NTR-UHS]
3. Indications of gingivectomy. [RGUHS]
4. Differentiate between gingivectomy and gingivoplasty. [RGUHS]
5. What are the indications for gingival curettage? [MUHS]
6. Differentiate between area-specific and universal curette. [MUHS]
7. What are the causes of failure of gingivectomy? [MUHS]
8. Enumerate the different means of taking a gingivectomy incision. [MUHS]
9. Differentiate between gingivectomy and gingivoplasty. [MUHS]
10. Indications of mucogingival surgery. [MUHS]
11. Preprosthetic periodontal surgery. [MUHS]
12. Operations of removal of frenum. [MUHS]
13. Indications of mucogingival surgery. [MUHS]
14. Frenectomy or frenotomy. [GOA]
15. Electrosurgery. [GOA]
16. Curettage. [GOA]
17. Periodontal dressings. [RGUHS]

PERIODONTAL FLAP SURGERY

Long Essays

1. Classify flaps. Write in detail about the laterally positioned flap. [GOA]
2. Describe the various types of healing following periodontal surgical procedures. [RGUHS]
3. Enumerate various pocket elimination procedures. Give indications, contraindications and procedures of flap surgery in detail. [RGUHS]
4. Enumerate the various pocket elimination procedures. What are the indications for flap surgery? Describe the technique of modified Widman's flap. [RGUHS]

5. Define and give classification of periodontal flaps. What are the objectives and essential steps of modified Widman's flap? [MUHS]
6. Discuss the different therapeutic procedures available for the elimination of periodontal pocket. [MUHS]
7. What are the indications of conventional flap operation? Describe its technique in detail. [MUHS]
8. Define flap. Classify basic flaps. Give a step-by-step account of modified Widman's flap. [MUHS]
9. Give different therapeutic procedures available for evacuation of periodontal pockets. Discuss the healing process following subgingival curettage. [MUHS]
10. Define and give classification of periodontal flaps. What are objectives and essential steps of modified Widman's flap? [MUHS]
11. Define flap. Classify basic flap. Give a step-by-step account of modified Widman's flap. [MUHS]
12. Define and classify periodontal flap. Write the indications and technique of modified Widman's flap. [RGUHS]
13. Define and classify gingival recession. Mention the various surgical procedures for root coverage and describe in detail any one surgical procedure for root coverage. [RGUHS]
14. Enumerate periodontal surgical procedures. Write in detail indications, contraindications and technique of modified Widman's flap. [GOA]
15. Define and classify periodontal flap. Discuss the modified Widman's flap in detail. [NTR]
16. Define periodontal flap. Describe the indications, contraindications and technique of modified Widman's flap procedure. [NTR]
17. Define and classify periodontal flap. Describe the indications, advantages and step-by-step procedure of modified Widman's flap. [NTR-UHS]
18. Define and classify periodontal flap. Give indications and techniques of modified Widman's flap. [GOA]
19. List the causes of recession. Enumerate treatment options for recession. Give indications, contraindications and method of laterally positioned flap. [GOA]
20. Define periodontal flap. Write indications, contraindications step-by-step procedure of modified Widman's flap. [RGUHS]
21. Enumerate causes of recession. Describe procedure of the laterally positioned flap, indications and contraindications of the same. [GOA]

Short Essays

1. Types of periodontal flap surgical procedures. [RGUHS]
2. Indications for periodontal surgery. [RGUHS]
3. Modified Widman's flap. [RGUHS; GOA]
4. Papilla preservation. [NTR]
5. Describe the surgical procedure of modified Widman's flap. [GOA]
6. Modified Widman's flap technique. [GOA]
7. Papilla preservation flap. [RGUHS]
8. New attachment procedures. [RGUHS]

Short Notes

1. Excisional new attachment procedure (ENAP). [MUEIS]
2. ENAP. [MUHS]
3. Methods of pocket elimination. [MUHS]
4. Horizontal incisions for flap surgery. [RGUHS]
5. New attachment. [RGUHS; NTR-UHS]
6. Root resection in the management of furcation involvement. [GOA]

RESECTIVE OSSEOUS SURGERY

Long Essays

1. Steps in osseous resective surgery. [RGUHS]
2. Difference between ostectomy and osteoplasty. [RGUHS]
3. Define and give classification of periodontal flaps. What are objectives and essential steps of modified Widman's flap? [MUHS]
4. Define osseous surgery. Describe the steps in respective osseous surgery. [RGUHS; GOA]
5. Describe the various types of osseous defects. Describe the steps in osseous resective surgery. [GOA]

Short Essays

1. Resective osseous surgery.
2. Osteoplasty. [MUHS]
3. Repair, regeneration and new attachment. [NTR-UHS]
4. Root biomodification. [NTR-UHS]
5. Steps in osseous respective surgery. [GOA]
6. Bone swaging. [RGUHS]

Short Notes

1. Bone blend. [MUHS]

2. Bone swaging. [RGUHS]
3. Root planing. [RGUHS]
4. Reversed architecture. [NTR-UHS]
5. New attachment. [NTR-UHS]

6. Steps in osseous respective surgery. [NTR-UHS]
7. Osteoplasty. [GOA]
8. Ostectomy. [GOA]
9. Osseous coagulum. [RGUHS]

REGENERATIVE OSSEOUS SURGERY

Long Essay

1. Write in detail about rationale and objectives of bone graft. [RGUHS]
2. Define 'reattachment' and 'new attachment'. Describe the various factors that affect the likelihood of new attachment. [MUHS]
3. Describe non-graft associated reconstructive periodontal surgical techniques. [MUHS]
4. Define periodontal regeneration. Enumerate the different methods used to achieve the same. Discuss the principles of guided tissue regeneration. [RGUHS]
5. Define gingival recession. Describe its aetiology and classification. Explain any one root coverage procedure. [RGUHS]
6. Define osseous surgery. Discuss various osseous grafting procedures. [NTR-UHS]
7. Classify bone grafts. Discuss rationale and uses of GTR. [GOA]

Short Essays

1. Allograft. [RGUHS; GOA]
2. Guided tissue regeneration. [RGUHS; NTR-UHS]
3. Autogenous bone grafts. [MUHS]
4. Non-bone graft materials. [MUHS]
5. Factor affecting healing in periodontal therapy. [MUHS]
6. Bone autografts. [RGUHS]
7. Alloplastic bone graft materials. [RGUHS]
8. Free gingival autograft. [RGUHS]
9. GTR. [RGUHS; GOA]
10. Classification of osseous grafts. [NTR-UHS]
11. Subepithelial connective tissue graft (SCTG). [NTR-UHS]

12. Osseous coagulum. [NTR-UHS]
13. Define new attachment. What are GTR membranes and rational of use of the same? [GOA]
14. Bone grafts. [GOA]
15. Membranes in guided tissue regeneration. [RGUHS]

Short Notes

1. Autogenous bone graft. [RGUHS; GOA]
2. Non-bone graft material. [RGUHS]
3. Definition of guided tissue regeneration. [RGUHS]
4. Guided tissue regeneration. [MUHS]
5. Describe in short the various forms of obtaining bone grafts from intraoral sites. [MUHS]
6. Commercial allografts. [MUHS]
7. Describe in short the various methods of obtaining bone grafts from intraoral sites. [MUHS]
8. Bone graft materials. [MUHS]
9. What are the guidelines for preparing splint? [MUHS]
10. Periodontal splints. [MUHS]
11. Rationale of GTR. [GOA]
12. Define regeneration and repair. [RGUHS]
13. Pedicle grafts. [RGUHS]
14. Osseous coagulum. [RGUHS]
15. Tissue bank. [NTR-UHS]
16. Guided bone regeneration (GBR). [NTR-UHS]
17. Platelet-rich plasma (PRP). [NTR-UHS]
18. Allografts. [NTR-UHS; GOA; RGUHS]
19. Bone fill. [NTR-UHS]
20. Bone blend. [NTR-UHS]
21. Alloplasts. [GOA]
22. GTR. [GOA]
23. Buttressing bone formation. [GOA]

FURCATION INVOLVEMENT AND ITS MANAGEMENT

Long Essays

1. Classify furcation involvement. Describe in detail treatment of class I furcation involvement. [RGUHS]

2. Classify furcation involvement. Write the treatment of grade furcation involvement in lower first molar. [RGUHS]

3. Describe furcation involvement, types of furcation and various treatment procedures in the management of

furcation. [RGUHS]

4. Define furcation involvement. Describe the classification, clinical and radiographic features and treatment of furcation involvement. [MUHS 2005,1993,1995]

5. Define furcation involvement. Describe the classification and give the different modalities of treatment of a grade furcation involvement with periapical lesion. [MUHS 2002]

6. Define and classify furcation defects. Discuss in detail about the treatment modalities of grade II furcation defect. [NTR- UHS Jul 2011]

7. Define and classify furcation involvement. Describe the treatment of grade II furcation involvement. [GOA 2000]

Short Essays

1. Give the management of the furcation involvement. [MUHS]

2. Give the aetiology management of the furcation involvement. [MUHS]

3. Treatment of grade II furcation involvement. [MUHS]

4. Aetiology and classification of furcation involvement. [RGUHS]

5. Root biomodification. [RGUHS]

6. Root resection in the management of furcation involvement. [GOA]

7. Discuss furcation involvement. [GOA]

Short Notes

1. Hemisepta. [RGUHS]
2. Root conditioners. [RGUHS; NTR-UHS]
3. Furcation involvement. [RGUHS]
4. Classify furcation involvement. [RGUHS; NTR-UHS]
5. Name common root conditioners. [RGUHS]
6. Furcation involvement and management. [RGUHS]
7. Management of true pulpo-periodontal problems. [MUHS]
8. Indications for root resection. [MUHS]
9. Furcationoplasty. [NTR-UHS]
10. Classification of furcation. [RGUHS]
11. Hemisection. [GOA; NTR-UHS]
12. Root resection. [NTR-UHS; GOA]

ENDODONTIC PERIODONTAL LESIONS AND THEIR MANAGEMENT

Long Essay

1. Classify the pulpo-periodontal problems. Describe its aetiology, diagnosis and management. [RGUHS]

Short Essay

2. Retrograde periodontitis. [NTR-OR; RGUHS]

Short Notes

1. Retrograde periodontitis. [RGUHS; GOA]
2. Pulpo-periodontal lesion. [RGUHS]
3. Pulpal and periodontal lesions. [RGUHS]
4. Retrograde. [RGUHS]
5. Dental endoscope. [NTR-UHS]
6. Influence of restorations on gingival health. [GOA]

ORTHODONTIC PERIODONTAL INTERRELATIONSHIP

Short Essays

1. Effects of orthodontics treatment in periodontal tissues. [RGUHS]

2. Describe features of fixed and removable appliances which affect periodontal health. [GOA]

3. Rationale for orthodontic tooth movement in periodontal therapy. [GOA]

PERIOPROSTHODONTICS/OCCLUSAL EVALUATION

Long Essay

1. Enumerate occlusal prematurities and describe steps of occlusal adjustments. [RGUHS Apr 2002]

Short Essays

1. Bruxism. [RGUHS Mar 2004]
2. Enumerate occlusal prematurities and describe the steps of occlusal adjustments.
3. Detection of premature occlusal contacts. [MUHS 1996]
4. Coronoplasty. [MUHS 1997]
5. Coronoplasty and its role in control of periodontal diseases. [MUHS 2003]
6. Coronoplasty. [NTR-OR Nov 1994, Oct 1998, 2005]
7. Occlusal interferences. [NTR-OR Apr 1995]
8. Indications for occlusal adjustments. [NTR-OR Nov 1992]

Short Notes

1. Bruxism. [RGUHS Aug 1995]
2. Parafunctional habits and periodontium. [RGUHS]
3. Aetiology, clinical features and management of bruxism. [MUHS 2005]
4. Define coronoplasty. What are its indications? [MUHS]
5. Define occlusal adjustment. Mention the various procedures by which it is achieved. [MUHS 2004]
6. Indications of coronoplasty and enumerate the steps of coronoplasty. [MUHS 2006]
7. Facets. [NTR-NR Apr 2002, May 2004]
8. Supra contacts. [NTR-NR Apr 2006]
9. Occlusal adjustments. [NTR-NR Apr 2000]
10. Indications for coronoplasty. [NTR-NR Oct 2002]

SUPPORTIVE PERIODONTAL TREATMENT (MAINTENANCE PHASE)

Long Essay

1. Discuss the rationale and importance of maintenance phase of treatment planning in periodontics. [MUHS]

Short Essays

1. Supportive periodontal therapy and its importance. [RGUHS]
2. Desensitizing agents. [MUHS]
3. Gingival depigmentation procedures. [RGUHS]
4. Objectives of supportive periodontal therapy. [RGUHS]
5. Rationale of supportive periodontal therapy. [RGUHS]

6. Maintenance phase of periodontal treatment. [NTR-UHS]
7. Supportive periodontal therapy. [GOA]

Short Notes

1. SPT. [RGUHS]
2. Maintenance phase. [RGUHS]
3. Describe in short the important factors to prevent recurrence of periodontal disease. [MUHS]
4. Recurrence of periodontal disease. [MUHS]
5. Rationale of supportive periodontal therapy. [RGUHS]
6. Phases of treatment plan. [NTR-UHS]
7. Supportive periodontal treatment. [GOA]

Frequently Asked Questions
PERIODONTICS

Frequently Asked Questions

PERIODONTICS

A free companion to
Essential Quick Review: Periodontics

Editor-in-Chief
Priya Verma Gupta MDS FPFA
Professor
Department of Pedodontics and Preventive Dentistry
Divya Jyoti College of Dental Sciences and Research
Ghaziabad, Uttar Pradesh, India

Co-Author
Vinita Ashutosh Boloor MDS
Associate Professor
Department of Periodontics
Yenepoya Dental College
Yenepoya University, Deralakatte
Mangalore, Karnataka, India

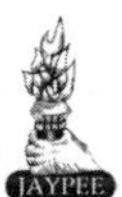

The Health Sciences Publisher

New Delhi | London | Philadelphia | Panama

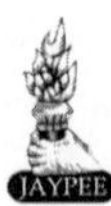

Jaypee Brothers Medical Publishers (P) Ltd

Headquarters

Jaypee Brothers Medical Publishers (P) Ltd
4838/24, Ansari Road, Daryaganj
New Delhi 110 002, India
Phone: +91-11-43574357
Fax: +91-11-43574314
Email: jaypee@jaypeebrothers.com

Overseas Offices

J.P. Medical Ltd
83 Victoria Street, London
SW1H 0HW (UK)
Phone: +44 20 3170 8910
Fax: +44 (0)20 3008 6180
Email: info@jpmedpub.com

Jaypee-Highlights Medical Publishers Inc.
City of Knowledge, Bld. 235, Clayton
Panama City, Panama
Phone: +1 507-301-0496
Fax: +1 507-301-0499
Email: cservice@jphmedical.com

Jaypee Medical Inc.
325 Chestnut Street
Suite 412, Philadelphia,
PA 19106, USA
Phone: +1 267-519-9789
Email: support@jpmedus.com

Jaypee Brothers Medical Publishers (P) Ltd
17/1-B Babar Road, Block-B, Shaymali
Mohammadpur, Dhaka-1207
Bangladesh
Mobile: +08801912003485
Email: jaypeedhaka@gmail.com

Jaypee Brothers Medical Publishers (P) Ltd
Bhotahity, Kathmandu, Nepal
Phone: +977-9741283608
Email: kathmandu@jaypeebrothers.com

Website: www.jaypeebrothers.com
Website: www.jaypeedigital.com

Inquiries for bulk sales may be solicited at: jaypee@jaypeebrothers.com

Frequently Asked Questions: Periodontics

First Edition: **2016**

ISBN: 978-93-86056-24-5

Printed at Rajkamal Electric Press, Plot No. 2, Phase-IV, Kundli, Haryana.

Editorial Board

Preface

I am very pleased to introduce you to the first edition of Essential Quick Review; A series for final year undergraduate students.

The series will be available in eight subjects. I.e., Periodontics, Pedodontics, Prosthodontics, Endodontics and Conservative Dentistry, Oral Surgery, Oral Medicine Radiology and Public Health Dentistry covering essential parts of each subject. This book will not only help the student to attain the knowledge, but will also give an idea how to attempt a question during the examination, covering entire syllabus in a limited period of time.

It is a supplementary booklet for each subject that contains three sections, i.e., definitions, classifications and viva voce covering the entire syllabus enabling the student to undergo a quick revision. The language used is very simple for better understanding.

The study material provided in this book is an attempt to provide an additional help to students for easy retention and reproduction of subject in the examination. This book is in no way a replacement to standard text book.

I thank all my subject matter experts for their valued suggestions and contributions. A very special word of thanks to my family for being the source of constant encouragement.

I profusely thank Shri Jitender P Vij (CEO), Mr Ankit Vij (Group President), and production team of M/S Jaypee Brothers Medical Publishers (P) Ltd, New Delhi for their enthusiasm and constant efforts in bringing out this book.

Priya Verma Gupta

Contents

Definitions

Gingiva

Gingiva is defined as that part of oral mucosa that covers the alveolar processes of the jaws and surrounds the necks of the teeth in a collar like fashion.

Periodontal ligament

It is a complex vascular and highly cellular connective tissue that surrounds the tooth root and connects it to inner wall of the alveolar bone.

Alveolar bone

It is defined as that portion of the maxilla and mandible which forms and supports the tooth socket.

Cementum

The calcified, avascular mesenchymal tissue that forms the outer covering of the anatomic root.

Plaque

It is a specific but highly variable structural entity, resulting from sequential colonization of microorganisms on tooth surfaces, restorations and other parts of oral cavity, composed of salivary components like mucin, desquamated epithelial cells, debris and microorganisms, all embedded in extracellular gelatinous matrix.

Calculus

An adherent calcified or calcifying amorphous mass that forms on the surface of natural teeth, restorations and dental prosthesis.

Inflammation

The local response of living tissues to injury due to any agent. It is the body's defense mechanism in order to eliminate or reduce the spread of injurious agent as well as to remove the consequent necrosed cells and tissues.

Host

The organism from which a micro-organism obtains its nourishment and modulation.

Diabetes

Diabetes is defined as clinically and genetically heterogeneous group of metabolic disorders manifested by high levels of glucose in blood.

Oral malodor/halitosis/breath malodor

The unpleasant subjective perception after smelling someone's breath due to some pathological cause.

Gingival abscess

Gingival abscess is a localized, acute inflammatory lesions that can arise due to various number of sources such as microbial, trauma and foreign body compactions.

Desquamative gingivitis

Desquamative gingivitis is a clinical term used to describe red, painful, glazed and friable gingiva, which may be a manifestation of some mucocutaneous conditions such as lichen planus or similar disorders.

Periodontal pocket

A pathologically deepened gingival sulcus.

Trauma from occlusion

When the forces exceed the adaptive capacity of the tissues, tissue injury results. The resultant injury is termed as trauma from occlusion.

Chronic periodontitis

An infectious disease resulting in inflammation within the supporting tissues of the teeth, causing attachment loss and bone loss.

Wasting diseases

Any gradual loss of tooth substance characterized by deformation of smooth and polished surfaces, without regard to the possible mechanism of this loss.

Erosion/corrosion

It is a wedge shaped depression which is sharply defined in the cervical area of the facial region of the tooth.

Attrition

It is the occlusal wear caused due to functional contacts with opposite teeth.

Risk assessment

Risk is the probability that an individual will develop a specific disease in a given period. There are numerous components which define risk assessment.

Prognosis

Prognosis is defined as the prediction of the probable course, duration and outcome of a disease based on the general knowledge of the pathogenesis of the disease and the presence of risk factors for the disease and the likelihood of its response to treatment.

New attachment

It is the formation of new periodontal ligament into cementum.

Reattachment

The establishment of an organic connection between connective tissue and cementum in the area of gingival or periodontal pocket.

Dental Plaque

It can be defined as the soft deposits that form the biofilm adhering to the tooth surface or other hard surfaces in the oral cavity, including removable and fixed restorations.

Plaque control

It is the removal of microbial plaque and the prevention of its accumulation on the teeth and adjacent gingival surfaces.

Gingivoplasty

It is reshaping of the gingiva to create physiologic gingival contours, with the main purpose of recontouring of gingiva.

Curettage

The scraping of the gingival wall of a periodontal pocket to separate diseased soft tissue.

Gingivectomy

Excision of the gingiva.

Periodontal flap

A section of gingiva or mucosa surgically separated from the underlying tissue to provide visibility of and access to the bone and root surfaces.

Osseous surgery

The procedure by which changes in the alveolar bone can be accomplished to rid it of deformaties induced by the periodontal disease process or other related factors, such as exostosis and tooth supraeruption.

Furcation involvement

The invasion of bifurcation or trifurcation of multirooted tooth by periodontitis.

Dental implants

A prosthetic device of alloplastic material(s) implanted into the oral tissues beneath the mucosal and/or periosteal layer, and on/or within the bone to provide retention and support for a fixed or removable prosthesis.

Osseointegration

The apparent direct attachment or connection of osseous tissue to an inert and alloplastic material without intervening connective tissue.

Acquired pellicle

It is a homogenous, membranous and acellular film that covers the tooth surfaces and frequently forms the interface between the surface of the dental plaque and calculus.

Active eruption

Active eruption is the movement of the teeth in the direction of the occlusal plane.

Actual position

It is the level of the epithelial attachment on the tooth.

Adult periodontitis

A form of periodontitis that usually has an onset beyond the age of 35 years. Bone resorption usually progresses slowly and predominantly in the horizontal direction.

Aggressive periodontitis

It is a periodontal destruction that becomes clinically significant around adolescence or early adulthood.

Allograft

A graft between genetically dissimilar members of the same species.

Alloplastic graft

A graft of inert synthetic material, which is sometimes called, implant material.

Alveolar bone proper

It is a plate of compact bone, the radiographic image of which is termed as lamina dura.

Alveolar mucosa

Mucosa covering the basal part of the alveolar process of continuing without demarcation into the vestibular fornix and the floor of the mouth. It is loosely attached to the periosteum and is movable.

Ankylosis

Fusion of the cementum and the alveolar bone with the obliteration of the periodontal ligament is termed as ankylosis.

Antibiotics

These are naturally occurring, semisynthetic or synthetic type of antimicrobial agents that destroy or inhibit the growth of selective microorganisms, generally at low concentrations.

Antibody

A class of serum proteins that are induced following interaction with an antigen. They bind specifically to the antigen that induced their formation.

Antigen

Any material that is specifically bound by antibody. A structure recognized as foreign by the immune system.

Antimicrobial agent

It is a chemotherapeutic agent that works by reduction in bacterial number.

Apparent position

It is the level of the crest of the gingival margin.

Attached gingival width

It is the distance between the mucogingival junction and the projection on the external surface of the bottom of the gingival sulcus or the periodontal pocket. The attached gingiva is continuous with the marginal gingiva. It is firm, resilient and tightly bound to the underlying periosteum of the alveolar bone.

Autograft

Tissue transferred from one position to another within the same individual.

Biofilm

It is defined as matrix enclosed bacterial population adherent to each other and/or to surface or interface.

Biointegration

Bonding of the living bone to the surface of an implant, usually independent of any mechanical interlocking mechanism.

Biologic depth

It is the distance between the gingival margin and the base of the pocket (coronal end of the junctional epithelium).

Biologic width

The dimension of space that the healthy gingival tissues occupy above the alveolar bone.

Bruxism or occlusal necrosis

The clenching or grinding of the dentition during non-functional movements of the masticatory system.

Bulbous bone contours

These are bony enlargements caused by exostosis, adaptation to function and buttressing bone formation. They are commonly found in maxilla.

Bullous pemphigoid

It is a chronic autoimmune subepidermal, bullous disease with tense bullae that rupture and become flaccid.

Bundle bone

The layer of the alveolar bone into which the principal fibers (Sharpey's fibers) are inserted.

Buttressing bone formation/lipping bone formation

Occurs in an attempt to buttress bony trabeculae that are weakened by resorption. If it occurs within the jaw, it is termed central buttressing bone formation. When it occurs on external surface, it is referred to as peripheral buttressing bone formation.

Cell-mediated immunity

An immune reaction mediated by activated T lymphocytes, involving release of biologic response modifiers (lymphokines) on exposure to antigen.

Secondary cementum

Cementum that forms after tooth eruption and in response to functional demand.

Chemotaxis

It is the locomotion of cells, which is directed along an increasing chemical gradient of a soluble substance.

Chemotherapeutic agent

Chemical substance that provides chemical therapeutic benefit.

Chronic periodontitis

An infectious disease resulting in inflammation within the supporting tissues of the teeth, leading to progressive attachment loss accompanied with bone loss.

Clenching

It is the closure of the jaws under vertical pressure.

Complement

A group of serum proteins involved in the control of inflammation, the activation of phagocytes and lytic attack on cell membranes. It can be activated by interaction with antigen-antibody complexes or bacterial substances.

Compromise osseous reshaping

It indicates a bone pattern that cannot be improved without significant osseous removal that would be detrimental to overall result.

Contact inhibition

Inhibition of movement and division caused by physical contact between cells of the same type. The process by which the graft material prevents apical proliferation of the epithelium.

Coronal cementum

Cementum that is found deposited on the occlussal areas above the enamel.

Cuticle

It is thin, acellular structure with a homogenous matrix, sometimes enclosed within clearly demarcated and linear borders.

Cyst

Cyst is a swelling consisting of fluid, semi-fluid and gaseous content, which may or may not be lined by epithelium or endothelium.

Cytokines

A small protein messengers released by cells, which affects the division, differentiation and function of various other cells.

Debridement

The removal of inflamed, devitalized or contaminated tissue/foreign material from the adjacent site alongwith the lesion to improve the healing potential of the remaining healthy tissue.

Degree of separation

It is the angle of separation between two roots.

Dental epidemiology

The study of pattern (distribution) and dynamics of dental diseases in a human population.

Dental splint

An appliance designed to immobilize and stabilize loose teeth.

Dental stain

Pigmented deposits on tooth surface.

Dentifrice

Agent that aids in cleaning and polishing tooth surfaces.

Desmosome

A specialized attachment between epithelial cells, to impart strength to epithelium.

Diagnosis

It may be defined as identifying disease from an evaluation of the history, signs and symptoms, laboratory tests and procedures.

Disclosing agents

They are solutions or wafers capable of staining bacterial deposits on the surface of teeth, tongue and gingiva.

Disinfectant

An antimicrobial agent that is generally applied to inanimate surfaces to destroy microorganisms.

Displaced flap

It is placed apically, coronally or laterally to their original position.

Disuse or functional atrophy

The thinning of periodontal ligament, with reduced number as well as thickness of trabeculae pertaining to reduced occlusal forces .

Divergence

It is the distance between two roots (cones). This distance normally tends to increase with age in apical direction.

Down syndrome

It is a congenital disease caused by a chromosomal abnormality and characterized by mental deficiency and growth retardation.

Ecological niche

The functional position, which bacterial species occupies within a complex ecosystem such as plaque.

Electrocoagulation

The process which provides a wide range of coagulation or hemorrhage control using electrocoagulation current. Electrosection electrotomy or acusection is used for incision, excision and tissue planing.

Electrofulguration

A method of electrosurgery used to produce superficial desiccation of tissue, which employs a highly or moderately damped alternating current that is radiated through a monoterminal active electrode that is held close to the patient, so that the sparks spray over the lesion being treated.

Electrosurgery (radiosurgery)

It is currently used to identify surgical techniques performed on soft tissue using controlled high frequency electrical current in the range of 1.5–7.5 million cycles/second or MHz.

Electrosurgery

The process of division of tissue by high frequency electrical current applied locally with a metal instrument or needle.

Endodontic-periodontal lesions

The periapical lesions in which necrosis may drain to the oral cavity through periodontal ligament and adjacent alveolar bone perceding pulpal inflammation.

Endotoxin

A complex heat stable toxin usually with an active component, such as lipopolysaccharide (a structural component of gram-negative bacterial cell wall).

Epidemiology

The study of the distribution and determinants of health-related states or events in specified populations.

Epithelial adaptation

It is the close apposition of the gingival epithelium to the tooth surface without obliteration of the pocket.

Epulis

It is the generic term to designate all discrete tumor and tumor-like mass of gingiva.

Erosion (cuneiform defect)

It is a sharply defined wedge-shaped depression in the cervical area of the facial tooth surface.

Etiology

The cause of disease, for instance, in the case of microbial dental plaque, gingivitis and periodontal disease.

Excisional new attachment

It is a definitive subgingival curettage performed with a knife.

Excursive movement

Any movement of the mandible away from intercuspal position.

Exostosis

It is the outgrowth of the bone of varied size and shape.

Exploratory stroke

It is a light 'feeling' stroke performed with probe and explorer to evaluate the dimensions of the pocket and to detect calculus and irregularities on the tooth surface.

Exposure

It is defined as a factor that may possibly lead to cause of disease or may be protective against a disease.

Extrusion

Pathologic migration in the occlusal or incisal direction is termed as extrusion.

Fc

The part of an immunoglobulin molecule, which binds to specific receptors on neutrophils and macrophages, except an antigen.

Fibronectin

A connective tissue protein, which binds cells to the extracellular matrix.

Fibro-osseous integration

An integration in which soft tissues such as fibers and/or cells are interposed between the two surfaces.

Fimbriae

A fine filamentous surface appendage on a bacterium. These are important for attachment and adhesion.

Finger rest

The finger rest serves to stabilize the hand instrument by providing a firm fulcrum, as movement is made to activate the instrument.

Flat architecture

It is reduction of the interdental bone to the same height as radicular bone.

Food impaction

It is the forceful wedging of food into the periodontium by occlusal forces.

Fremitus

A palpable or visible movement of teeth when subjected to occlusal forces. It is the measurement of the vibratory patterns of the teeth when teeth are placed in contacting positions and movements.

Frenectomy

It is complete removal of the frenum, including its attachment to underlying bone and may be required in correction of an abnormal diastema between maxillary central incisors.

Frenotomy

It is the incision of frenum.

Frenum

It is a fold of mucous membrane usually with enclosed muscle fibers that attaches the lip and cheeks to the alveolar mucosa and/or gingiva and underlying periosteum.

Full thickness flap

All the soft tissue, including the periosteum is reflected to expose the underlying bone.

Furcational entrance

It is the transitional area between the divided and undivided part of the root.

Furcational fornix

The roof of the furcation.

Furcation invasion

Pathologic resorption of bone within the furcation.

Furcation involvement

Furcation involvement refers to the invasion of the bifurcation and trifurcation of multirooted teeth by periodontal disease.

Generalized aggressive periodontitis

Clinically characterized by generalized interproximal attachment loss affecting at least three permanent teeth other than first molars and incisors.

Genetic marker

Genetic marker refers to any gene or nucleotide sequence that can be mapped to a specific location or region on a chromosome.

Genotype

The generic composition of an organism.

Gingival abscess

It is a localized, painful and rapidly expanding lesion, which is usually of sudden onset. It is generally limited to the marginal gingiva or interdental papilla. It can be localized in the gingiva, caused by injury to the outer surface of the gingiva not involving the supporting structures.

Gingival crevicular fluid (GCF)

It is an altered serum transudate found in the gingival sulcus.

Gingival enlargement

Increase in the size of the gingiva.

Gingival hyperplasia

An enlargement of gingiva due to the increase in the number of cells.

Gingival pocket (pseudopocket)

This type of pocket is formed by gingival enlargement without destruction of the underlying periodontal tissues.

Gingival sulcus

It is the shallow crevice or space around the tooth bounded by the surface of the tooth on one side and the epithelial lining the free margin of the gingiva on the other side.

Gingivoplasty

It is the reshaping of the gingiva to create physiologic gingival contour, with the sole purpose of recontouring the gingiva in the absence of periodontal pocket.

Glycosaminoglycan

A molecule of repeating sugar subunits, which forms a major component of ground substance of connective tissue.

Graft

It is a viable tissue/organ which after its removal from donor site, is either implanted or transplanted within the host tissue, where it is than repaired, restored and remodelled.

Guided tissue regeneration

An epithelial exclusionary technique that promotes new connective tissue attachment without the use of any implant material.

Habit

An act of repeated performance, almost automatic, such as bruxism or tongue thrusting.

Hemisection

It is surgical removal of a root with the associated part of crown. It is the splitting of the two-rooted tooth into two separate portions. The process has been called bicuspidization or separation.

Hemiseptum

The one walled defect is called hemiseptum.

Homeostasis

The production of a stable equilibrium in a body system by means of feedback mechanisms.

Horizontal bone loss

The common pattern of bone loss in which bone is reduced in height, but the bone margins are roughly perpendicular to the tooth surface.

Hydrolytic enzymes

A class of enzymes, which cleaves various types of bonds including peptide, ester and glycosidic bonds by addition of water. For e.g., many degradative and lysosomal enzymes.

Hypercementosis

It refers to the prominent thickening of the cementum. It may be localized or generalized.

Hyperfunction

It is a functional adaptation in which additional structural elements are formed on cementum and in bone to withstand the added forces, expressed clinically and microscopically as a thickened lamina dura, buttressing bone formation, osteosclerosis and cemental spurs.

Hypersensitivity

The root surfaces exposed by gingival recession may be hypersensitive to thermal changes or tactile stimulation.

Iatrogenic factors

Inadequate dental procedures that contribute to the deterioration of the periodontal tissues.

Immune complex

A complex of antigen and antibody molecules that are bound to each other and later together.

Immunogenicity

It is the capacity to induce a detectable immune response such as the production of antibody or the stimulation of cellular immunity.

Immunoglobulin

A glycoprotein composed of heavy and light peptide chains; functions as antibody in serum and secretions.

Inadvertent curettage

Some degree of curettage is done unintentionally, while scaling and root planing is performed.

Intercuspal position (ICP)

The position of the mandible when there is maximum intercuspation between the maxillary and mandibular teeth (Synonym Centric occlusion).

Interdental gingiva

The type of gingiva which occupies the gingival embrasure i.e., the interproximal space beneath the area of tooth contact.

Intermediate cementum

It is an ill-defined zone near cementodentinal junction of certain teeth that appears to contain cellular remnants of Hertwig's sheath embedded in calcified ground substance.

Intrabony defects

The three-walled vertical defect was originally called intrabony defect.

Junctional Epithelium

A single or multiple layers of non-keratinizing cells adhering to the tooth surface at the base of the gingival crevice. It denotes the tissue that joins to the tooth on one side and to the oral sulcular epithelium and connective tissue on the other.

Juvenile periodontitis

A disease of periodontium occurring in an otherwise healthy adolescent, which is characterized by a rapid loss of alveolar bone, involving more than one tooth of the permanent dentition.

Lamina dura

The compact bone (alveolar bone proper), which lines the tooth socket and in a radiograph appears as a dense opaque line.

Lateral pressure

The pressure created when force is applied against the surface of a tooth with the cutting edge of a bladed instrument.

Ledges

These are plateau-like bone margins caused by resorption of thickened bony plates.

Leukemia

It is a malignant neoplasia of white blood cell (WBC) precursors.

Leukoplakia

A white patch or plaque that does not rub off on scraping and cannot be diagnosed as any other disease.

Lichen planus

It is a relatively common, chronic dermatosis characterized by the presence of cutaneous, violaceous papules that may coalesce to form plaques. It is defined as unique cutaneous entity consisting of an eruption of papules usually distinct in color, configuration, patterns, location of appearance, microscopic and gross structure.

Lipopolysaccharide

The active component of bacterial endotoxins.

Localized gingivitis

It is confined to the gingiva of a single tooth or group of teeth.

Localized aggressive

It is characterized as a disease with proximal periodontitis attachment loss on at least two permanent teeth, particularly first molar and incisors.

Localized diffuse gingivitis

It extends from the gingival margin to the mucobuccal fold, but is limited in area.

Localized marginal gingivitis

It is confined to one or more areas of the marginal gingiva.

Localized periodontitis

It is considered localized when less than 30% of the sites assessed in the mouth, demonstrate loss of bone attachment.

Loci

Loci are defined as the specific location on the chromosomes.

Lymphokines

Cytokines secreted by lymphocytes. Cytokines is not a preferred term for this group of substances because these are secreted by many other types of cells.

Malnutrition

Any disorder of nutrition, it may be due to imbalance or insufficient diet or to defective assimilation or utilization of foods.

Marginal gingiva

The terminal edge or border of the gingiva surrounding the teeth in a collar-like fashion.

Marginal gingivitis

Inflammation of the gingival margin which may include a portion of the contiguous attached gingiva.

Marginal plaque

It is the supragingival plaque that is in direct contact with the gingival margin.

Masticatory mucosa

The gingival and mucosal covering of hard palate.

Materia alba

It is a yellowish or whitish, soft, sticky deposit and is somewhat less adherent than dental plaque. It is a concentration of microorganisms, desquamated epithelial cells, food debris, leukocytes and mixture of salivary proteins and lipids.

McCall's festooning

These are life preserver-shaped enlargements of the marginal gingiva that occurs most frequently in the canine and premolar areas on the facial surface.

Mediotrusive side

The side of either dental arch corresponding to the side of mandible moving towards the midline (Synonym Balancing side, non-working side).

Metalloproteinases

Enzymes, which degrade protein in the presence of metal ions, usually calcium and magnesium.

Mobility

It is a measurement of horizontal and vertical tooth displacement created by examiner's force.

Moderate periodontitis

Periodontal destruction is generally considered moderate if 3–4 mm of clinical attachment loss has occurred.

Modified pen grasp

The thumb, index finger and middle finger are used to hold the instrument as a pen is held, but the middle finger is positioned so that the side of the pad next to the fingernail is resting on the instrument shank. The index finger is bent at the second joint from the fingertip and is positioned well above the middle finger on the same side of the handle.

Modified widman flap

A scalloped, replaced, mucoperiosteal flap, accomplished with an internal bevel incision that provides access for root planing.

Monocyte

A large mononuclear phagocytic leukocyte—the circulating precursors of macrophages.

Mucogingival deformity

It is defined as a significant departure from the normal

shape of gingiva and alveolar mucosa, and may involve the underlying alveolar bone.

Mucogingiva

It is defined as a generic term used to describe the mucogingival junction and its relationship to the gingiva, alveolar mucosa, frenula, muscle attachments, vestibular fornices and the floor of the mouth.

Mucogingival surgery

It is defined as periodontal surgical procedures designed to correct defects in the morphology, position, and/or amount of gingiva.

Mucous membrane pemphigoid

It is a chronic, vesiculobullous and an autoimmune disorder of unknown cause that predominantly affects women in the 5th decade of life, also known as cicatricial pemphigoid.

Necrotizing ulcerative periodontitis

It is an extension of necrotizing ulcerative gingivitis (NUG) into the periodontal structures, leading to bone and attachment loss. It is defined as severe and rapidly progressive disease that has a distinctive erythema of the free gingiva, attached gingiva and alveolar mucosa; extensive soft tissue necrosis; severe loss of periodontal attachment; deep pocket formation is not evident.

Negative architecture

It refers to a condition, in which interdental bone is more apical than radicular bone.

Neutrophil

A phagocytic polymorphonuclear leukocyte.

Non-displaced flap

When the flap is returned and sutured in its original position.

Non-thrombocytopenic purpura

It occurs as a result of either vascular wall fragility or thrombasthenia.

Occlusal trauma

An injury to the attachment apparatus as a result of excessive occlusal force.

Offset blade

The term used to describe Gracey curettes, as they are angled approximately 60–70 degrees from the lower shank.

Opsonin

A substance, which facilitates phagocytosis when bound to the surface of a bacterium or other particle. A substance capable of enhancing phagocytosis.

Oral candidiasis

Infection of oral mucous membrane by a fungus of the genus Candida.

Oral epithelium

The epithelium which covers the crest and outer surface of marginal gingiva alongwith the surface of attached gingiva.

Oral mucosa

The tissue lining the oral cavity.

Osseous craters

The concavities in the crest of the interdental bone, confined within the facial and lingual walls.

Osseous defects

Various types of bone deformities that can result from periodontal disease.

Ostectomy

It is defined as the excision of bone or portion of bone in periodontics; ostectomy is done to correct or reduce deformities caused by periodontitis and includes removal of the supporting bone.

Osteoclast activating factor (OAF)

A mixture of cytokines, including interleukin-1 (IL-1), tumor necrosis factor (TNF), TNF-β and platelet-derived growth factor (PDGF), which induces bone resorption. It was previously considered to be a distinct cytokine.

Osteoconduction

It is a physical effect by which the matrix of the graft forms scaffold that favors outside cells to penetrate the graft and form new bone. The graft material acts as passive material, like a trellis for new bone to cover.

Osteogenesis

The formation or development of new bone by cells contained in the graft.

Osteoinduction

A process by which graft material is capable of promoting cementogenesis, osteogenesis and new periodontal ligament. It is a chemical process by which molecules contained in the graft (BMPs) convert the neighboring cells into osteoblast, i.e., the bone forming cells .

Osteoplasty

The reshaping of alveolar process to achieve a more physiologic form without removal of the supporting bone.

Passive eruption

Passive eruption is the exposure of the teeth by apical migration of the gingiva.

Pathologic migration

This refers to tooth displacement that results when the balance among the factors that maintain physiologic tooth position is disturbed by periodontal disease.

Pellicle

An organic coating formed when the crown of the tooth erupts and is exposed to saliva, which is called dental pellicle.

Peri-implant mucositis

Inflammatory changes confined to the soft tissue surrounding an implant.

Peri-implantitis

A term used to describe inflammation around a dental implant and/or its abutment.

Periodontal abscess

It is a localized accumulation of pus within gingival wall of a periodontal pocket. Localized purulent inflammation in the periodontal tissues. Periodontal abscess are acute lesions that may result in very rapid destruction of the periodontal tissues. These are purulent infections localized to the gingival, periodontal or pericoronal regions.

Periodontal cyst

A small cyst of periodontal ligament found most often in the mandibular canine and premolar area; associated with a vital tooth and postulated to originate from the rests of Malassez, the rests of the dental lamina or a supernumerary tooth bud.

Periodontal disease

A group of inflammatory conditions of the supportive tissues of the teeth that are caused by bacteria.

Periodontal dressing/pack

A protective material applied over the wound created by periodontal surgical procedures.

Periodontology

The branch of dentistry concerned with prevention and treatment of periodontal disease. In other words, the clinical science that deals with the periodontium in health and disease is called periodontology and its practice is termed periodontics.

Phagocytosis

It is the process by which cells ingest particles of a size visible by light microscopy.

Phase I therapy

The process to alter or eliminate the microbial etiology and other contributing factors responsible for gingival and periodontal diseases.

Plasma cell

A mature B lymphocyte, which secretes antibody.

Positive architecture

This refers to radicular bone located apical to interdental bone.

Primary herpetic gingivostomatitis

It is an infection of the oral cavity caused by the herpes simplex virus type-1.

Primary trauma from occlusion

It is the injury resulting from excessive occlusal forces applied to a tooth or teeth with normal support. It includes a tissue reaction, which is elicited around a tooth with normal height of the periodontium. When trauma from occlusion is the result of alteration in the occlusal forces, it is called primary trauma from occlusion.

Probing depth

It is a distance to which an ad hoc instrument (probe) penetrates into pocket.

Proteoglycan

A protein with numerous glycosaminoglycan side chains usually a component of connective tissue ground substance.

Puberty gingivitis

A higher prevalence and severity of gingivitis and gingival enlargement is found in the circumpubertal period.

Pyogenic granuloma

It is a tumor-like gingival enlargement that is considered an exaggerated conditioned response to minor trauma.

Pyorrhea

An archaic term for several periodontal diseases.

Radicular cementum

Cementum that covers the root.

Radius of action

Range of effectiveness of about 1.5–2.5 mm within which bacterial plaque can induce loss of bone.

To attach again

The reunion of epithelial and connective tissue with root surfaces and bone, which occurs after an incision or injury.

Redox potential

A measure of the ease with which oxidation and reduction reactions will occur.

Refractory periodontitis

According to American Academy of Periodontology, it has been defined as, those cases, which do not respond to any treatment provided, whatever be the thoroughness or frequency. It includes patients who are unresponsive to any treatment provided, whatever be the thoroughness or frequency; as well as patients with recurrent disease at single or multiple sites.

Regeneration

It is the growth and differentiation of new cells and intercellular substances to form new tissue and parts of lost or injured tissue.

Repair

Healing of a wound by scar formation that does not fully restore the architecture or function of the part. It restores the continuity of the diseased marginal gingiva and re-establishes a normal gingival sulcus at the same level on the root as the base of the pre-existing periodontal pocket.

Risk factor

It is defined as an aspect of personal behavior or lifestyle, an environmental exposure, alongwith an inborn or inherited characteristic, on the basis of epidemiologic evidence. It is known to be associated with health conditions considered important for prevention.

Risk indicator

A probable or putative risk factor that has been associated with the disease through cross-sectional studies.

Risk marker

A factor that is associated with increased probability of future disease.

Risk

It is the probability that an individual will get a specific disease in a given period of time.

Root amputation

The removal of a root from multirooted teeth.

Root planing stroke

It is a moderate to light pull stroke that is used for final smoothening and planing of the root surface.

Root planing

It is the process by which residual embedded calculus and portion of cementum are removed from the roots to produce a smooth, hard and clean surface.

Hemisection

It is the splitting of two rooted tooth into two separate portions.

Root resection

It is the surgical removal of all or a portion of root before or after endodontic treatment.

Root separation/bicuspidization

It is the sectioning of the root complex and maintenance of all roots.

Saliva

The fluid secreted by the salivary glands that aids in the digestion of food.

Scaling stroke

It is short, powerful pull stroke that is used with bladed instruments for the removal of supragingival and subgingival calculus.

Scaling

The process by which plaque and calculus are removed from both supragingival and subgingival tooth surface.

Secondary trauma from occlusion

When the trauma results from reduced ability of the tissues to resist the occlusal forces. Tissue reaction elicited around a tooth by occlusal forces, with reduced height of periodontium. Injury resulting from normal occlusal forces applied to tooth/teeth with inadequate support.

Segregation analysis classic twin study

The study in which, reared together monozygotic and dizygotic twins, are compared to estimate the effects of shared genes. The observed pattern of disease in families is compared with patterns expected under various models of inheritance.

Sensitivity

The ability of a test or observation to detect the incidence of disease.

Serumal calculus

Calculus formed apical to gingival margin, often brown or black, hard and tenacious.

Severe periodontitis

Periodontal destruction is considered severe when 5 mm or more of clinical attachment loss has occurred.

Splint

It is an appliance used for immobilization of injured or diseased parts.

Stillman's clefts

These are apostrophe-shaped indentations extending from and into the gingival margin for varying distances on the facial surfaces.

Stippling

A form of adaptive specialization or reinforcement to function.

Subgingival calculus

It is located below the crest of the marginal gingiva and not visible in routine clinical (serumal calculus) examination.

Subgingival curettage

The procedure that is performed apical to the epithelial attachment severing the connective tissue attachment down to the osseous crest.

Subgingival plaque

The community of microorganisms that develops on tooth surfaces that are apical to the gingival margin. Subgingival plaque is found below the gingival margin, between the tooth and gingival sulcular tissue.

Subclinical gingivitis

The initial response of the gingiva to bacterial plaque is not apparent.

Subtraction radiography

It is a technique that facilitates both qualitative and quantitative visualization of even minor density changes in bone by removing the unchanged anatomic structures from the image.

Traumatic occlusion

An occlusion, which causes an injury is called traumatic occlusion.

Treatment plan

It is the blueprint for case management. It includes all procedures required for the establishment and maintenance of oral health.

Tunnel preparation

A surgical procedure performed on a multirooted tooth, usually a mandibular molar, resulting in a completely opened furcation to provide access for hygiene.

Ultrasonic scaler

An instrument vibrating in the ultrasonic range, which accompanied by the stream of water, can be used to remove adherent deposits from teeth.

Universal curette

One curette designed for all area and surfaces.

Vitalometer

A device that measures the response of a tooth to an electric stimulus to aid in determining pulp vitality.

Vertical/angular defects

The defects that occur in an oblique direction, leaving out a hollowed-out trough in the bone alongside the root; the base of the defect is located apical to the surrounding bone.

Vincent's angina

It is a fusospirochetal infection of the oropharynx and throat.

Xenograft or heterograft

The donor of the graft is from different species from the host.

Classifications

Types of Principal Fibres of Periodontal Ligament

Six groups of principal fibres of periodontal ligament:

❑ Transseptal group
❑ Alveolar crest group
❑ Horizontal group
❑ Oblique group
❑ Apical group
❑ Interradicular group.

Types of Cementum

According to Schroeder, cementum has been classified as follows:

S.No	Types of Cementum	Disease characteristics
1.	Acellular Afibrillar-Cementum (AAC)	• Type of cementum neither contains cells nor collagen fibres • Consists of mineralized ground substance • Produced by cementoblats with a thickness of 1–15 μm

2.	Acellular extrinsic Fibre Cementum (AEFC)	• Consists of mainly Sharpey's fibres and does not contain any cells • Produced by fibroblasts and cementoblasts. • Found in the apical third of the roots • Thickness around 30–230 µm
3.	Cellular Mixed Stratified Cementum (CMSC)	• Consists of both extrinsic fibres and intrinsic fibres and also consists of cells • Produced by fibroblasts and cementoblasts • Found in the apical third of the roots and apex and in furcation areas
4.	Cellular Intrinsic Fibre Cementum (CIFC)	• Consists of cells and intrinsic fibres • Does not contain extrinsic fibres • Formed by cementoblasts
5.	Intermediate Cementum	• Consists of cellular remnants of Hertwig's epithelial sheath, embedded in a calcified ground substance • Seen near the cemento-dentinal junction

Classifications of Periodontitis

Various classifications of various forms of periodontitis are as follows:

❑ American Academy of Peridontology (AAP) world workshop in clinical Periodontics (1989)

S.No	Forms of periodontitis	Disease characteristics
1.	Adult periodontitis	• Age of onset > 35 years • Slow rate of disease progression • No defect in host defences
2.	Early onset periodontitis (may be prepubertal, juvenile, or rapidly progressive)	• Age of onset < 35 years • Rapid rate of disease progression • Defect in host defences. • Associated with specific microflora
3.	Periodontitis associated with systemic disease	• Systemic disease that predispose to rapid rates of periodontitis • Diseases are: Diabetes Down's syndrome, HIV infection, Papillon-Lefevre syndrome
4.	Necrotizing ulcerative periodontitis	• Similar to Acute Necrotizing Ulcerative Gingivitis (ANUG), but with associated clinical attachment loss
5.	Refractory periodontitis	• Recurrent periodontitis that does not respond to treatment

❑ European Workshop in Periodontology (1993)

S.No	Forms of periodontitis	Disease characteristics
1.	Adult periodontitis	• Age of onset: fourth decade of life • Slow rate of disease progression • No defects in host response

2.	Early – onset periodontitis	• Age of onset: before fourth decade of life • Rapid rate of disease progression • Defect in host defense
3.	Necrotizing periodontitis	• Tissue necrosis with bone and attachment loss

❑ American Academy of Peridontology (AAP) International Workshop for Classification of Periodontal Diseases (1999)
  • Chronic periodontitis
    – Localized (<30% of sites involved)
    – Generalized (>30% of sites involved)
  • Aggressive periodontitis
    – Localized
    – Generalized
  • Periodontitis as a manifestation of systemic disease.

❑ Chronic Periodontitis: Following characteristics can be seen in a patient of chronic periodontitis.
  • Prevalent in adults, but can occur in children
  • Amount of destruction consistent with local factors
  • Associated with a variable microbial pattern
  • Subgingival calculus frequently found
  • Slow to moderate rate of progression with possible periods of rapid progression.

❑ Possible modified by or associated with the following:
  • Systemic diseases such as Diabetes mellitus and HIV infection
  • Local factors predisposing to periodontitis
  • Environmental factors such as cigarette smoking and emotional stress.

❏ Chronic periodontitis may be further subclassified into localized and generalized forms and characterized based on the common features as:
  - Slight: 1–2 mm of clinical attachment loss
  - Moderate: 3 to 4 mm of clinical attachment loss
  - Severe: >= mm of clinical attachment loss.

❏ Aggressive Periodontitis: Following characteristics can be seen in the patient suffering from aggressive periodontitis:
  - Otherwise clinically healthy patient
  - Rapid attachment loss and bone destruction
  - Amount of microbial deposits inconsistent with disease severity
  - Familial aggregation of diseased individuals.

❏ The following characteristics are common but not universal:
  - Diseased sites infected with *Actinobacillus actinomycetemcomitans*
  - Abnormalities in phagocyte function
  - Hyperresponsive macrophages, producing increased prostaglandin E_2 (PGE_2) and interleukin 1β
  - In some cases , self – arresting disease progression.

❏ Aggressive periodontitis may be further classified into localized and generalized forms based upon the common features as:
  - Localized form:
    - Circumpubertal onset of disease
    - Localized first molar or incisor disease with proximal attachment loss of at least two permanent teeth , one of which is a first molar
    - Robust serum antibody response to infecting agents.
  - Generalized form:
    - Usually affecting persons under 30 years of age (however , may be older)

- Generalized proximal attachment loss affecting at least three teeth other than first molars and incisors
- Pronounced episodic nature of periodontal destruction
- Poor serum antibody response to infecting agents.
- Periodontitis as a manifestation of systemic disease: It may be observed as a manifestation of the following systemic diseases.

❑ Heamatologic disorders
  - Acquired neutropenia
  - Leukemias
  - Others.

❑ Genetic disorders
  - Familial and cyclic neutropenia
  - Down syndrome
  - Leukocyte adhesion deficiency syndromes
  - Papillon–lefevre syndrome
  - Histiocytosis syndromes
  - Glycogen storage disease
  - Infantile genetic agranulocytosis
  - Chediak–Higashi syndrome
  - Cohen syndrome
  - Ehlers–Danlos syndrome (types IV and VII AD)
  - Hypophosphatasia
  - Others.

❑ Not otherwise specified.

International Workshop Classification of Periodontal Diseases and Conditions 1999

❑ Gingival Diseases
  - Dental plaque induced
    - Associated with dental plaque only with or without other local contributing factors.

- o Gingival diseases modified by systemic factors:
- o Associated with endocrine system: puberty associated gingivitis, menstrual cycle associated gingivitis, pregnancy associated gingivitis, pyogenic granuloma and Diabetes Mellitus associated gingivitis
- o Associated with blood dyscrasias: Leukaemia associated gingivitis and others.
- – Gingival diseases modified by medications:
  - o Drug induced gingival enlargements
  - o Drug influenced gingivitis, e.g., oral contraceptives, etc.
- – Gingival diseases modified by malnutrition, e.g., vitamin C and others

❑ Non Plaque induced gingival lesions
- • Specific bacterial origin: *Neisseria gonorrhoeae, Treponema pallidum, Streptococcal* species and others.
  - – Viral origin : Herpes virus infections and others.
  - – Fungal origin : Candida species infections, Linear gingival erythema, Histoplasmosis and others
  - – Genetic origin : Hereditary gingival fibromatosis and others.
    - o Manifestations of systemic conditions:
    - o Mucocutaneous disorders: Lichen planus, Pemphigus and Pemphigoid, etc.
    - o Allergic reactions

1. Dental restorative materials- mercury, acrylic, etc.

2. Reactions attributed to toothpastes/dentifrices, mouth rinses/washes, chewing gum additives, food and additives

3. Others.
   - – Traumatic lesions: chemical, physical, thermal, factitious, iatrogenic, accidental
   - – Foreign body reactions
   - – Not otherwise specified (NOS)

❏ Chronic periodontitis: Based on clinical radiographic, historic and laboratory characteristics
- Localized (<30% of sites involved)
- Generalized (>30% of sites involved)

❏ Aggressive periodontitis
- Localized
  - ○ Circumpubertal onset
  - ○ First molar or incisor has proximal attachment loss
  - ○ Robust serum antibody response to infective agents
- Generalized
  - ○ Affects below 30 years of age
  - ○ Generalized proximal attachment loss
  - ○ Poor serum antibody response to infective agents
  - ○ Episodic nature of periodontal disease.

❏ Periodontitis as a manifestation of systemic disease
- Associated with haematological disorders: acquired neutropenia , leukaemia ,and others
- Associated with genetic disorders: LAD deficiency syndromes and others.

❏ Necrotizing periodontal diseases
- Necrotizing ulcerative gingivitis (NUG)
- Necrotizing ulcerative periodontitis (NUP).

❏ Abscesses of the periodontium
- Gingival
- Periodontal
- Pericoronal.

❏ Periodontitis associated with endodontic lesions
- Combined periodontal–endodontic lesion

❑ Developmental or acquired deformities and conditions
  • Localized tooth related factors that modify or predispose to plaque induced gingival diseases/periodontitis
    o Tooth anatomic factors
    o Dental restorations/appliances
    o Root fractures
    o Cervical root resorption and cemental tears.

  • Mucogingival deformities and conditions around teeth
    o Gingival/soft tissue recession on facial/lingual/ interproximal/papillary
    o Lack of keratinized gingiva
    o Decreased vestibular depth
    o Aberrant frenum/muscle position.
  • Gingival excess
  • Pseudo pockets, inconsistent gingival margin, excessive gingival display, gingival enlargement, abnormal colour, mucogingival deformities and conditions on edentulous ridges
    o Vertical and/or horizontal ridges deficiency
    o Lack of gingival/keratinized tissue
    o Gingival/soft tissue enlargement
    o Aberrant frenum/muscle position
    o Decreased vestibular depth
    o Abnormal colour.
  • Occlusal trauma
    o Primary occlusal trauma
    o Secondary occlusal trauma.

Classification of Plaque

❑ Supragingival
  • Coronal plaque-it is in contact with only the tooth surface

- Marginal plaque–it is in contact with tooth surface at the margin of gingiva
- ❏ Subgingival plaque
  - Attached plaque
    - o Tooth associated
    - o Epithelium associated
    - o Connective tissue associated.
  - Unattached plaque.

Classification of Dental Calculus

❏ Supragingival calculus: Microscopically, it is heterogeneous in nature. It is a layered structure in which the degree of calcification varies with each layer

❏ Subgingival calculus: Microscopically, it is homogeneous as it is built in layers with almost equal quality of minerals.

Types of Inflammation

❏ Acute
- Relatively short duration (lasting from a few minutes to a few days)
- Characterized by fluid, plasma protein exudation, and by mainly neutrophilic leukocyte accumulation.

❏ Chronic
- Longer duration (days to years)
- Manifested by infiltration of lymphocytes and macrophages.

Types of Diabetes

❏ Type I–Insulin dependent diabetes
❏ Type II–Non-Insulin dependent diabetes .

Classification of Gingival Enlargements

❏ Inflammatory enlargement

- Chronic
- Acute.

❑ Drug induced enlargement

❑ Enlargements associated with systemic disease or conditions
  - Conditioned enlargements
    - Pregnancy
    - Puberty
    - Vitamin C deficiency
    - Plasma cell gingivitis
    - Non specific conditioned enlargements (pyogenic granuloma).
  - Systemic disease causing gingival enlargements
    - Leukaemia
    - Granulomatous diseases (e.g., Wegener's granulomatosis).

❑ Neoplastic enlargement (gingival tumours)
  - Benign tumours
  - Malignant tumours.

❑ False enlargements

❑ Depending upon the location and distribution, gingival enlargement can be given the following designations:
  - Localized: Limited to gingiva adjacent to a single tooth or group by teeth
  - Generalized: Involving the gingiva throughout the mouth
  - Marginal: Confined to the marginal gingiva
  - Papillary: Confined to the interdental papilla
  - Diffuse: It involves the marginal attached gingiva and papilla
  - Discrete: It is an isolated sessile or tumor like enlargement.

Classification of Acute Gingival Lesions

❑ Traumatic lesions of gingiva
  - Physical injury
  - Chemical injury.
❑ Viral infections
  - Acute herpetic gingivostomatitis
  - Herpangina
  - Measles
  - Herpes varicella/ Herpes zoster viral infections
  - Glandular fever.
❑ Bacterial infection
  - ANUG
  - Tuberculosis
  - Syphilis.
❑ Fungal disease
  - Candidiasis.
❑ Gingival abscess
❑ Aphthous ulcers
❑ Erythema multiform
❑ Drug surgery and contact hyper sensitivity.

Classification of Periodontal Pocket

❑ Depending on the number of surfaces involved:
  - Simple - Involving one tooth surface
  - Compound-Two or more tooth surfaces. The base of the pockets is in direct communication with the gingival margin along each of the involved surface
  - Complex-Spiral type pocket that originates on one tooth surface and twists around the tooth to involve one or more additional surfaces. The only communication with gingival margin is at surface where the pocket originates.

❑ Depending on Morphology:
- Gingival/pseudo pocket
- Periodontal pocket
  - Suprabony pocket
  - Infrabony pocket
    - According to number of walls
    - 3 walled defects
    - 2 walled defects
    - 1 walled defects
    - According to its depth and width
    - Type I shallow narrow
    - Type II shallow wide
    - Type III deep narrow
    - Type IV deep wide.
- Combined pocket.

❑ Depending on disease activity:
- Active pocket
- Inactive pocket.

❑ Depending on the nature of soft tissue wall:
- Edematous
- Fibrotic.

Classification of Trauma From Occlusion

❑ Acute
- It is caused by an abrupt occlusal impact which can result from biting over a hard object such as stone or a olive pip
- It can also result from restorations or prosthetic appliances that may interfere with or alter the direction of occlusal force
- Various features of acute trauma from occlusion are:
  - Tooth pain
  - Sensitivity to percussion
  - Increased tooth mobility

- Cemental tears can also lead to acute trauma from occlusion.
❑ Chronic
  - Chronic trauma from occlusion is more common than acute trauma from occlusion and has more clinical importance
  - It results from gradual changes in occlusion produced by tooth wear, drifting movement and extrusion of teeth, combined with a parafunctional habit such as bruxism and clenching, rather than as a sequel of acute periodontal trauma
  - It can be divided into:
    - Primary
      o It may be caused by alterations in occlusal forces, reduced capacity of the periodontium to withstand occlusal forces or both
      o When it results from alteration in occlusal forces, it is referred to as primary trauma from occlusion
      o The main aetiological factors in primary trauma from occlusion are the local alterations in the occlusion due to the following reasons:
        Because of insertion of a high filling or a prosthetic replacement that creates excessive force on the abutment and antagonist teeth
        The extrusion or the drifting movement of the teeth into spaces created by unreplaced missing teeth or the orthodontic movement of teeth into functionally unacceptable position.
      o Changes produced by primary trauma do not alter the level of connective tissue attachment and do not initiate pocket formation because supracrestal gingival fibres are not affected. Therefore, prevents apical migration of the junctional epithelium.

- Secondary
    - It occurs when the adaptive capacity of the tissues to withstand occlusal forces is impaired by bone loss resulting from marginal inflammation. This diminishes the periodontal attachment area and alters the leverage on the remaining tissues
    - The periodontium becomes more vulnerable to injury and previously well tolerated occlusal forces becomes traumatic
- Combined trauma from occlusion
    - When the injury results from abnormal occlusal forces applied to teeth or teeth with inadequate periodontal support.

Classification of Periodontal Instruments

❑ Non-surgical instruments:
- According to the purpose they serve–
    - Periodontal probes–locate, measure and mark pocket
    - Explorers–locate calculus deposits and caries
    - Scaling, Root planing and Curettage instruments
        - Hand instruments
        - Sickle scalers
        - Curette
        - Hoe
        - Chisel
        - File scalers
        - Ultrasonic and sonic
        - Rotating instruments
        - Reciprocating instruments
        - Lasers.
    - Periodontal endoscope–to visualize deposits subgingivally in pocket and furcation.

- Cleaning and polishing instruments–to clean and polish tooth surface.
    o Rubber cups
    o Brushes
    ◊ Dental tape.
❑ **Surgical instruments:**
  - According to the purpose they serve –
    - Excisional and Incisional instruments
        o Gingivectomy knives–used for excision and incision during gingivectomy. Kirkland 15–16, Crane-Kaplan 3–4, Interdental–Orbans 1–2, Waerhaug, Merrifield 1, 2, 3 and 4
        o Surgical blades–used for incisional purpose Surgical blades No. 11,12,15 and 15C
        o Electrosurgical instruments.
    - Surgical curettes and sickle scaler–used for removing granulation tissue, subgingival deposits and inter-dental tissues during surgery
        o Kramer curettes and Kirkland surgical instruments
        o Ball scaler.
    - Periosteal elevators–used to reflect periodontal flap
        o Goldman fox 14
        o Glickman 24G
        o Prichard
        o Molt
    - Surgical chisel and hoes–used for removing and reshaping bone.
        o Wiedelstadt
        o Todd-Gilmore
        o Ochsenbein 1–2
        o Rhodes 36–37
        o Fedi.
    - Surgical files–used for smoothening rough bony edges and removing bone

- o Sugarman
- o Schluger.
- – Scissors and Nippers-used for removing tissue tags during gingivectomy and trimming the margins of flap
  - o Goldman fox 16
  - o LaGrange
  - o Dean Scissors.
- – Needle holders-used to suture the flap.
  - o Crile wood
  - o Castroviejo
  - o Thomas Walker
  - o Osler Hegar
  - o Mathieu
  - o Mayohegar
  - o Kilner
  - o Halsey
  - o Rayden vascular.

Classification of Periodontal Probes

Probes can be classified into 5 generations:

❏ First generation probes: e.g., manual probes (hand-held probes)

❏ Second generation probes: pressure sensitive probes, e.g., true pressure sensitive probes.

- 30g of probing pressure is sufficient to determine the probing pocket depth
- 50g of probing pressure is required to detect alveolar bone defects
- These probes lack tactile sensitivity.

❏ Third generations probes: Computerized probes e.g., Florida probe, foster miller probe and Toronto automated probes.

- Drawbacks of automated probes:
  - Tactile sensitivity is less
  - Patient discomfort is more
  - Intensive.
- Fourth generation probes: They are still under development.
  - This probes, attempt to extend linear probing in a serial manner to take account of the continuous and three dimensional topography of the pocket being examined
- Fifth generation probe: Without penetrating, they aim at identification of attachment level.
  - They are non invasive
  - Eg are ultrasound probes.

Probes are further classified into various types:

- Marquis probe: Calibrations are in 3 mm sections
- UNC–15 probe: 15 mm long probe with mm markings at each mm and color at 5th, 10th and 15th mm
- University of Michigan 'O' probe with Williams marking at 1, 2, 3, 5, 7, 8, 9 and 10 mm
- Michigan 'O' probe with marking at 3, 6 and 8 mm
- WHO probe: 0.5 mm ball at the tip and mm markings at 3.5, 8.5 and 11.5 and color coding from 3.5–5.5
- Goldman fox probe: Flat, rectangular probe with markings at 1, 2, 3, 5, 7, 8, 9 and 10 mm
- Nabers probe: Curved probe used for furcation areas
- Moffitt/Maryland probe: WHO design with Williams marking
- NIDR probe: It is a color coded and is graduated in 2 mm increments at 2, 4, 6, 8, 10 and 12 mm with alternating increments colored in yellow
- Florida probe: The criteria given by NIDR were met by florida research group. Gibbs et al in the year 1988 developed the Florida

- Probe system. This incorporates constant probing force, precise electrical measurement, computer storage of data. The parts are Probe Hand piece, Digital readout, Switch, Computer Interface and Computer. Two models have been developed which differ in their fixed reference point
    - Stent model: The probe has 1 mm metal collar that rests on a prepared ledge on a prefabricated vacuoform stent
    - Disk model: Has a 11 mm disk which rests on the occlusal surface or incisal edge of the tooth
- Shortcomings are: Lack tactile sensitivity, forces the operatorm to predetermine the point of insertion, underestimation of deep probing depths, measurement taken with this system are less variable than with conventional probing.

❑ Toronto automated probe: Developed by researchers at the University of Toronto. Like the Florida probe, it uses the occlusal–incisal surface to measure clinical attachment levels. The sulcus is probed with 0.5 mm nickel-titanium wire that is extended under air pressure. It controls angular discrepancies by means of a mercury tilt sensor that limits angulation within ± 30°, but it requires reproducible positioning of the patient's head and can't easily measure third and second molars

❑ Interprobe: Developed by Goodson and Kondon in 1988. This has an optical encoder transduction element

❑ Briek probe: Developed by Briek et al. in 1987. Works by constant air pressure and uses the occlusal surface as its reference point

❑ The Jeffcoat probe (or Foster Muller Probe): Developed by Jeffcoat in 1986. It is capable of coupling pocket depth measurement with detection of the CEJ. The probe extends a thin metal fiber along the tooth surface into the sulcus and detects a slight acceleration rise when encountering the CEJ and then undergoes final extension, under constant force, on reaching the base of the pocket.

Various Types of Explorers

❑ 17–Orbans Explorer: Single ended instrument is ideal for calculus detection interproximally and in deep periodontal pocket. Long, thin shank and less than 2 mm fine tip allow easy access to deep, narrow pockets. Tip is right angle to shank

❑ 23–Shepherd's hook Explorer: Single ended/paired with 17. It has thicker shank and working end than other explorers which makes it more rigid. Rigidity enhances the role in caries detection, but limits its role in calculus detection

❑ Pigtail/Cowhorn/3CH Explorer no. 21 and 22: Double ended instrument that is easily adapted throughout the mouth. Working end is curved and shank is thin for calculus detection. Because shank is curved and relatively short, instrument is best used in children/adults with minimal periodontal pocket depth less than 1 mm. It can also be used for detecting calculus in areas of furcation involvement (similar instrument design to Naber's probe), detecting proximal and cervical caries. Ineffective in evaluating occlusal caries because the instrument's design limits the force needed to determine occlusal caries

❑ 3A Explorer : It has a long, fine, arc like tip. It adapts well in deep pocket and furcation areas. Its fine tip allows for good tactile sensitivity, especially for calculus detection

❑ Old Dominion University (ODU) 11/12 Gracey Type Explorer or EXD 11–12: Shank design of ODU is similar to that of Gracey 11/12 curette. It was developed by faculty of Old Dominion University, thus name ODU 11/12. It is a double ended, paired instrument for calculus detection.

Types of Dental mirror surfaces

❏ Plane/Flat surface mirror: Reflecting surface on the back of the mirror lens which produces double image
❏ Concave surface mirror: Produces magnified image that may be distorted
❏ Front surface mirror: Reflecting surface on the front of the lens that eliminates double image, producing a clear image.

Classification of Pulpal Periodontal Problems

❏ Pulps periodontal problems can be classified as:
  • Primary endodontic lesions
  • Primary periodontal lesion
  • Independent periodontal and endodontic lesions
  • Combined periodontal and endodontic
  • Primary endo secondary
  • Primary perio secondary.

Classification of Periodontal Flaps

Flaps can be classified as follows:

❏ Bone exposure after flap reflection
❏ Placement of the flap after surgery
❏ Management of the papilla
  • Based on bone exposure after reflection
    – They can be either full thickness flap also known as mucoperiosteal or they could be partial thickness also known as split thickness flap
    – In a full thickness flap, complete reflection of epithelium and connective tissue is done
    – In a partial thickness flap only epithelium and part of connective tissue is reflected leaving behind some part of connective tissue and the periosteum
    – Bone exposure is not there

- It is indicated when the flap apically or when the operator decreased want to expose the bone.

❑ Based on placement of slap after surgery
  - Nondisplaced flap
    - These are returned back of their original position and sutured.
  - Displaced flaps
    - They can be displaced either coronally or laterally depending upon the requirement of the case, and sutured in the desired position

❑ Based on management of the papilla
  - Conventional flap.
  - Papilla preservation flap.

Types of Suture Materials

❑ Nonabsorbable (Non resorbable)
  - Silk-braided
  - Nylon-monofilament (ethilion)
  - EPTFE-monofilument
  - Poly ester-braided (ethibond).

❑ Absorbable (resorbable)
  - Surgical: Gut
  - Plain gut: Monofilament (30 days)
  - Chronic gut: monofilament (45–60 days).

❑ Synthetic
  - Polyglycolic-braided (16–20 days)
  - Vicryl
  - Polygbe comprone-monofilament (90–12 days)
  - Monocryl (ethicon)
  - Polyglyconate-monofilament.

Types of Bone Grafts

❑ Autografts
❑ Allografts
❑ Alloplasts
❑ Xenografts.

Classification of Furcation Defects

Classification: in 4 grades:-

❑ Grade 1: It is an early stage of furcation involvement. Only soft tissue is involved. Early bone loss may be seen because of increased in probing depth but there are n radiological signs
❑ Grade 2: In this the lesion is *cul de sac* having a definite horizontal component. This implies that the bone loss has occurred at one side of the tooth. If multiple defects are present, they do not communicate with each other as the alveolar bone remains attached to the tooth. Radiographically it may or may not be depicted
❑ Grade 3: In this the bone is not attached to the dome of the furcation, therefore a multiple defects communicate with each other. In early Grade 3, the opening may be filled with soft tissue which is generally not visible. A periodontal probe also cannot be passed through and through completely because of interference with the bifurcational ridges or facial/lingual bony margins
❑ Grade 4: In this grade the interdental bone is destroyed and the soft tissue recedes apically, so the furcation can be seen clinically. Therefore, a probe is easily passed through and through in the furcation area.

Classification of Recession

❑ Class I: Marginal tissue recession does not enters to the mucoginginal junction There is no loss of bone or soft tissue in the interdental area

- ❑ Class II: Marginal tissue recession extends to or beyond the mucogingival junction
- ❑ There is no loss of have or say tissue in interdental area
- ❑ Class III: Marginal tissue recession to or beyond the mucogingival junction There is interdental bone and tissue loss along with malpositioning of the teeth
- ❑ Class IV: Marginal tissue recession extends to or beyond the mucogingival junction There is severe bone loss and soft tissue loss interdentarly along with severe malpositioning.

Classification of Dental Implants

Based on placement within the tissues

- ❑ Transosteal Implants:
  - A dental implant that penetrates both cortical plates and passes through the entire thickness of the alveolar bone.
- ❑ Sub Periosteal Implant:
  - An implant that is placed beneath the periosteum of the bone, It receives it's primary bone support by resting on it. This implant does not osseointegrate.
- ❑ Endosseous Implant:
  - An implant that is present within the bone, extends into basal bone for support. Types: Screw form, Cyclinder form (Hollow,Solid), Blade form.

Depending on the materials used:

- ❑ Metallic Implants:
  - Titanium
  - Titanium alloy
  - Cobalt chromium molybdenum.

Depending on their reaction with bone (Meffert)

- ❑ Bioactive: HA coated, CaP coated
- ❑ Bio-inert implants: Metals

Classification of Plaque Control Agents

❏ First generation:
- Triclosan–it is a phenol derivative, non ionic compound which is used as a topical antimicrobial agent.
  - It has a broad spectrum of action against both ram positive and gram negative bacteria
    ○ It acts on the microbial cytoplasmic membrane and uses bacteriolysis
  - It delays plaque maturation and inhibits formation of prostaglandins and leukotrienes.
- Metallic ions
  - Zinc and copper salts are most commonly used .
  - They act by reducing the glycolytic activity in micro organisms and inhibit bacterial growth.
- Quaternary ammonium compounds
  - These are antiseptics and surface active agents
  - They are more effective against gram positive rather than gram negative organisms
  - They are effective in reducing the development of plaque as it contains mainly contains gram positive micro organisms
  - They act by distrupting the cell wall structure of micro organisms
  - Examples benzethoniom chloride, benzalkoniom chloride and cetyl peridinium chloride.
- Sanguinarine
  ○ This is an alkaloid which is derived from a plant, sanguinaria canadensis.
- These inhibit mainly the gram negative organisms.
  - It has good retentive property when used as a mouth rinse.
- Antibiotics
  - Vancomycin, erythromycin, nidamycin and canamycin are the commonly used antibiotics for plaque control

- Enzymes
  - Example-mucinase, dextranase, lactoperoxidase and thiocynate synthase enzymes have shown bacteriocidal activity when applied topically in the mouth
  - They are able to break down already formed matrix of plaque and calculus.
- ❑ Second generation
  - Bisbiguinides –
    - Example–0.2 % chlorhexidine gluconate
    - It is a cationic bisbiguinide which has a very broad spectrum of action against a wide area of organisms including gram positive, gram negative, fungi, yeast, and viruses
    - It shows both anti plaque and anti bacterial action.
    - Anti plaque action:
    - Chlorhexidine shows antiplaque activity, because of the property of sustained availability that is chlorhexidine is slowly released form all oral surfaces resulting in bacterio static activity in oral cavity
    - Chlorhexidine inhibits plaque by the following mechanisms:
      - o Prevention of pellicle formation- it blocks acidic groups on salivary glycoprotein thus reducing glycoprotein adsorption on tooth surface
      - o It binds to the bacteria thus preventing the adsorption of bacterial cell wall on tooth surface
      - o It displaces calcium from the plaque matrix thus preventing binding of mature plaque
      - o Note : chlorhexidine prevents the formation of new plaque but has little effect on preexisting plaque.
    - Anti bacterial action:
    - Exhibits a wide spectrum of activity against gram positive, gram negative bacteria, fungi, yeast and viruses

- – Chlorhxidine is bacteriostatic in low concentrations and bacteriocidal in high concentrations
  - – After a single mouth rinse with chlorhexidine, saliva exhibits bacteriocidal activity for five hors and bacteriostatic activityfor more than twelve hours
  - – Regular use of chlorhexidine can reduce the aerobic and anerobic bacterial poppulations in saliva by 80-90 %.
- Indications
  - – In moderate to severe inflammation, as an adjunct to mechanical oral hygiene
  - – Post periodontal therapy or oral surgical procedures
  - – In physicaly, mentally and medivally challenged individuals
  - – Patients undergoing fixed or removable orthodontic treatment
  - – In patients who have undergone intermaxillary fixation.
- Adverse effects of chlorhexidine
  - o Reversable brownish staining of teeth or restotaions
  - o Loss of taste sensation specially bitter and salt sensation
  - o Some individuals have reported hypersensitivity to chlorhexidine
  - o The dead bacteria due to use of chlorhexidine may act as the initiator for supragingiva; calculus formation
  - o Can cause oral mucal erossons when used in high concentrations.
- Third generation
  - – Delmopinol-it inhibits plaque growth and reduce gingivitis
  - – It targets dextran producing streptococci by blocking synthesis.

- It reduces bacterial adherence by causing weak binding of the plaque to the tooth surface, thus aiding in easy removal by mechanical procedures
- It is used as a pre brushing mouth rinse
- It can cause transient staining of tongue and teeth
- Taste alteration and mucosal erosions have also been reported.

Classification of Chemicals used for Supragingival Plaque Control

❑ Addy's Classification
- Antibiotics:
    - Penicillin
    - Vancomycin
    - Kanamycin
    - Erythromycin
    - Spiramycin
    - Metronidazole.
- Enzymes:
    - Mucinase
    - Protease
    - Lipase
    - Amylase
    - Elastase
    - Lactoperoxidase
    - Hypothiocynase
    - Mutanase.
- Quaternary Ammonium Compounds:
    - Cetylpyridinium chloride
    - Benzethonium chloride
    - Benzalkonium chloride
    - Domiphen bromide

- Bisbiguanide:
  - Chlorhexidine
  - Alexidine
  - Octenidine/bispyridines.
- Metallic salts:
  - Copper
  - Tin
  - Zinc.
- Herbal extracts:
  - Sanguinarine.
- Fluorides
  - Strontium fluoride.
- Oxygenating agents:
  - Hydrogen peroxide.
- Phenolic compounds:
  - Thymol
  - Menthol
  - Eucalyptol.
- Other antispetics:
  - Iodine
  - Povidine Iodine
  - Sodium hypochlorite
  - Hexetidine
  - Triclosan.

Viva-Voce

1. **The most common dental disease evidenced in the embalmed bodies of the ancient Egyptians was:**

Ans: Periodontal disease

2. **Who is regarded as the 'Father of the Dental profession?'**

Ans: Pierre Fauchard

3. **The inventor of dental floss is:**

Ans: Levi Spear Parmly

4. **Anesthesia was discovered by:**

Ans: Horace Wells

5. **Local anesthesia was developed by:**

Ans: Carl Koller

6. **Periodontics was recognized as a specialty of dentistry by the American Dental Association in:**

Ans: 1947

7. Radiograph was discovered by:

Ans: Wilhelm Rontgen

8. The covering mucosa of the hard palate is:

Ans: Masticatory mucosa

9. The soft tissue wall of the gingival sulcus is formed by:

Ans: Marginal gingiva

10. The V-shaped space around the tooth bounded by free gingival margin on one side and the tooth surface on the other is known as:

Ans: Gingival sulcus

11. The depth of the gingival sulcus in absolutely normal or ideal condition is about:

Ans: 0 mm

12. The depth of a clinically healthy gingival sulcus in histologic section is:

Ans: 1.8 mm

13. The probing depth of a clinically normal gingival sulcus in human is:

Ans: 2–3 mm

14. The various anatomical areas of gingiva are:

Ans: Marginal, attached and interdental areas

15. The most keratinized areas of the oral mucosa is:

Ans: Palate

16. The junctional epithelium is:

Ans: Nonkeratinized

17. **The length of junctional epithelium ranges from:**

Ans: 0.25–1.35 mm

18. **The connective tissue of gingiva is known as:**

Ans: Lamina propria

19. **Three types of gingival fibers are:**

Ans: Collagen, reticular and elastic

20. **The color of the alveolar mucosa is:**

Ans: Red

21. **Water content in the ground substance of the periodontal ligament is approximately:**

Ans: 70 %

22. **The shape of periodontal ligament is:**

Ans: Hourglass

23. **With age permeability of cementum:**

Ans: Decreases

24. **Reimplanted tooth that become ankylosed usually exfoliate after:**

Ans: 4–5 years

25. **Radiographically, the inner socket wall of the alveolar process is regarded as:**

Ans: Lamina dura

26. **Which part of tooth is highly vascular:**

Ans: Cervical third

27. **The electronic device used to measure the gingival cervicular fluid collected on a 'blotter paper' employing an electronic transducer is:**

Ans: Periotron

28. **Organic compounds found in gingival cervicular fluid are:**

Ans: Glucose hexosamine and hexuronic acid

29. **Which component of the saliva is helpful in tooth integrity maintenance?**

Ans: Glycoprotein

30. **The immunoglobulin primarily found in saliva is:**

Ans: IgA

31. **Saliva contains the following coagulation factors, except:**

Ans: Factor VII

32. **The most common form of gingival disease associated with dental plaque is:**

Ans: Gingivitis

33. **Which medication does not modify gingival diseases?**

Ans: Phenytoin

34. **The characteristics of individuals that place them at increased risk for getting a disease is called:**

Ans: Risk factor

35. **Gingival indices are used in epidemiologic studies:**

Ans: To compare prevalence of gingivitis in various population groups

36. **Which instrument is not required to assess periodontal tissues applying Russell's Periodontal index?**

Ans: Periodontal probe

37. **The extent and severity of periodontal disease in individuals and populations are assessed separately by which index:**

Ans: Extent and severity index (ESI)

38. **A nearly mature microbiota is established in the gut of a newborn within:**

Ans: 2 weeks

39. **Which bacteria is often called an 'obligate periphyte?'**

Ans: Streptococcus mutans

40. **In a healthy gingival crevice, bacterial count is approximately:**

Ans: 1000

41. **Supragingival plaque and tooth associated subgingival plaque are critical in formation of calculus and:**

Ans: Root caries

42. **Inorganic components of the subgingival plaque are derived from:**

Ans: Gingival cervicular fluid

43. **Subgingival calculus is typically dark green or dark brown because of the presence of:**

Ans: Blood products

44. Which microorganism possesses fimbriae that helps binding to the dental pellicle?

Ans: *A. viscosus*

45. Most of the coaggregations among the strains of different genera can be inhibited by:

Ans: Lactose

46. After 3 days of accumulation, plaque attains thickness of:

Ans: 20–30 μm

47. In general, early plaque formation occurs faster in areas of:

Ans: Molar

48. Gram-positive microorganisms in plaque use sugars as an energy source and saliva as a source of:

Ans: Carbon

49. The etiology of periodontitis involves three groups of factors which determines the occurrence of active periodontitis. These factors include all of the following, except:

Ans: Good oral hygiene

50. Which of the following virulence factors possessed by A. actinomycetemcomitans plays a significant role in its pathogenicity?

Ans: Leukotoxin

51. The primary cause of gingival inflammation is:

Ans: Plaque

52. **The most common location for supragingival calculus to develop is:**

Ans: Buccal surface of maxillary molars

53. **Subgingival calculus is located:**

Ans: Below the crest of the marginal gingiva

54. **The location and extent of the subgingival calculus may be evaluated clinically by:**

Ans: Explorer

55. **Calculus attaches to the tooth surface through the mode:**

Ans: Chemical bonding to the hydroxyapatite

56. **Calcifying plaques may become 50% mineralized within:**

Ans: 2 days

57. **In pathogenesis of periodontal disease, calculus acts as:**

Ans: Contributing factor

58. **A smoker is defined as heavy if he consumes:**

Ans: 20 cigarettes/day

59. **Chronic inflammation is dominated by the migration of:**

Ans: Lymphocytes and macrophages

60. **The normal count of neutrophils in blood (per mm^3) ranges from:**

Ans: 4000–8000

61. **Macrophages are precursors of:**

Ans: Monocytes

62. **The source of the neutrophil chemotactic factor is:**

Ans: Mast cells

63. ***Actinobacillus actinomycetemcomitans*** **can only be controlled by neutrophils when opsonized by antiboby:**

Ans: IgG

64. **The concentration of IgG1 in serum is:**

Ans: 9 mg/ml

65. **The initial step of periodontitis is:**

Ans: Colonization of the periodontal tissues by pathogenic bacterial species

66. **Coaggregation refers to:**

Ans: Adherence between different bacterial strains

67. ***A. actinomycetemcomitans*** **evades host defenses by:**

Ans: Producing leukotoxin

68. **The first leukocyte to arrive at the site of periodontal inflammation is:**

Ans: Neutrophils

69. **Coating of bacteria with host proteins for the purpose of phagocytosis is referred to as:**

Ans: Opsonization

70. **The classic form of localized aggressive periodontitis was initially referred to as:**

Ans: Periodontosis

71. **The dominant serum antibody isotype specific for A. actinomycetemcomitans in localized aggressive periodontitis is:**

Ans: IgG_2

72. **Which inflammatory condition is an early indication of the toxic effect of folic acid antagonists:**

Ans: Ulcerative stomatitis

73. **The periodontal fibers that are least affected by vitamin C deficiency are:**

Ans: Those just below the junctional epithelium

74. **The change observed in gingiva during pregnancy in the absence of local factors is:**

Ans: Not notable

75. **Aggravation of the gingivitis in pregnancy is principally due to:**

Ans: An increased level of progesterone

76. **A narrow, bluish black discoloration of gingival margin in the areas of preexisting gingival inflammation is characteristic pigmentation of:**

Ans: Bismuth

77. **Periodontal disease is a/an:**

Ans: Infectious

78. **Acute thromboembolic events may be promoted by:**

Ans: *S. Sanguis*

79. **The sixth complication of diabetes is:**

Ans: Periodontal disease

80. Which antibiotic suppresses the glycation of proteins and reduces the activity of matrix metalloproteinase?

Ans: Tetracyclines

81. Infants are classified as low birth weight (LBW) if the weight at birth is below:

Ans: 2500 gm

82. Typical smell associated with candidiasis is produced by:

Ans: Acrylic dentures, especially when kept in the mouth at night

83. Synonym for hairy tongue is:

Ans: Lingua villosa

84. Tonsillolith is:

Ans: Formation of calculus in the crypts of tonsils

85. In patients with liver insufficiency, which compound accumulates in the blood and exhaled to cause malodor:

Ans: Ammonium

86. Which oral malodorous compound has highest volatility?

Ans: Skatole

87. Which is an irrelevant self examination method to detect oral malodor?

Ans: Smelling one's own breath by expiring in the hands kept in front of the mouth

88. The "gold standard" in the examination of breath malodor is:

Ans: Organoleptic assessment by a trained judge

89. The smell of "rotten apples" is indicative of

Ans: Insulin-dependent diabetes

90. The concentration of chlorhexidine in halitosis is:

Ans: 0.05%

91. Mouth spray reduces oral malodor by means of:

Ans: Masking the oral malodor

92. Stage I gingivitis is also referred to as:

Ans: Initial lesion

93. A key feature that differentiates the established lesion is the increased number of:

Ans: Plasma cells

94. Inflammation of gingival margin and a portion of contiguous attached gingiva is regarded as:

Ans: Marginal gingivitis

95. The two earliest symptoms of gingival inflammation preceding established gingivitis are:

Ans: Increased gingival cervicular fluid production and bleeding on probing

96. The most common cause of abnormal gingival bleeding on probing is:

Ans: Chronic inflammation

97. Gingival bleeding may follow the administration of excessive amounts of drugs undermentioned, except:

Ans: Cyclosporine

98. The color changes of gingiva is diffuse in case of:

Ans: Acute herpetic gingivostomatitis

99. The severity of gingival recession is determined by:

Ans: Level of epithelial attachment

100. Recession tends to be more frequent and severe in patients with:

Ans: Good oral hygiene

101. In case of combined gingival enlargement, inflammation is usually a:

Ans: Secondary complication

102. Drug-induced gingival enlargement starts at:

Ans: Interdental papilla

103. Name the drug, which causes highly vascularized gingival enlargement:

Ans: Cyclosporine

104. Systemic administration of phenytoin:

Ans: Accelerates healing of gingival wound

105. The drug which can replace cyclosporine is

Ans: Tacrolimus

106. Gingival enlargement has been described in 'tuberous sclerosis'. Patient with 'tuberous sclerosis' do not present:

Ans: Bleeding disorder

107. Bacterial plaque is not necessary for the initiation of gingival enlargement in:

Ans: Wegener's granulomatosis

108. The microorganism associated with pregnancy gingivitis is:

Ans: *P. intermedia*

109. Name a non-neoplastic gingival enlargement?

Ans: Pregnancy tumor

110. Puberty gingivitis affects:

Ans: Male and female adolescents

111. Gingival enlargement is associated with the deficiency of:

Ans: Vitamin C

112. Atypical gingivitis is another name for:

Ans: Plasma cell gingivitis

113. Pyogenic granuloma is a:

Ans: Nonspecific conditioned gingival enlargement

114. Among the all malignant tumors in the body, oral cancer constitute:

Ans: < 3%

115. The characteristic lesions of necrotizing ulcerative gingivostomatitis (necrotizing ulcerative gingivitis) are:

Ans: Punched-out lesion

116. Craterlike punched out lesions of interdental gingiva are characteristic of:

Ans: Necrotizing ulcerative gingivitis

117. Diffuse erythema of the gingiva with no ulcers is seen in:

Ans: Streptococcal gingivostomatitis

117. Necrosis of gingiva is not a feature of:

Ans: Streptococcal gingivostomatitis

118. Necrotizing ulcerative gingivitis is caused by:

Ans: Spirochetes and Fusiform bacilli

119. Herpetic gingivostomatitis is a:

Ans: Viral infection

120. Herpetic gingivostomatitis occurs mostly in:

Ans: Infants/children

121. Characteristic feature of herpetic gingivostomatitis is:

Ans: Vesicles

122. The vesicles in herpetic gingivostomatitis rupture approximately after:

Ans: 24 hrs

123. Multiple, small painful ulcers with elevated halo-like margin and depressed grayish white central portion are seen in:

Ans: Herpetic gingivostomatitis

124. Tzanck cells are seen in:

Ans: Herpetic gingivostomatitis

125. Healing of the lesions with scarring is seen in:

Ans: Large aphthous ulcers

126. Pericoronitis refers to inflammation of the gingiva in relation to the crown of an incompletely erupted:

Ans: Any tooth of the dentition

127. The localized complication of acute pericoronitis is:

Ans: Pericoronal abscess

128. The drug of choice in necrotizing ulcerative gingivitis is:

Ans: Amoxicillin

129. The pseudomembrane in necrotizing ulcerative gingivitis should be removed at:

Ans: First visit

130. Patients with necrotizing ulcerative gingivitis are advised to rinse with:

Ans: Equal mixture of 3% H_2O_2 and warm water

131. Herpes infection of a clinician's finger is referred to as:

Ans: Herpetic whitlow

132. The normal color of gingiva of deciduous dentition is:

Ans: Pale pink

133. The most common sites for eruption cyst are:

Ans: Permanent lower incisors and first molar

134. Most prevalent type of gingival disease in childhood is:

Ans: Chronic marginal gingivitis

135. The incidence of marginal gingivitis in children peaks at the age of:

Ans: 11–13 years

136. The pocket formed by gingival enlargement is referred to as:

Ans: Pseudopocket

137. The pocket that occurs due to destruction of the supporting tissues of a tooth is called as:

Ans: Periodontal pocket

138. The cells capable to phagocytize collagen fibres in periodontal disease are:

Ans: Fibroblasts

139. The presence of pus in the periodontal pocket signifies:

Ans: Nature of inflammation

140. Periodontal abscess is also known as:

Ans: Parietal abscess

141. Periodontal cyst is commonly seen in the region of:

Ans: Mandibular canine and premolar

142. 'Radius of action' of plaque to induce bone loss is:

Ans: 1.5–2.5 mm

143. The response of alveolar bone to inflammation includes:

Ans: Bone formation and bone resorption

144. Trauma from occlusion can cause bone loss:

Ans: Regardless of inflammation

145. The term 'lipping' refers to:

Ans: Peripheral buttressing bone formation

146. The most common pattern of bone loss in periodontal disease is:

Ans: Horizontal bone loss

147. **'Combined osseous defect' refers to combination of:**

Ans: Angular defects with varying number of walls at cervical and apical part

148. **Three-walled defects are most commonly found on the:**

Ans: Mesial surfaces of the molars

149. **The other term for 'hemiseptum' is:**

Ans: One-walled defect

150. **How many walls are destroyed in the one-walled defects?**

Ans: Three

151. **Traumatic occlusion refers to:**

Ans: Occlusion that produces injury to periodontium

152. **Trauma from occlusion refers to:**

Ans: Injury in the periodontium from occlusion

153. **Restoration/prosthetic appliances that alter the direction of occlusal forces on teeth may induce:**

Ans: Acute trauma

154. **Trauma from occlusion is:**

Ans: Reversible

155. **The most common clinical sign of trauma from occlusion is:**

Ans: Tooth mobility

156. **The maximal interdigitation and occlusal contact between mandibular and maxillary teeth is termed as:**

Ans: Centric occlusion

157. Clinical attachment loss of 1–2 mm is considered as:

Ans: Mild periodontitis

158. Occlusal adjustment is:

Ans: An irreversible intervention

159. Clinical attachment loss of 1–2 mm is considered as:

Ans: Mild periodontitis

160. Periodontal destruction is considered as severe when clinical attachment loss is of equal or more than:

Ans: 5 mm

161. Chronic periodontitis is a disease of:

Ans: Age-associated

162. Generalized aggressive periodontitis encompasses the disease previously classified as:

Ans: Generalized juvenile periodontitis and rapidly progressive periodontitis

163. Localized aggressive periodontitis has a localized presentation affecting mainly:

Ans: First molars/incisors

164. A striking clinical feature of localized aggressive periodontitis is:

Ans: Lack of clinical inflammation despite of presence of deep periodontal pockets

165. The classic radiographic sign of localized aggressive periodontitis is:

Ans: Arc-shaped loss of alveolar bone in relation to first molar

166. Clinically, generalized aggressive periodontitis is characterized by:

Ans: Generalized interproximal attachment loss affecting at least three permanent teeth other than first molars and incisors

167. Human immunodeficiency virus (HIV) was identified in:

Ans: 1984   168.   HIV has a strong affinity for:

Ans: T lymphocytes

169. After initial exposure, the acute symptoms experienced by HIV-infected individuals usually last for:

Ans: 2 weeks

170. Oral hairy leukoplakia in HIV-infected individuals is found exclusively on:

Ans: Lateral borders of the tongue

171. The most common oral lesion in AIDS patients is:

Ans: Candidiasis

172. The systemic therapy required for treatment of candidiasis in HIV-infected patients is:

Ans: Ketoconazole

173. Periodontal maintenance recall visit for AIDS patients should be conducted at the interval of:

Ans: 2–3 month

174. The key factor in both the development and the treatment of furcation involvement is:

Ans: Root trunk length

175. Basis for the diagnosis of a dental disease is constituted by:

Ans: Clinical findings

176. The Loss of tooth substance induced by mechanical wear other than that of mastication is termed as:

Ans: Abrasion

177. Dentoalveolar ablation refers to:

Ans: Loss of tooth substance due to forceful frictional actions between the oral soft tissues and the adjacent hard tissues

178. Toothbrushing with an abrasive dentifrice is a common cause of:

Ans: Abrasion

179. Which method is used clinically to measure the tooth mobility?

Ans: Tooth is held firmly between the handles of two metallic instruments

180. Systematic periodontal examination should start at the:

Ans: Molar region either in the maxilla or mandible

181. In the edematous type of tissue response, gingiva is:

Ans: Glossy

182. The only reliable method of detecting periodontal pocket is:

Ans: Probing

183. When the gingival margin is located apical to the cementoenamel junction, the loss of attachment is determined by:

Ans: Distance between the CEJ and gingival margin is added to pocket depth

184. The width of keratinized gingiva is:

Ans: Distance between the mucogingival junction and gingival margin

185. The amount of attached gingiva is determined by:

Ans: Subtracting the sulcus or pocket depth from the total width of gingiva

186. Radiologic name for the alveolar bone proper is:

Ans: Lamina dura

187. The line drawn between cementoenamel junction (CEJ)s of the approximating teeth and the crest of the interdental septum is generally :

Ans: Parallel

188. The earliest radiographic change seen in periodontitis is:

Ans: Fuzziness or break in the continuity of the lamina dura

189. Widening of PDL is seen in:

Ans: Scleroderma

190. How much bone mass to be lost at the alveolar crest to be detected radiographically:

Ans: 30%

191. The conventional radiographs are :

Ans: Highly specific but lack sensitivity

192. Superimposition of digital images obtained from the serial radiographs is the principle of:

Ans: Subtraction radiographs

193. In subtraction radiographs, the lighter areas indicate:

Ans: Bone gain

194. The disadvantage of subtraction radiography is:

Ans: Requires an identical projection in serial radiographs

195. PerioTemp probe is used to measure:

Ans: Subgingival temperature

196. The amount of probing force required to diagnose a periodontal osseous defects is:

Ans: 50 gm

197. The diameter of the Florida probe tip is:

Ans: 0.4 mm

198. Which is an automated probe for recording pocket depth?

Ans: Florida probe

199. The automated probe that detect CEJ is:

Ans: Foster-Miller probe

200. The advantage of the bacterial culture technique is that:

Ans: It can assess antibiotic susceptibility of the microbes

201. Evalusite is:

Ans: Chairside membrane immunoassay

202. Periotron is used for to measure:

Ans: Gingival cervicular fluid volume

203. Periogard is a:

Ans: Chairside test kit for aspartate aminotransferase (AST)

204. Periocheck is a:

Ans: Chairside test kit to detect neutral proteases in gingival cervicular fluid

205. Matrix metalloproteinases (MMPs) are members of a large subfamily of proteolytic enzymes, which are:

Ans: Zinc and calcium-dependent

206. Name the protective antibody whose response to A. actinomycetemcomitans in patients with aggressive periodontitis is controlled by genetics:

Ans: IgG2

207. Loss of attachment in men as compared to women is:

Ans: More

208. The best clinical indicator for gingival inflammation is:

Ans: Bleeding on probing

209. The Prognosis is established:

Ans: After making the diagnosis and before establishing the treatment plan

210. **The characteristics that predict the outcome of a disease present are called:**

Ans: Prognostic factor

211. **The prognosis that allows the clinician to initiate treatment of teeth that have doubtful outlook in the hope that a favorable response may tip the balance and allow teeth to be retained is regarded as:**

Ans: Provisional prognosis

212. **For two patients with comparable levels of remaining connective tissue attachment and alveolar bone, the prognosis is generally:**

Ans: Better in the older

213. **If the contour of the existing bone and the number of osseous walls are favorable, regeneration of bone to the level of alveolar crest is excellent in case of:**

Ans: Angular defects

214. **The prognosis of a smoker with slight to moderate periodontitis is generally:**

Ans: Fair to poor

215. **The most important local factor in periodontal diseases is:**

Ans: Plaque and calculus

216. **Flat, ectopic extension of enamel that extends beyond the normal contour of the cementoenamel junction is:**

Ans: Cervical enamel projection

217. **The tooth which offers the greatest difficulties in accessibility of mesiodistal furcation is:**

Ans: Maxillary first premolar

218. **The likelihood of restoring tooth stability is related to the extent of mobility caused by the loss of supporting alveolar bone and it is:**

Ans: Inversely proportional

219. **The healing after periodontal surgery is not delayed by which local factor:**

Ans: Adequate plaque control

220. **Which hormone does not impair healing?**

Ans: Progesterone

221. **Which term is employed to described a natural renewal of structure by growth and differentiation of new cells and intercellular substances to form new tissues?**

Ans: Regeneration

222. **What term is employed to describe a situation where close apposition of gingival epithelium to tooth surface is attained after periodontal therapy?**

Ans: Epithelial adaptation

223. **What changes can occur if the populated cells of a periodontal wound is originated from alveolar bone?**

Ans: Root resorption and ankylosis

224. **The function of an explorer is to:**

Ans: Locate caries

225. **The sickle scalers are used to remove:**

Ans: Supragingival calculus

226. **The instrument used for removal of tenacious subgingival calculus and altered cementum is:**

Ans: Hoe

227. **The instrument used to visualize deeply into subgingival pockets and furcations:**

Ans: Perioscope

228. **The most commonly used alloy to manufacture dental instruments is:**

Ans: Stainless steel

229. **Furcation areas can be best evaluated by using:**

Ans: Nabers probe

230. **UNC-15 probe is having markings at each millimeter and color coding at:**

Ans: At 5, 10 and 15 mm

231. **The smoothness of the root surfaces after root planing is checked by:**

Ans: Explorer

232. **The sickle scalers are used with:**

Ans: Pull stroke

233. **The instrument of choice for removal of deep subgingival calculus and soft tissue lining of a periodontal pocket is:**

Ans: Curette

234. **The cutting edge of a curette is present:**

Ans: On both sides of the working end

235. **The more flexible shanked, finishing** *Mini Five curettes* **are appropriate for:**

Ans: Light scaling and deplaquing

236. Langer and Mini-Langer curettes is the combination of:

Ans: Standard Gracey and Universal curettes

237. The Schwartz Periotrievers are designed for:

Ans: Removal of broken instruments from deep pockets

238. The primary function of a periodontal file is to:

Ans: Fracture or crush large deposits of tenacious calculus

239. Vibrations at the tips of the ultrasonic units ranges from:

Ans: 20,000–45,000 Hz

240. In the magnetostrictive ultrasonic units, the pattern of vibration of the tip is:

Ans: Elliptical

241. In the piezoelectric ultrasonic units, the pattern of vibration of the tip is:

Ans: Back and forth

242. Vibration at the sonic tip ranges from:

Ans: 2000–6500 cycles per second

243. The water spray used in sonic and ultrasonic scalers contains tiny vacuum bubbles that quickly collapse and release energy. The process is known as:

Ans: Cavitation

244. Prophy-jet delivers an air-powered slurry of warm water and:

Ans: Sodium bicarbonate

245. The Kirkland knife is:

Ans: Kidney-shaped

246. Electrotomy is also referred to as:

Ans: Electrosection

247. The instrument used to remove tabs of tissue during gingivectomy and to remove the muscle attachments in mucogingival surgery is:

Ans: Nippers

248. The cutting edge of an instrument can be evaluated for its sharpness:

Ans: By drawing lightly across an acrylic rod

249. During sharpening of a curette, the angle between the face of the blade and the surface of the sharpening stone should be:

Ans: 100–110°

250. Effective instrumentation is governed by all of the following, except:

Ans: Application of high amount of pressure

251. During instrumentation, the feet of the clinician should be:

Ans: Flat on the floor

252. Careful lip retraction during scaling is especially important for patients with the history of:

Ans: Recurrent herpes labialis

253. **Factors that provide stability to the instruments during instrumentation are:**

Ans: Instrument grasp and finger rest

254. **The most effective and stable grasp for all periodontal instruments is:**

Ans: Modified pen grasp

255. **The instrument grasp where shank of an instrument rests on the side of the middle finger is regarded as:**

Ans: Standard pen grasp

256. **The finger preferred by most of the clinicians for finger rest is:**

Ans: Fourth finger

257. **In which technique, finger rest is established on the teeth surfaces immediately adjacent to the working area:**

Ans: Conventional

258. **The two most commonly used extraoral fulcrums are:**

Ans: Palm up and palm down

259. **The manner of placing a periodontal instrument against the tooth surface is called:**

Ans: Adaptation

260. **The correct method for precise adaptation of bladed-instruments against the tooth surface is:**

Ans: The lower third of the working end adjacent to the toe or tip must be kept in constant contact with the tooth

261. The tooth-blade angulation during gingival curettage should be:

Ans: > 90°

262. The direction, length, pressure and number of strokes required for either scaling or root planing are not determined by which factor:

Ans: Nature of gingival/periodontal disease

263. The scaling stroke should be initiated in the:

Ans: Forearm

264. In which stroke, instrument engages the lateral or coronal border of the calculus and the fingers provide a thrust motion to dislodge it:

Ans: Push stroke

265. The most effective and versatile instruments for root planing procedure are:

Ans: Curettes

266. Vibrations of the scaler tip of sonic instruments ranges from:

Ans: 6000–9000 Hz

267. The major advantage of sonic scalers over the ultrasonic regarding plaque and calculus removal is:

Ans: Tapping motion

268. The forces on scaler tip of sonic instruments should not exceed:

Ans: 2.0 N

269. Minimum flow rate of cooling irrigation fluid during ultrasonic scaling ranges from:

Ans: 14–23 ml/min

270. The unidirectional fluid flow caused by ultrasound waves is:

Ans: Acoustic streaming

271. Plaque formation begins on:

Ans: Interproximal surfaces

272. The range of dimensions of acceptable toothbrush head according to the American Dental Association is:

Ans: 1–1.25 inches long and 5/16–3/8 inches wide

273. Bristle materials used in the toothbrushes are:

Ans: Natural bristles from hogs and artificial filament made of nylon

274. Advantages of natural bristles is:

Ans: Removes plaque efficiently

275. Bristle hardness of a toothbrush is:

Ans: Directly proportional to square of the bristle diameter and inversely proportional to square of bristle length

276. Diameter of the bristles in medium tooth brush is:

Ans: 0.012 inch

277. The number of bristles per tuft in a toothbrush ranges from:

Ans: 80–86

278. Electrically powered toothbrushes were invented in:

Ans: 1939

279. Dentifrice enhances the abrasive action of a toothbrush by:

Ans: 40 times

280. In which part of the dental arch, abrasion is more frequent?

Ans: Maxillary left

281. For caries reduction fluoride in a toothpaste ranges from:

Ans: 1000–1100 ppm

282. `Tartar control toothpastes' are effective against the:

Ans: Formation of new supragingival calculus

283. The simplest and most common method of toothbrushing is:

Ans: Scrub technique

284. The recommended technique in areas with gingival recession and root exposure is:

Ans: Modified Stillman

285. The recommended brushing technique in areas of healing wounds after periodontal surgery is:

Ans: Charters

286. The purpose of interdental cleaning is:

Ans: To remove plaque

287. The most widely recommended tool for interproximal cleaning is:

Ans: Dental floss

288. Type of dental floss recommended is based on:

Ans: Ease of use and personal preference

289. Dental floss is the most effective dental hygiene aid for:

Ans: Narrow gingival embrasures that are occupied by intact papillae

290. The suitable aid for cleaning large, irregular, or concave tooth surfaces adjacent to wide interdental spaces is:

Ans: Interdental brush

291. The diameter of interdental brush should be:

Ans: Larger than the gingival embrasure to be cleaned

292. The way in which wooden tip or plastic alternative is placed in interdental space is that:

Ans: Base of the triangle rests on gingiva and sides in contact with proximal tooth surfaces

293. Which motion should be used with the rubber tips in gingival embrasure?

Ans: Circular

294. Which part of the gingiva shows increased keratinization in response to gingival massage?

Ans: Oral epithelium

295. The contents of an essential oil mouth rinse are:

Ans: Thymol, eucalyptol, menthol and methyl Salicylate

296. Triclosan is more effective in combination with:

Ans: Zinc citrate

297. Chemical agents capable of staining bacterial deposits on the surfaces of teeth, tongue and gingiva are:

Ans: Disclosing agents

298. Naturally occurring, semisynthetic or synthetic antiinfective agent capable of destroying and inhibiting the growth of selective microorganisms at low concentration is called:

Ans: Antibiotic

299. Which is an active ingredient of antiplaque and antigingivitis mouth rinses and dentifrices?

Ans: Antiseptic

300. Metronidazole, an antiinfective agent against anaerobic bacteria, falls under the category of:

Ans: Nitroimidazole

301. The minimum concentration of tetracycline required in gingival cervicular fluid to be effective against the periodontal pathogens is:

Ans: 2–4 µg/m

302. Mechanism of action of metronidazole is:

Ans: Disrupt bacterial DNA synthesis

303. Mechanism of action of penicillin is:

Ans: Inhibits bacterial cell wall production

304. Penicillin is:

Ans: Bactericidal

305. Pseudomembranous colitis with diarrhea or cramping is a common side effect of:

Ans: Clindamycin

306. The antibiotic to which all strains of A. actinomycetemcomitans are susceptible is:

Ans: Ciprofloxacin

307. Mechanism of action of erythromycin is:

Ans: Inhibits protein synthesis by binding to 50S ribosomal subunit

308. Atridox used for subgingival delivery of:

Ans: Doxycycline

309. Up to what percentage of the depth of a periodontal pocket mouth rinses penetrate:

Ans: 4%

310. In subgingival irrigation, up to what percentage of the depth of a periodontal pocket, an irrigant penetrates:

Ans: 75–93%

311. The irrigator used for subgingival irrigation is:

Ans: Blunted cannulae with end or side parts

312. In supragingival irrigation, the position of the jet stream to the long axis of the teeth should be:

Ans: Perpendicular

313. The minimum effective dosage of supragingival irrigation with chlorhexidine digluconate once daily is:

Ans: 400 ml of 0.02%

314. The alteration of function or status in response to a stimulus or an altered chemical or physical environment is called:

Ans: Modulation

315. Host modulatory therapy restores the balance between:

Ans: Proinflammatory and Anti-inflammatory Mediators

316. Group of patients with abundant plaque and calculus but minimal pocket depth is regarded as:

Ans: Periodontal disease resistant

317. Host modulatory therapy (HMT) is used:

Ans: As adjuncts to conventional periodontal Therapy

318. Host modulatory therapy (HMT) usually:

Ans: Ameliorate excessive or pathologically elevated inflammatory processes

319. Which is not a systemically administered host modulation agent?

Ans: Bone morphogenic proteins

320. The subantimicrobial-dose of doxycycline (Periostat) is:

Ans: 20 mg

321. **The only FDA-approved, systemically administered host modulatory therapy indicated for the treatment of periodontitis is:**

Ans: Subantimicrobial dose doxycycline

322. **Subantimicrobial-dose doxycycline on continuous dosing can be prescribed up to a maximum of:**

Ans: 9 months

323. **Where does the mandibular canal divides into the incisive and mental canal:**

Ans: Premolar

324. **The lingual nerve is a branch of:**

Ans: Posterior division of the mandibular nerve

325. **The muscle which separates sublingual space from submandibular space is:**

Ans: Mylohyoid

326. **Which of the processes of the maxilla determines the depth of vestibular fornix?**

Ans: Zygomatic

327. **The terminal branches of the nasopalatine nerves and vessels pass through the:**

Ans: Incisive canal

328. **The greater palatine foramen opens:**

Ans: 3–4 mm anterior to the posterior border of the hard palate

329. Maxillary sinus is measured on an average:

Ans: $30 \times 30 \times 25$ mm

330. The base of the maxillary sinus is lined by:

Ans: Ciliated columnar epithelium

331. The maxillary sinus opens superiorly into the:

Ans: Middle nasal fossa

332. The most common location of the mandibular torus is the:

Ans: Lingual area of canine and premolars

333. Maxillary tori are usually located in the:

Ans: Midline of the hard palate

334. Swelling of the face, severe trismus and pain occur due to infection in the:

Ans: Masticator space

335. Raising of the floor of the mouth with displacement of the tongue is seen in the infection of:

Ans: Sublingual space

336. Which nerve is most susceptible to damage during extraction of a mandibular third molar?

Ans: Lingual nerve

337. Infection of which anatomic space results in Ludwig's angina?

Ans: Submandibular space

338. Infection of which anatomic space can lead to asphyxiation?

Ans: Submandibular

339. **Minimum of how long a smoker should stop smoking, if not quit, to facilitate periodontal healing?**

Ans: 3 weeks

340. **In Coe-Pak, the reaction is based on:**

Ans: ZnO and fatty acid

341. **Retention of a periodontal pack is obtained:**

Ans: Mechanically

342. **Working time for the Coe-Pak is:**

Ans: 15–20 min

343. **As a general rule, a periodontal pack over a periodontal wound is placed for:**

Ans: 7 days

344. **Immediately after surgery tooth mobility:**

Ans: Increases

345. **Desensitizing agents are not effective unless used continuously for at least:**

Ans: 2 week

346. **How long a patient should avoid eating after desensitizing treatment?**

Ans: 1 hour

347. **The surgical procedures for periodontal pocket that limited to the gingival tissues without involving the underlying osseous structures include:**

Ans: Gingival curettage and Gingivectomy

348. The word 'curettage' in periodontics refers to the:

Ans: Scraping of the gingival wall of a periodontal pocket to separate diseased soft tissue

349. Scraping of the gingival wall of a periodontal pocket apical to the epithelial attachment, severing the connective tissue attachment down to the osseous crest is called:

Ans: Subgingival curettage

350. During curettage, an instrument is inserted to engage the inner lining of the pocket wall and the stroke is used:

Ans: Horizontally

351. The motion of the curette in subgingival curettage is:

Ans: Scooping

352. The excisional new attachment procedure (ENAP) is performed with:

Ans: Knife

353. The incision used in excisional new attachment procedure is:

Ans: Internal bevel

354. Instrument(s) used for ultrasonic curettage is:

Ans: Morse scaler-shaped

355. The main reason for discarding the use of caustic drugs in gingival curettage is:

Ans: Extent of tissue destruction cannot be controlled

356. For restoration and epithelialization of the sulcus after gingival curettage requires:

Ans: 2–7 days

357. Immediately after the scaling and curettage, the color of gingiva is:

Ans: Bright red

358. How many weeks of scaling and curettage, gingiva attain its normal color, consistency, surface texture and contour?

Ans: 2

359. Which condition is an indication of gingivectomy?

Ans: Elimination of the suprabony pockets with fibrous and firm pocket wall

360. The gingivectomy incision apical to the pocket markings should be directed:

Ans: Coronally

361. The sole purpose of gingivoplasty is the:

Ans: Recontouring of gingiva in the absence of periodontal pocket

362. Complete epithelial repair after gingivectomy takes about:

Ans: 1 month

363. Complete repair of connective tissue after gingivectomy takes about:

Ans: 7 weeks

364. Gingival crevicular fluid flow reached the maximum level after how many days of gingivectomy:

Ans: 7

365. The surgical section of the gingiva and/or mucosa separated from the underlying tissues to provide visibility and accessibility is regarded as:

Ans: Periodontal flap

366. The apically displaced flaps cannot be performed in:

Ans: Palatal aspect of the maxillary posterior teeth

367. The unattached gingiva is absent in:

Ans: Palatal aspect of the maxillary posterior teeth

368. Transformation of the pocket wall into the attached gingiva is an important advantage of:

Ans: Apically displaced flap

369. Widening of the attached gingiva as well as the pocket elimination are accomplished by:

Ans: Apically displaced flap

370. The internal bevel incision is also called:

Ans: Reverse bevel incision

371. The second incision in periodontal flap is:

Ans: Crevicular incision

372. The interdental incision in periodontal flap is also called:

Ans: Third incision

373. The flaps reflected using only horizontal, with no vertical incisions are termed as:

Ans: Envelope flaps

374. Horizontal, internal bevel, nonscalloped incisions are used to remove gingival papillae in the procedure called:

Ans: Interdental denudation procedure

375. Healing of the interdental denudation procedure occurs by:

Ans: Secondary intention

376. After how many days of periodontal flap surgery, a fully epithelialized gingival crevice with a well-defined epithelial attachment forms?

Ans: 1 month

377. Which type of the suture material alleviate the 'wicking effect'?

Ans: Chromic gut

378. Natural, plain gut suture is processed from:

Ans: Purified collagen of either sheep or cattle intestines

379. The suture used in the wide interdental spaces to properly adapt the tissues to the bone is:

Ans: Horizontal mattress

380. Closing of the flap in distal wedge procedures is best accomplished by:

Ans: Anchor suture

381. The surgery designed to restore the form of pre-existing alveolar bone to the level present at the time of surgery is called:

Ans: Subtractive osseous surgery

382. The goal of osseous resective therapy is to:

Ans: Reshape the marginal bone

383. Treatment technique used for the correction of osseous defects largely depends on:

Ans: Morphology of the osseous defect

384. The resective osseous surgery is performed in combination with:

Ans: Apically displaced flap

385. The interproximal bone normally is:

Ans: Pyramidal in form

386. Level of interdental bone is same as that of the radicular bone in:

Ans: Flat architecture

387. The bone reshaping procedure that refers no improvement in overall result even further bone is removed is called:

Ans: Definitive osseous reshaping

388. Reshaping of the bone involving bone removal to the level, which is detrimental to the overall result is referred to as:

Ans: Compromise osseous reshaping

389. The buccolingual contour of the interdental bone in osseous crater appears as that of:

Ans: Opposite to the CEJ

390. The treatment modality for a tooth with significant loss of bone both horizontally and vertically in one or more furcations is:

Ans: Periodontal surgery, endodontic therapy and restoration of the tooth

391. The process of splitting of a two-rooted tooth into two halves and both retained is called:

Ans: Bicuspidization

392. The most commonly performed root resection is the:

Ans: Distobuccal root of maxillary first molar

393. If a vital root resection is to be performed, a more horizontal cut through the root is advisable, because:

Ans: It exposes a relatively small surface area of radicular pulp

394. Type of attachment gain after reconstructive periodontal surgery can only be determined by:

Ans: Histological analysis

395. Cells having potentiality for regeneration of the attachment apparatus of a tooth resides in:

Ans: Periodontal ligament

396. Gore-Tex is a:

Ans: PTFE membrane

397. Biobrane is:

Ans: Synthetic skin

398. Emdogain is:

Ans: Enamel matrix protein

399. Enamel matrix protein is:

Ans: Osteoconductive

400. Obtaining graft materials from a different individual of the same species is termed as:

Ans: Allograft

401. The chemical process by which molecules contained in the graft convert the neighboring cells into osteoblasts, which inturn form bone is known as:

Ans: Osteoinduction

402. The flap technique best suited for grafting purposes is:

Ans: Papilla preservation flap

403. Osseous coagulum is a mixture of:

Ans: Bone dust and blood

404. The technique where bone is triturated to a workable, plastic-like mass before placing into a bony defect is known as:

Ans: Bone blend technique

405. Boplant is a:

Ans: Xenograft

406. Plaster of Paris resorbs completely in:

Ans: 1–2 weeks

407. A composite of Polymethylmethacrylate and Polyhydroxyethylmethacrylate (HTR) polymer is:

Ans: Nonresorbable

408. The Vestibular depth is measured from the:

Ans: Gingival margin to the bottom of the vestibule

409. Surgical removal of the frenum is indicated when:

Ans: Tension on frenum may tend to open the sulcus

410. The most common etiologic factor of the marginal gingival tissue recession is:

Ans: Traumatic tooth brushing

411. In comparison to the desired width of attached gingiva, size of the free gingival autograft should be:

Ans: Twice

412. Ideal thickness of a free gingival autograft is:

Ans: 1.0–1.5 mm

413. Revascularization of a free gingival autograft starts from:

Ans: 2nd or 3rd day

414. Which portion of the free gingival autograft is last to vascularize?

Ans: Central section

415. How much time is required to replace the epithelium of a free gingival autograft undergoing degeneration with a new epithelium?

Ans: 4–7 day

416. Healing of a free gingival autograft of intermediate thickness (0.75 mm) is completed by:

Ans: 10.5 weeks

417. After 24 weeks, free gingival autograft placed on denuded bone shrink by:

Ans: 25%

418. The flap technique which is used to increase the width of keratinized gingiva but cannot predictably deepen the vestibule with attached gingiva is:

Ans: Apically positioned flap

419. Orthodontic correction of the marginal ridge discrepancy produces a hemiseptal defect in the bone if:

Ans: Bone level is flat between the adjacent teeth and marginal ridges are at significantly different levels.

420. One of the most important factors that determine the outcome of orthodontic therapy is:

Ans: The location of bands and brackets

421. Orthodontic brackets on the posterior teeth are positioned relative to the:

Ans: Marginal ridges and cusps

422. Orthodontic brackets on the anterior teeth are positioned relative to the:

Ans: Incisal edges

423. How much of a tooth should be erupted orthodontically for the purpose of restoration, if a tooth fracture extends to the level of alveolar bone?

Ans: 4 mm

424. To avoid relapse and reintrusion of a orthodontically erupted tooth, how much time period is necessary for stabilization?

Ans: 6 months

425. The most common cause of pulpal disease is:

Ans: Dental caries

426. The organisms being cultured predominantly from the infected root canals are:

Ans: Gram-negative anaerobes

427. If the inflammatory lesion of the pulp cannot be resolved, even after elimination of the source of trauma, the resulting progressive degeneration of the pulp is described as:

Ans: Irreversible pulpitis

428. The process by which bacteria and the inflammatory products of periodontitis gain access to the pulp is called:

Ans: Retrograde pulpitis

429. Sensation from the core of the pulp is initiated by:

Ans: Unmyelinated C fibers

430. The true combined periodontal and endodontic lesion results from the development and extension of an endodontic lesion into:

Ans: Existing periodontal pocket

431. While treating a combined periodontal and endodontic lesion, the attempts should be first made to treat:

Ans: Endodontic lesion

432. A dental abscess with a draining sinus tract indicates a lesion of:

Ans: Endodontic origin

433. How long one should wait after soft tissue grafting technique before initiation of restoration?

Ans: 2 months

434. Biologic width is defined as the physiologic dimensions of:

Ans: Junctional epithelium and connective tissue attachment

435. The biologic width is the distance between:

Ans: The coronal end of junctional epithelium to the alveolar crest

436. Placement of the margin of a restoration that has least impact on periodontium is:

Ans: Supragingival

437. **In order to correct the violation of the biologic width after rapid orthodontic extrusion of a tooth, supracrestal fibrotomy is performed every:**

Ans: 1 week

438. **For placement of a restorative margin in relation to the periodontal attachment, which structure may be used as a guideline:**

Ans: Existing gingival sulcus depth

439. **At the time of final impression of a prepared tooth, the cords used for gingival retraction should be:**

Ans: Removed coronal one and left behind the apical one

440. **Name one ideal pontic design?**

Ans: Ovate

441. **The epithelial cell attaches with implant surface by:**

Ans: Hemidesmosomes

442. **The probing depth with no bleeding around an implant presumed to be healthy is:**

Ans: 3.0 mm

443. **The arrangement of collagen fibers around an implant is:**

Ans: Parallel and unattached

444. **The term which is a synonym of osseointegration:**

Ans: Functional ankylosis

445. **The critical temperature for bone cells is:**

Ans: 47°C for 1 min

446. The critical temperature for bone cells is 47ºC at an exposure time of 1 minute. Because it leads to:

Ans: Denaturation of alkaline phosphatase

447. Osteoclasts are derived from:

Ans: Monocytes

448. The oxide layer on titanium surface mainly consists of:

Ans: Titanium dioxide

449. The probable reason for poorer clinical outcome with implants in posterior maxilla is:

Ans: Deficiency in primary stability

450. Periotest device is used for detecting mobility of:

Ans: Both of the implants and teeth

451. The vascular supply of the peri-implant gingival tissue is:

Ans: Less than that of gingival tissues around teeth

452. The inflammatory reaction in the soft tissues around implants is regarded as:

Ans: Periimplantitis

453. The term 'osseoperception' refers to:

Ans: Tactile sensitivity at bone-implant interface

454. The noninvasive method to assess the implant mobility is:

Ans: Resonanace frequency analyser

455. An absolute contraindication for implant therapy is:

Ans: Radiotherapy of head and neck

456. The minimum amount of bone required all around an implant after its placement is: ?

Ans: 1.0–1.5 mm

457. Modification of implant surfaces using the additive technique includes:

Ans: HA-coating and oxidation process

458. The subtractive implant surface modifications include:

Ans: Acid itching and sand blasting

459. Recommended speed for drilling the surgical site for implant placement is:

Ans: 800–1200 rpm

460. The surgical technique which increases the visuality more than 10x with the use of a microscope is called as:

Ans: Microsurgery

461. Dental loupes are fundamentally:

Ans: Telescopes

462. To produce a color correct image in compound loupes, lenses are made achromatic by:

Ans: The specific density of each lens counteracts the chromatic aberration of its paired lens

463. Microsurgical instruments are manufactured from:

Ans: Titanium

464. The first laser device was invented by:

Ans: Maiman

465. The active medium for the excimer lasers used for hard tissue ablation is:

Ans: Argon-fluoride) (ArF)

466. Which types of lasers are used for caries and calculus detection?

Ans: Diode

467. Between spouses and other family members, bacteria associated with periodontitis can be:

Ans: Transmitted

468. Return of pathogens to pretreatment levels after pocket debridement, generally occurs in approximately:

Ans: 9–11 weeks

469. What is considered as 'gold standard' for evidence?

Ans: Systemic reviews and meta-analysis

470. The maximum level of evidence associated with question about therapy or prevention is derived from systemic reviews of:

Ans: Randomized controlled trial studies

471. The highest level of evidence associated with questions about diagnosis is derived from systemic reviews of:

Ans: Controlled trials

472. **The highest level of evidence associated with question about etiology, causation, harm is derived from systemic reviews of:**

Ans: Cohort studies

473. **The primary type of evidence-based sources include:**

Ans: Original research publications

474. **The purpose of CASP (Critical Appraisal Skill Program) is to:**

Ans: Review randomized controlled trials, systemic reviews, and several other types of studies

475. **The purpose of QUOROM (Quality of Reporting of Meta-analyses) is to:**

Ans: Improve the reporting and review of systematic reviews

476. **Who is regarded as the 'Father of Dentistry'?**

Ans: Pierre Fauchard

477. **Who is regarded as the 'Father of Oral hygiene'?**

Ans: Levi Spear Parmly

478. **Who is known as the 'Father of Non surgical periodontal therapy'?**

Ans: Isadore Hirschfeld

479. **Who is considered as the 'Father of periodontal plastic surgery'?**

Ans: Preston D Miller

480. **Who is regarded as the 'First periodontist' in the history?**

Ans: John W Riggs

481. Who invented the hydraulic dental chair and when?

Ans: Wilkerson, 1877

482. Who described gingivectomy with scalloped incision?

Ans: Zentler

483. Who first placed bone graft materials for reconstruction of osseous defects produced by periodontal disease?

Ans: Hegedus

484. Who gave the term 'mucogingival surgery'?

Ans: Nathan Friedman

485. Who introduced the term 'periodontosis'?

Ans: Orban and Weinmann

486. Who introduced gingival graft?

Ans: Nabers

487. Who first described the relationship between periodontal and pulpal disease?

Ans: Simring and Goldberg

488. Which is a zinc oxide noneugenol periodontal dressing available in the form of paste-gel, whose setting occurs by chemical reaction?

Ans: Periocare

489. The fluid volume collected on a paper strip from gingival sulcus can be quantified by:

Ans: Periotron

490. A rapid chair side test kit developed to detect Aspartate aminotransferase in gingival cervicular fluid is:

Ans: Periogard

491. The instrument tips for scaling and root planing designed for removal of minimal tooth structures are:

Ans: Perio-tor

492. When should we give appointment for hypertensive patient?

Ans: Afternoon

493. What should be the position of a pregnant lady on dental chair during treatment?

Ans: Left lateral

494. After how much time period of myocardial infarction dental treatment can be carried out?

Ans: 6 month

495. Which drugs should be avoided in breastfeeding patient?

Ans: Tetracycline, ciprofloxacin and vancomycin

496. Periodontal treatment in the patient undergoing chemotherapy should be done

Ans: The day before chemotherapy

497. The Instrument used for detecting the tooth mobility is:

Ans: Periodontometer

498. Simplified oral hygiene index (OHI-S) was given by:

Ans: Green and Vermillion

499. Original Widman flap was modified by:

Ans: Ramfjord and Nissle

500. Periodontal index was developed by:

Ans: Russel